Updates in Surgery

SOCIETÀ ITALIANA DI CHIRURGIA
FONDATA A ROMA NEL 1882

Giovanni de Manzoni (Ed.)

Treatment of Esophageal and Hypopharyngeal Squamous Cell Carcinoma

In collaboration with
Simone Giacopuzzi
Andrea Zanoni

Forewords by
Gianluigi Melotti
Claudio Cordiano

Springer

Editor
Giovanni de Manzoni
Dept. of Surgery
Upper G.I. Surgery Division
University of Verona
Verona, Italy

In collaboration with
Simone Giacopuzzi
Andrea Zanoni

The publication and the distribution of this volume have been supported by the Italian Society of Surgery

ISBN 978-88-470-5613-8 ISBN 978-88-470-2330-7 (eBook)

DOI 10.1007/978-88-470-2330-7

Springer Milan Dordrecht Heidelberg London New York

Softcover re-print of the Hardcover 1st edition 2012

9 8 7 6 5 4 3 2 1 2012 2013 2014

Cover design: Simona Colombo, Milan, Italy
Typesetting: Graphostudio, Milan, Italy

Springer-Verlag Italia S.r.l. – Via Decembrio 28 – I-20137 Milan
Springer is a part of Springer Science+Business Media (www.springer.com)

To my teacher Prof. Cordiano to whom
I owe most of my knowledge about esophageal cancer

Foreword

What each of us, as surgeons, would like to have available at our fingertips is a comprehensive and state-of-the-art answer to any pathology we expect to be confronted with. Now, in this remarkable work by Giovanni de Manzoni on squamous cell carcinoma of the esophagus and hypopharynx, our wishes, at least in terms of these pathologies, have come true.

Instructive texts are, almost by definition, never produced casually, especially those addressing surgical issues. Indeed, the order, clarity, accuracy, and exhaustiveness of this work reveal the author's many years of experience, developed at the prestigious School of Verona led by Claudio Cordiano.

This is not a textbook on surgical technique: nowadays, educational cartoons, drawings, and photographs have become nearly obsolete given all the readily available, top-quality visual aids we have quickly grown used to. Rather, the subject matter is scrutinized from all medical standpoints: epidemiology, classification, staging, pre-operative evaluation protocols, and pre- and postoperative oncology, including molecular-biology-based information. In addition, comments on the accreditation of the facilities and surgeons best qualified to treat these conditions are–duly and boldly–provided.

Thanks to its careful method, effective synthesis, and explanatory clarity, this text is not only useful, it is also a pleasure to read. The explanations it provides are easily incorporated into everyday practice.

This work is a significant contribution to the publishing goals of the Società Italiana di Chirurgia, whose approach and mission are to disseminate state-of-the art surgical knowledge. I am confident that works such as this one are an important step in communicating, in Italy and abroad, the high-quality achieved by Italian surgery.

A surgeon's job today is less and less based on manual dexterity and instead increasingly dependent on the ability to lead teams of specialists–a strategy that ensures the best results, especially in the field of oncology.

This book, by de Manzoni and collaborators, is a powerful teaching instrument of particular interest to young surgeons completing their specialty training;

in addition, residents will undoubtedly appreciate the knowledge it contains and readily use the information provided.

I congratulate and thank Professor de Manzoni for his work, and sincerely hope that he will continue to produce such high-quality contributions as this one.

Rome, October 2011

Gianluigi Melotti
President, Italian Society of Surgery

Foreword

To read a book on esophageal cancer is, for me, a journey through my own life as a surgeon. My first contact with the Japanese experience was during a meeting, held in Rome in 1968, on esophagogastroplasty. In a single lecture, Nakayama made all previous reconstructive techniques essentially obsolete, from the Gavriliu procedure to jejunoplasty to the Ivor Lewis esophagogastrectomy.

I performed my first esophagectomy in 1971, reported the use of the pull-through technique in Catania in 1977, during the Congress of the Italian Society of Surgery, and then engaged in a challenging but fruitful surgical competition with Alberto Peracchia, a master of esophageal surgery, and his pupil Ermanno Ancona, whom I remember with affection.

After 1986, following a report by Girolamo Fracastoro, neoadjuvant treatment was introduced at our institution, based on the experience from Wayne State University (Detroit, MI, USA). The successful development of this approach was largely due to the enthusiasm and clinical skills of Felice Pasini. Surgery of the hypopharynx was accordingly standardized, in collaboration with Walter Mozzo and Oreste Mosciaro. In our institution my studies on end-to-end esophagogastric anastomosis contributed to the routine application of this technique beginning in the late 1990s.

My highly rewarding involvement in research on the diagnosis and treatment of esophageal cancer was interrupted in 2005. In 2004, Ernesto Laterza, who had joined me in this work, left to become director of a surgical unit. This led me to reorganize the activity in my own department, such that Professor Giovanni de Manzoni, who was already in charge of gastric surgery, also took over responsibilities for esophageal surgery. In 2009, I asked Professor Enrico De Antoni and the Directive Council of the Society to promote a biennial lecture series on esophageal cancer.

In Italy, esophageal surgery is a low-volume operation and research is carried out by only a few specialized surgical groups. Moreover, there have been only marginal gains over the past few years and the influence of those findings on practical clinic is still limited.

Giovanni de Manzoni intended this book to be a review of current information as well as an informative review at ongoing studies. It is aimed not only at surgeons but also at oncologists, radiotherapists, and radiologists. I am grateful to him not only for his acceptance of this enormous task but also because he has carried on the work I did in Verona for many years. Those very difficult and risky surgical activities trained and inspired me, and I am confident that his experience will be the same.

I would like to thank once again the President of the Italian Society of Surgery, Professor Gianluigi Melotti, its directive council and its 2009 President for their acceptance of my proposal for this Biennial Conference, and for having assigned to Giovanni de Manzoni the realization of this event.

Verona, October 2011 **Claudio Cordiano**

Contents

Contributors

Valentina Ambrosini, Dept. of Nuclear Medicine, "Sant'Orsola" Hospital, University of Bologna, Bologna, Italy

Franco Barbieri, Otoiatric Surgery Unit, Borgo Trento Hospital, Verona, Italy

Paola Caroli, Dept. of Nuclear Medicine, "Sant'Orsola" Hospital, University of Bologna, Bologna, Italy

Francesco Casella, Dept. of Surgery, Upper G. I. Surgery Division, University of Verona, Verona, Italy

Filippo Catalano, Surgical Endoscopy Unit, Borgo Trento Hospital, Verona, Italy

Daniela Cenzi, Radiology Unit, Borgo Trento Hospital, Verona, Italy

Angelo Cerofolini, Surgical Endoscopy Unit, Borgo Trento Hospital, Verona, Italy

Giovanni de Manzoni, Dept. of Surgery, Upper G. I. Surgery Division, University of Verona, Verona, Italy

Alberto Di Leo, General Surgery Unit, Arco Hospital, APSS of Trento, Trento, Italy

Walid El Kheir, Dept. of Surgery, Upper G. I. Surgery Division, University of Verona, Verona, Italy

Stefano Fanti, Dept. of Nuclear Medicine, "Sant'Orsola" Hospital, University of Bologna, Bologna, Italy

Anna Paola Fraccon, Service of Medical Oncology, "Dott. Pederzoli" Polyspecialist Private Clinic, Peschiera del Garda (VR), Italy

David Fuster, Dept. of Nuclear Medicine, Hospital Clinic of Barcelona, Barcelona, Spain

Simone Giacopuzzi, Dept of Surgery, Upper G. I. Surgery Division, University of Verona, Verona, Italy

Antonio Grandinetti, Radiation Oncology Unit, Borgo Trento Hospital, Verona, Italy

Milena Gusella, Dept. of Medical Oncology, "Santa Maria della Misericordia" Hospital, Rovigo, Italy

Jun Isogaki, Dept. of Surgery, Fujita Health University, School of Medicine, Nagoya, Japan

Francesco Lombardo, Surgical Endoscopy Unit, Borgo Trento Hospital, Verona, Italy

Gerardo Mangiante, Dept. of Surgery, Upper G. I. Surgery Division, University of Verona, Verona, Italy

Maria Cristina Marzola, Dept. of Nuclear Medicine, "Santa Maria della Misericordia" Hospital, Rovigo, Italy

Stefania Montemezzi, Radiology Unit, Borgo Trento Hospital,Verona, Italy

Massimiliano Motton, Radiology Unit, Borgo Trento Hospital, Verona, Italy

Felice Pasini, Dept. of Medical Oncology, "Santa Maria della Misericordia" Hospital, Rovigo, Italy

Michele Pavarana, Oncology Unit, Borgo Trento Hospital, Verona, Italy

Corrado Pedrazzani, Surgery Division, Rovereto Hospital, Rovereto (TN), Italy

Francesca Pons, Dept. of Nuclear Medicine, Hospital Clinic of Barcelona, Barcelona, Spain

Thomas J. Re, Radiology Unit, Borgo Trento Hospital, Verona, Italy

Luca Rodella, Surgical Endoscopy Unit, Borgo Trento Hospital, Verona, Italy

Domenico Rubello, Dept. of Nuclear Medicine, "Santa Maria della Misericordia" Hospital, Rovigo, Italy

Teodoro Sava, Oncology Unit, Borgo Trento Hospital, Verona, Italy

Francesca Steccanella, Dept. of Surgery, Upper G. I. Surgery Division, University of Verona, Verona, Italy

Ichiro Uyama, Dept. of Surgery, Fujita Health University, School of Medicine, Nagoya, Japan

Giuseppe Verlato, Unit of Epidemiology and Medical Statistics, University of Verona, Verona, Italy

Jacopo Weindelmayer, Dept. of Surgery, Upper G. I. Surgical Division, University of Verona, Verona, Italy

Andrea Zanoni, Dept. of Surgery, Upper G. I. Surgery Division, University of Verona, Verona, Italy

Section I

General Issues

Epidemiology of Esophageal and Hypopharyngeal Squamous Cell Carcinoma

1

Giuseppe Verlato and Giovanni de Manzoni

1.1 Incidence

1.1.1 Incidence of Esophageal Cancer, Irrespective of Histology

Esophageal cancer is the eighth most common cancer worldwide, with 481,000 new cases (3.8% all newly diagnosed cancers) estimated in 2008, and the sixth most common cause of death from cancer, with 406,000 deaths (5.4% of all cancer deaths) [1]. These figures encompass both of the major histological types, squamous cell carcinoma (SCC) and adenocarcinoma (AC).

New cases occur twice as often in men (n = 326,000 in 2008) as in women (n = 155,000). In different countries, esophageal cancer is two to four times more common among men than women [1]; for example, in Sweden, the incidence is about four times higher in men than in women (3.4 vs. 0.9/100,000 person-years) [2]. However, in the Iranian Caspian littoral region, the incidence is the same in the two sexes [3].

More than 80% of the cases and the related deaths occur in developing countries. The highest rates (approximately 15/100,000 person-years) are recorded in Asia, particularly in the "central Asian esophageal cancer belt." Intermediate rates of 8–14 new cases per 100,000 person-years are found in parts of Southeast Africa, South America, and Europe, especially Eastern Europe and the UK (10/100,000 person-years). The lowest rates are recorded in Sweden, Norway, South Europe, North Africa, and some countries of South America [1].

The highest mortality rates occur in both sexes in Eastern and Southern

G. Verlato (✉)
Unit of Epidemiology and Medical Statistics, University of Verona,
Verona, Italy

G. de Manzoni (Ed.), *Treatment of Esophageal and Hypopharyngeal Squamous Cell Carcinoma*,

Africa and in Eastern Asia. Within Europe, Scotland has the highest mortality, for both men and women (10.9 and 4 per 100,000 person-years), followed by England and Wales, while the lowest mortality among men is recorded in Greece, Bulgaria, Italy, and Finland (< 3 per 100,000 person-years) [4].

1.1.2 Incidence of Esophageal Squamous Cell Carcinoma

Official statistics usually report overall incidence and mortality of esophageal cancer, so that data by histological subtypes are sparse. Figure 1.1 shows the risk of esophageal cancer (SCC or AC) in men during the first 75 years of life, according to the Five-Continent database [5]. It can be appreciated that the cumulative incidence of esophageal SCC (blue columns) is the lowest in Kuwait (0.07–0.12% in different ethnicities), Israel (0.06–0.13%), and Peru (0.15%) and the highest in Porto Alegre, Brazil (1.84%). The risk of developing esophageal AC (pink columns) is about null in Korea and Thailand and peaks among Scottish men (0.6%). The cumulative incidence of esophageal SCC in women (ages 0 to 74 years) is the lowest (0.03%) in the Czech Republic, Slovakia, and Spain (0.03%) and the highest in India (0.84%) [5].

The incidence of esophageal SCC exceeds that of esophageal AC in all developing countries and in most developed countries [5]. In the Iranian

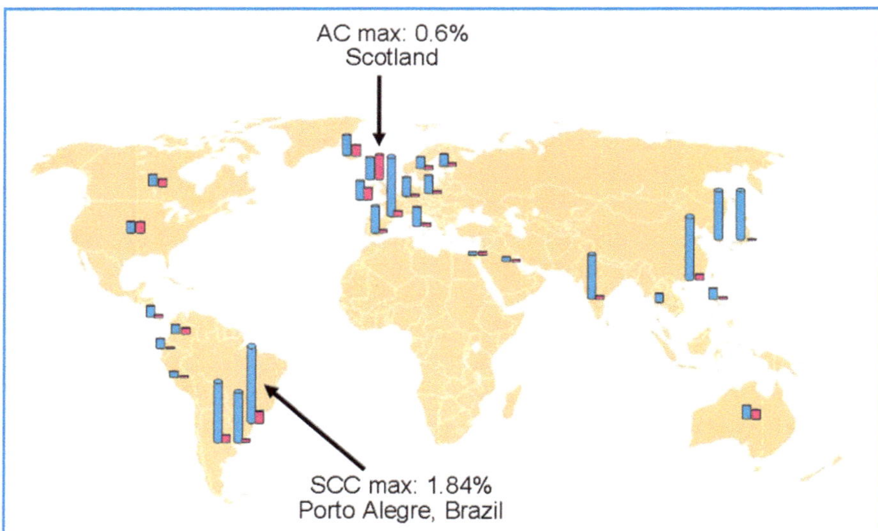

Fig. 1.1 Cumulative incidence (0-74 years of age) of esophageal cancer in men according to the Cancer Incidence in Five Continents database [5]. Blue columns indicate squamous cell carcinoma (SCC) and pink columns adenocarcinoma (AC). Data of Israel, Kuwait, and the USA refer, respectively, to white men, Kuwaitis, and Jews born in Israel. Within the UK, only figures for Scotland are reported

Caspian littoral population, and specifically, adults over 30 years of age, the incidence of SCC was 12.7 per 100,000 person-years between 1994 and 2003, while the incidence of AC was much lower (1.9); hence, SCC accounted for 86.9% of all esophageal cancers and AC for only 12.8% [3]. Similarly, in Italy, SCC represented 63% of all esophageal cancers in men and 66% of those in women in the period 1998–2002, while the proportion of AC was 21% in men and 15% in women [6]. By contrast, the incidence of AC has recently approached that of SCC in Scotland, the USA, and Israel. In Scotland, the cumulative incidence of AC in the first 75 years of life is higher than that of SCC in men (0.6% vs. 0.53%) but not in women (0.15% vs. 0.42%) [5]. In the USA, at the beginning of the 21st century (1998–2003), AC rates were higher than those of esophageal SCC among white and non-Hispanic men, while in men and women of all other ethnicities esophageal SCC rates were similar to, or greater than, AC rates [7]. Among Jews living in Israel, AC now accounts for 72.6% of the esophageal cancers in men [8].

Both histological types of esophageal cancer usually prevail in men: however, the male-to-female incidence ratio is much higher for AC (7–10) than for SCC (2–3) [9, 10]. As an exception, in the Iranian Caspian littoral, where the incidence of SCC is slightly higher in women than in men (14.0 vs. 11.4 per 100,000 person-years in those over 30 years of age, respectively), while the incidence of AC is 2–3 times higher in men (2.6 vs. 1.1) [3].

The incidence of esophageal SCC steadily increases with age both in developed [11] and developing [3] countries. In the USA, incidence rates increase in adults up to 70 years of age, after which they level out or even decrease in all ethnicities. For instance, the incidence rates are very low in whites under 50 years of age (0.13 and 0.07 per 100,000 person-years in men and women, respectively) and peak in white men over 80 years of age (12.04 per 100,000 person-years, 95% CI 11.05–13.11) and in white women 70–79 years of age (7.24 per 100,000 person-years, 6.77–7.74) [11].

Large variations in the incidence of esophageal SCC have been recorded also within the same country among different ethnicities [5]. Incidence rates of esophageal SCC in males in the USA during the period 1996–1998 were highest among blacks (8.8 per 100,000 person-years), intermediate among Asians/Pacific Islanders (3.9), and lowest among whites, Hispanics, and Native Americans (1.8). Among women, the highest rates were again recorded among blacks (3.4) and the lowest among Hispanics (0.4) [12].

Differences among ethnicities living in the same country are often larger than those recorded among people of the same ethnicity living in different countries. For instance, in Singapore, the cumulative incidence of esophageal SCC in the first 75 years of life is 30 times higher among Chinese men (0.92%) than among Malay men (0.03%), while the variability between Indians living in mainland India or in Singapore is much lower (1.07% vs. 0.60%) [5].

1.1.3 Incidence of Hypopharyngeal Cancer

Data on the incidence of hypopharyngeal cancer are sparse, as official statistics usually include cancer of the hypopharynx (coded as C13 in the International Classification of Diseases for Oncology) among cancers of the upper aerodigestive tract (UADT) or, at best, among cancers of the lip-oral cavity-pharynx (C00-C14).

In the 1990s, the incidence of hypopharyngeal cancer varied among men, ranging from 0.3 per 100,000 person-years in Iceland to 17 in Bas-Rhin, France, while in women the differences were less pronounced [13]. Between 2000 and 2004, the incidence of hypopharyngeal cancer in France, which comprises areas with the world's highest risk, is 1.89 per 100,000 person-years among men and 0.13 among women, with the values standardized according to the world population. Nearly all these cancers are SCC or transitional cell carcinomas. As a percentage, hypopharyngeal cancer represents 5.7% of all UADT cancers in men and 2.4% of those in women [14]. Based on these numbers, it can be concluded that cancer of the hypopharynx is rather rare, representing 0.40% of all cancers in men and 0.06% of those in women. In Sweden, the standardized incidence of hypopharyngeal carcinoma is five- to six-fold higher among male immigrants from the Indian Subcontinent [15].

Of note, a strong association has been found between SCC of the hypopharynx and the esophagus, with synchronous esophageal cancer observed in 16% of patients with hypopharyngeal cancer [16] and metachronous esophageal cancer in more than 20% of patients [17].

1.2 Survival

The prognosis of patients with esophageal cancer is rather poor, as the 5-year survival is only 12% in Europe [18] and 16% in the USA [19]. In Italy, the prognosis of esophageal cancer has slightly increased during the last decades in men but not in women, with 5-year survival increasing from 7% during 1986–1989 to 12% in 2000–2003 among men, while remaining stable among women (14% and 13%, respectively) [20, 21].

Survival of patients with hypopharyngeal cancer are also poor, 13% at 5 years, but improved survival was noted among Swedish men during the 1980s [22].

1.3 Risk Factors

The most important risk factors for SCC of the esophagus and hypopharynx are excessive alcohol consumption [23-25], tobacco smoking, low socioeconomic status, and nutritional deficiencies. The importance of alcohol consumption as a risk factor for esophageal [23, 24] and hypopharyngeal [25] cancers was confirmed in the Shanghai cohort study, in which regular drinkers of alcoholic beverages had a two-fold higher risk than non-drinkers of developing esophageal cancer, independent of tobacco smoke and other potential confounders [26].

Also tobacco smoking is a strong risk factor for esophageal cancer, and even more so for hypopharyngeal cancer. In a large multicenter European case-control study, in which the OR of current smokers vs. never smokers was 12.2 (95% CI 8.3–17.9) for hypopharyngeal and laryngeal cancers and three times lower for esophageal cancer (4.2, 2.45–7.1) [27]. The association between tobacco smoking and hypopharyngeal/laryngeal cancer becomes even stronger when considering only never alcohol drinkers (OR=47.3, 12.1–185.8), ruling out any confounding effect of alcohol consumption. Involuntary smoking exposure is a risk factor for hypopharyngeal/laryngeal cancer (OR=2.0, 0.8–5.1) but not for esophageal cancer (OR=0.8, 0.3–2.1) [27]. Moreover, even smokeless tobacco seems to be a risk factor for hypopharyngeal cancer [15]. In Europe tobacco and alcohol altogether explains 85% of hypopharyngeal/laryngeal cancer and 67% of esophageal cancer [28]. While smoking appears to be an independent risk factor, alcohol mainly potentiates the carcinogenic effect of tobacco smoke. Indeed, smoking alone was attributed 36.1% of hypopharyngeal/laryngeal cases and 24.1% of esophageal cases, alcohol alone 0.02% and 3.6%, and the joint effect of smoking and alcohol 48.8% and 38.9% respectively.

Nutritional deficiencies are also associated with esophageal and hypopharyngeal cancers. Esophageal SCC has been related to vitamin deficiency [29], low folate intake [30], consumption of salted meat and fish, excessive intake of hot beverages, and low socioeconomic status [24, 31], while the consumption of fruits (including oranges/tangerines), seafood, and milk is a protective factor [26]. Iron deficiency causes the so-called Plummer-Vinson syndrome, or sideropenic dysphagia, a precursor of hypopharyngeal and esophageal SCC.

People with a low socioeconomic status, a low level of education, or a low income have a higher incidence of esophageal [24, 31] and hypopharyngeal cancers [32]. This effect is not fully explained by behavioral risk factors, i.e., smoking, alcohol, and diet [32].

Human papillomavirus infection is an additional risk factor for hypopharyngeal cancer. In hypopharyngeal SCC, the prevalence of infection is 20–30% [33].

Of note, esophageal SCC, while sharing the most important risk factors with hypopharyngeal SCC, has a different risk profile than esophageal AC. Indeed, although AC is also associated with dietary deficiency and tobacco smoking, its most important predictor is gastroesophageal reflux and its major determinant is obesity [23, 24, 34].

1.4 Time Trends in Incidence and Mortality

1.4.1 Trends in Esophageal Cancer

Between 1990–1994 and 2000–2004, in the European Union, esophageal cancer mortality moderately decreased in men, from 5.7 to 5.4 per 100,000 person-years, while remaining stable in women at 1.1 [4]. A divergent pattern was observed within Europe, as mortality decreased in France, Spain, and Italy, while increasing in northern, central, and Eastern Europe [4]. In Italy, the incidence of esophageal cancer between1993–1995 and 2003–2005 has largely decreased in men (-23.1%), but has increased slightly in women (+3.1%) [35]. From 1980 to 2002, age-adjusted mortality from the disease decreased in Italy by 41% among men and by 36% among women [36].

In Jews living in Israel, the incidence of esophageal cancer in men has increased. The incidence in cancer involving the upper two-thirds of the esophagus has decreased such that 89% of these tumors in men now occur in the lower one-third [8].

1.4.2 Trends in Esophageal Cancers by Histology

Over the last several decades, the incidence of esophageal SCC has decreased, while the incidence of AC has markedly increased in Western countries, especially among whites. These trends are clearly evident in the USA [7, 37] and in many areas of Europe [38]. In developing countries, however, esophageal SCC is relatively stable or slightly decreasing [24].

Among white men in the USA, the incidence of esophageal SCC decreased by 35% between 1974–1976 and 1992–1994, from 3.4 to 2.2 per 100,000 person-years, while the incidence of esophageal AC increased by 350%, from 0.7 to 3.2 per 100,000 person-years. The increase in esophageal AC and the decrease in esophageal SCC were much less pronounced among black men [37]. The trend has continued into the 21st century, as evidenced by the 3.6%/year decrease in the incidence of esophageal SCC from 1998 to 2003 and the 2.1%/year increase in the incidence of esophageal AC during the same period [7]. SCC rates have decreased among both sexes in most racial or ethnic groups, whereas AC rates have increased, primarily among white non-Hispanic men. The percent annual variation in the incidence of esophageal SCC is -3.4% and -3.0% among white men and women, and -5.2% and -2.3% among black men and women. For esophageal AC, the values are 2.1% and 1.6%, and 0.4% and 9.3%, respectively [7]. These data imply that, in 1975, among white men in the USA, there were 4.7 cases of SCC for every case of AC; this ratio fell to 2.1:1 in 1995 and had completely reversed by 1996–1998 (0.43:1) [12, 37].

In most of Europe, between 1983 and 1997, there was a clear-cut annual increase in esophageal and gastric cardia AC of 1–7% whereas the trend in esophageal SCC was not homogeneous across the continent. Among men, the incidence of SCC rose mostly in Northern Europe and Slovakia, by 1–5% per year, but generally declined by the same amount in Southern and Western Europe. Among women an increasing trend was recorded all over Europe, with estimated annual percent changes of 1–8% [38].

1.4.3 Trends in Hypopharyngeal Cancer

Between 1990–1994 and 2000–2004, overall mortality from cancer of the oral cavity and pharynx declined in the European Union, from 6.6 to 6.0 per 100,000 person-years [4]. When considering only hypopharyngeal cancer, the age-standardized incidence significantly increased in Sweden from 1960 to 1989 by about 1.5% per year among men, while decreasing among women by about 2% per year [22]. More recently, an opposite trend was observed in France: from 1980–1985 to 2000–2004, standardized incidence rates decreased in men by 20.9%, from 2.39 to 1.89 per 100,000 person-years. In women, however, there was a large increase in incidence (+116.7%), although the absolute increase was quite small, from 0.06 to 0.13 per 100,000 person-years [14].

1.4.4 Trends in Risk Factors Can Explain Trends in Incidence

The decreasing trend in SCC of the esophagus and hypopharynx can be attributed, at least in part, to improvements in lifestyle, in particular to a reduction in smoking habits and alcohol consumption.

The role of tobacco smoke is reinforced by the divergent incidence pattern observed in men vs. women, decreasing in men and stable or increasing in women. This gender-specific pattern is typical of most smoking-related cancers [14]: in Italy, for instance, between 1993–1995 and 2003–2005, the incidence of cancers of the lung, UADT, and esophagus decreased, respectively, by 29.5%, 28%, and 23.1% in men, while increasing by 15.1%, 10.4%, and 3.1% in women [35]. Likewise, smoking has decreased in men over the last few decades, while remaining stable or increasing in women in many countries [39]. For instance, in France, the prevalence of regular smoking has decreased in men, from 72% in 1953 to 31.8% in 2010, but increased in women, from 17% to 25.7% [14].

Trends in alcohol consumption are less clear-cut. For instance, in Europe, alcohol consumption has generally increased in northern countries while decreasing in southern countries [40]. In France, since the 1930s, it has dropped by half in men and by two-thirds in women [14]. This divergent pattern may partly explain the divergent pattern of esophageal SCC incidence among European men, i.e., declining in southern countries while increasing in northern countries [38].

On the other hand, the increasing trend in the incidence of distal esophageal AC and gastric cardia cancer has been attributed to the simultaneous increase in the prevalence of gastroesophageal reflux disease and obesity.

References

1. Ferlay J, Shin HR, Bray F et al (2010) GLOBOCAN 2008, Cancer Incidence and Mortality Worldwide: IARC CancerBase No. 10 [Internet]. International Agency for Research on Cancer, Lyon, France. Available from: http://globocan.iarc.fr
2. Mousavi SM, Brandt A, Sundquist J, Hemminki K (2011) Esophageal cancer risk among immigrants in Sweden. Eur J Cancer Prev 20:71-76
3. Gholipour C, Shalchi RA, Abbasi M (2008) A histopathological study of esophageal cancer on the western side of the Caspian littoral from 1994 to 2003. Dis Esophagus 21: 322-327
4. La Vecchia C, Bosetti C, Lucchini F et al (2010) Cancer mortality in Europe, 2000-2004, and an overview of trends since 1975. Ann Oncol 21:1323-1360
5. Corley DA, Buffler PA (2001) Oesophageal and gastric cardia adenocarcinomas: Analysis of regional variation using the Cancer Incidence in Five Continents database. Int J Epidemiol 30:1415-1425
6. AIRT Working Group (2006) Italian cancer figures – Report 2006: Incidence, mortality and estimates. Epidemiologia & Prevenzione 30(1): Supplemento 2
7. Trivers KF, Sabatino SA, Stewart SL (2008) Trends in esophageal cancer incidence by histology, United States, 1998-2003. Int J Cancer 123:1422-1428
8. Rozen P, Liphshitz I, Barchana M (2009) The changing epidemiology of upper gastrointestinal cancers in Israel: clinical and screening implications. Eur J Cancer Prev 18:191-198
9. Vizcaino AP, Moreno V, Lambert R, Parkin DM (2002) Time trends incidence of both major histologic types of esophageal carcinomas in selected countries, 1973-1995. Int J Cancer 99: 860-868
10. Cook MB, Dawsey SM, Freedman ND et al (2009) Sex disparities in cancer incidence by period and age. Cancer Epidemiol Biomarkers Prev 18:1174-1182
11. Nordenstedt H, El-Serag H (2011) The influence of age, sex, and race on the incidence of esophageal cancer in the United States (1992—2006). Scand J Gastroenterol 46:597-602
12. Kubo A, Corley DA (2004) Marked multi-ethnic variation of esophageal and gastric cardia carcinomas within the United States. Am J Gastroenterol 99:582-588
13. Blot WJ, Devesa SS, McLaughlin JK, Fraumeni JR JF (1994) Oral and pharyngeal cancers. Cancer Surv 19/20:23-42
14. Ligier K, Belot A, Launoy G et al, for Network Francim (2011) Descriptive epidemiology of upper aerodigestive tract cancers in France: Incidence over 1980-2005 and projection to 2010. Oral Oncol 47:302-307
15. Mousavi SM, Sundquist J, Hemminki K (2010) Nasopharyngeal and hypopharyngeal carcinoma risk among immigrants in Sweden. Int J Cancer 127:2888-2892
16. Su YY, Fang FM, Chuang HC et al (2010) Detection of metachronous esophageal squamous carcinoma in patients with head and neck cancer with use of transnasal esophagoscopy. Head Neck 32:780-785
17. Wang WL, Lee CT, Lee YC et al (2011) Risk factors for developing synchronous esophageal neoplasia in patients with head and neck cancer. Head Neck 33:77-81
18. Berrino F, De Angelis R, Sant M et al (2007) Survival for eight major cancers and all cancers combined for European adults diagnosed in 1995-1999: results of the EUROCARE-4 study. Lancet Oncol 8:773-783
19. Jemal A, Siegel R, Ward E et al (2006) Cancer statistics, 2006. CA Cancer J Clin 56:106-130
20. Crocetti E, Capocaccia R, Casella C et al (2004) Cancer trends in Italy: figures from the Cancer Registries (1986-1997). Epidemiologia & Prevenzione 28:S1-S112
21. AIRTUM Working Group (2009) New incidence and mortality data: 2003-2005. Epidemiologia & Prevenzione 33(1-2): Supplemento 2

22. Wahlberg PCG, Andersson KE, Bjorklund AT, Moller TR (1998) Carcinoma of the hypopharynx: Analysis of incidence and survival in Sweden over a 30-year period. Head Neck 20:714-719
23. Falk GW (2009) Risk factors for esophageal cancer development. Surg Oncol Clin N Am 18:469-485
24. Hongo M, Nagasaki Y, Shoji T (2009) Epidemiology of esophageal cancer: Orient to Occident. Effects of chronology, geography and ethnicity. J Gastroenterol Hepatol 24:729-735
25. Lubin JH, Purdue M, Kelsey K et al (2009) Total exposure and exposure rate effects for alcohol and smoking and risk of head and neck cancer: a pooled analysis of case-control studies. Am J Epidemiol 170:937-947
26. Fan Y, Yuan J-M, Wang R et al (2008) Alcohol, tobacco, and diet in relation to esophageal cancer: the Shangai cohort study. Nutr Cancer 60:354-363
27. Lee YCA, Marron M, Benhamou S et al (2009) Active and involuntary tobacco smoking and upper aerodigestive tract cancer risks in a multicenter case-control study. Cancer Epidemiol Biomarkers Prev 18:3353-3361
28. Anantharaman D, Marron M, Lagiou P et al (2011) Population attributable risk of tobacco and alcohol for upper aerodigestive tract cancer. Oral oncology 47:725-731
29. Islami F, Malekshah AF, Kimiagar M et al (2009) Patterns of food and nutrient consumption in Northern Iran, a high-risk area for esophageal cancer. Nutr Cancer 61:475-483
30. Aune D, Deneo-Pellegrini H, Ronco AL et al (2011) Dietary folate intake and the risk of 11 types of cancer: a case-control study in Uruguay. Ann Oncol 22:444-451
31. Brown LM, Hoover R, Silverman D et al (2001) Excess incidence of squamous cell esophageal cancer among US black men: role of social class and other risk factors. Am J Epidemiol 153:114-122
32. Conway DI, McKinney PA, McMahon AD et al (2010) Socioeconomic factors associated with risk of upper aerodigestive tract cancer in Europe. Eur J Cancer 46:588-598
33. Hoffmann M, Gorogh T, Gottschlich S et al (2005) Human papillomaviruses in head and neck cancer: 8 year-survival-analysis of 73 patients. Cancer Letters 218:199-206
34. Corley DA, Kubo A, Zhao W (2008) Abdominal obesity and the risk of esophageal and gastric cardia carcinomas. Cancer Epidemiol Biomarkers Prev 17:352-358
35. Crocetti E, AIRTUM Working Group (2009) Per quali tumori l'incidenza sta cambiando più rapidamente? Epidemiol Prev 33:78
36. Centro Nazionale di Epidemiologia, Sorveglianza e Promozione della Salute, Istituto Superiore di Sanità. La mortalità per causa in Italia: 1980-2002. http://www.iss.it/site/mortalita/
37. Devesa SS, Blot WJ, Fraumeni JF Jr (1998) Changing patterns in the incidence of esophageal and gastric carcinoma in the United States. Cancer 83:2049-2053
38. Steevens J, Botterweck AAM, Dirx MJM et al (2010) Trends in incidence of oesophageal and stomach cancer subtypes in Europe. Eur J Gastroenterol Hepatol 22:669-678
39. Huisman M, Kunst AE, Mackenbach JP (2005) Educational inequalities in smoking among men and women aged 16 years and older in 11 European countries. Tob Control 14:106-113
40. World Health Organization Statistical Information System. Health topics. Alcohol drinking http://www.who.int/topics/alcohol_drinking/en/

Classification and Staging Systems

2

Giovanni de Manzoni, Francesca Steccanella, and Andrea Zanoni

2.1 Staging

An accurate staging system for cancer aims at providing an indication of prognosis that is as accurate as possible. It also aids in treatment planning, the evaluation of treatment results, and the exchange of information between different centers.

Both the Union Internationale Contre le Cancer (UICC) and the American Joint Committee on Cancer (AJCC) TNM classification and the Japanese classification of esophageal cancer are based on an assessment of the depth of esophageal wall infiltration, lymph node involvement, and presence of distant metastases [1, 2].

The 7th edition of the AJCC Cancer Staging Manual was published in 2010 [3]. Major modifications have been introduced for esophageal cancer, and only minor changes for hypopharyngeal carcinoma.

The location of esophageal cancer is defined by measuring the distance of the upper end of the cancer from the incisors. The esophagus is made up of three anatomic compartments: the cervical, thoracic, and abdominal esophagus.

The cervical esophagus begins at the hypopharynx and ends at the thoracic inlet. The thoracic esophagus is divided into three sections as well: upper thoracic, from the thoracic inlet to the azygos vein; middle thoracic, from the azygos vein to the inferior pulmonary veins; and lower thoracic, from the inferior pulmonary veins to the stomach.

G. de Manzoni (✉)
Dept. of Surgery, Upper G.I. Surgery Division, University of Verona,
Verona, Italy

G. de Manzoni (Ed.), *Treatment of Esophageal and Hypopharyngeal Squamous Cell Carcinoma*,

Table 2.1 Esophageal cancer staging system according to AJCC 7th end, 2010. (Reproduced from [3], with permission)

Stage	T	N	M	G	Location
0	is (HGD)	0	0	1	Any
IA	1	0	0	1	Any
IB	1	0	0	2-3	Any
	2-3	0	0	1	Lower
IIA	2-3	0	0	1	Upper, middle
	2-3	0	0	2-3	Lower
IIB	2-3	0	0	2-3	Upper, middle
	1-2	1	0	Any	Any
IIIA	1-2	2	0	Any	Any
	3	1	0	Any	Any
	4a	0	0	Any	Any
IIIB	3	2	0	Any	Any
IIIC	4a	1-2	0	Any	Any
	4b	Any	0	Any	Any
	Any	N3	0	Any	Any
IV	Any	Any	1	Any	Any

2.1.1 Hypopharyngeal SCC

In hypopharyngeal SCC, a T1 tumor is defined as being limited to one subsite (pyriform sinus, posterior wall, or postcricoid area) and/or ≤ 2 cm in its greatest dimension. The invasion of more than one subsite or a size > 2 cm but < 4 cm without fixation of the hemilarynx characterizes the T2 tumor. In T3, the tumor is > 4 cm in size or extends to the esophagus or causes fixation of the hemilarynx. T4 cancers invade adjacent structures: in T4a the tumor invades the thyroid/cricoid cartilage, hyoid bone, thyroid gland, or central compartment soft tissue, while in T4b the prevertebral fascia, carotid artery or mediastinal structures is involved. Considering N status, a metastasis of a single ipsilateral node less than 3 cm characterizes N1. A metastatic node > 6 cm is defined as N3. N2, then, consists of all intermediate cases: N2a is a single ipsilateral node 3–6 cm in size, N2b comprises multiple ipsilateral nodes, and N2c bilateral or contralateral metastatic nodes. As usual, M is defined as M0 or M1 if distant metastases are, respectively, absent or present.

2.1.2 Esophageal SCC

The previous AJCC staging system was based on a pattern of increasing T, followed by increasing N and then increasing M and was not data driven. Moreover, the statistical analysis was based on *P* values to test statistically significant differences among stage groups. In the current edition, the aim is to group cancer characteristics (both anatomic and non-anatomic) such that they reflect monotonicity, distinctiveness, and homogeneity of survival (Table 2.1).

Thirteen institutions worldwide collaborated to construct a database of 4627 patients, all of whom underwent surgery without induction or adjuvant chemotherapy or radiotherapy. Patients with squamous cell carcinoma (SCC) accounted for 40%, with a cancer location of upper-middle esophagus in 31% and lower third in 69%.

Stages 0 (tumor in situ) and stage IV (distant metastatic disease) are not data driven but are defined a priori. Data elaboration is based on risk-adjusted random forest analysis and the end-point is all-cause time-related mortality.

Major changes since the previous version are the following:

- T classification has changed for Tis and T4.
- All para-esophagel nodes are considered regional nodes and are classified based on the number of nodal metastasis.
- M classification is reserved for distant metastases, both lymphatic and hematological.
- Histologic grade, tumor location, and histologic type are incorporated as non-anatomic factors.

T Stage

Tis (high grade dysplasia), previously called carcinoma in situ, includes all types of non-invasive neoplastic epithelium. In the analysis by Rice and colleagues [1], there is an equivalence in survival between pTis and well-differentiated pT1a (tumor confined to the lamina propria). This is probably due to the absence of lymphatic vessels in the mucosal layer. As shown by Japanese researchers [4], the rate of lymph node metastases for m1 (intraepithelial) and m2 lesions (confined to the lamina propria) is very low (0-5%). If the tumor invades the muscularis mucosae, the nodal metastasis rate is not negligible (18% in their group of patients); in addition, other risk factors must be considered, such as histologic grade and vascular involvement, in therapeutic planning [4]. In the opinion of Rice's group, it is also difficult to distinguish between the different intramucosal lesions, so their classification is also clinically practical [5].

T4 is subclassified as T4a (resectable disease invading pleura, pericardium or diaphragm) and T4b (unresectable disease invading other adjacent structures). This subclassification was reached by consensus [1].

N Stage

A regional lymph node is redefined as "any para-esophageal node extending from cervical nodes to celiac nodes." The definition of non-regional lymph nodes was removed, because of the longitudinal nature of the intramural lymphatic plexus. Actually, there is an important difference in the definition of regional nodes between the AJCC-TNM and UICC-TNM systems. The former in fact considers regional nodes as those from the celiac trunk to the supraclavicular area, while the latter explicitly excludes supraclavicular nodes. N clas-

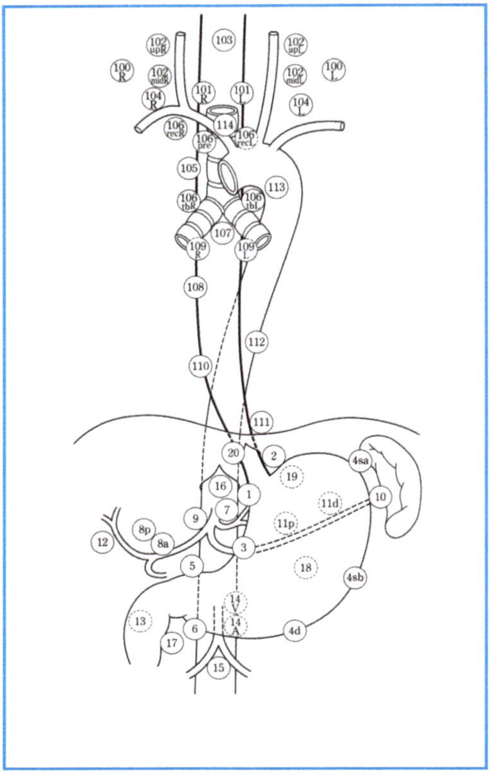

Fig. 2.1 Nodal stations according to the Japanese classification of Esophageal Cancer, 10th edn. (Reproduced from [2], with permission)

sification is now based on the number of positive lymph nodes, with N1: 1-2 nodes, N2: 3-6 nodes, N3: ≥ 7 nodes. The cut-off results from the analysis and is consistent with the classification used in gastric cancer [1].

Japanese Classification

The latest edition of the Japanese Society for Esophageal Cancer (10th edition) was published in 2008. Like the UICC/AJCC staging system, it is based on the depth of tumor infiltration in the esophageal wall (T), lymph node metastases (N), and distant metastases (M), but with some differences. Stage I does not include only N0 tumors, but also early esophageal cancers, i.e., T1a lesions, regardless of lymph node or distant metastases. Lymph node metastases are classified only on a location basis. Lymph nodes stations are numbered and divided into groups according to tumor location (Fig. 2.1). Stage IV does not include only distant metastases (IVb), but also locally advanced tumors (T4) and metastases to distant lymph nodes (N4) [2].

N Stage Controversies

Since the publication of the 6th edition of the AJCC staging manual, the influence of the number of lymph nodes resected and of metastatic lymph nodes on prognosis has been the subject of increasing attention in the literature. The number of nodes removed per operation differs because of different extents and methods of lymphadenectomy among different centers. There are various cut-off values in the literature for an optimal lymphadenectomy, but it is quite clear that the fewer the nodes harvested, the greater the likelihood that positive nodes will be missed, with the result that patients are often understaged, especially pT0 patients. For SCC, the impact of the total number of nodes removed on survival is controversial. Hsu et al., with a SCC-based database, found no survival difference between patients with more or less than 15 nodes removed. Nevertheless, the difference in the survival of patients with a low vs. a high rate of node metastasis was more evident in those undergoing extended lymphadenectomy [6]. Hu et al. demonstrated a worse survival experience for patients with < 6 nodes harvested, thus validating the previous cut-off [7]. In a study by Altorki et al., stage migration from early to more advanced stages diminished when > 25 nodes were resected for early stages and > 16 nodes for stage III and IV tumors. According to the authors, beyond a critical number of lymph nodes removed there is a prevalence of therapeutic effects [8]. The 7th edition of the AJCC/UICC classification states that optimum lymphadenectomy depends on T classification: for pT1, 10 nodes must be resected; for pT2, 20 nodes; for pT3-4, 30 nodes or more [1].

In a 2003 paper, Rice et al. demonstrated that classifying all node positive patients as N1 resulted in an inhomogeneous grouping, because survival decreased as the number of regional lymph node metastases increased. Instead, they subclassified N+ as N1 (≤ 2 LN) and N2 (≥ 3 LN) [5]. In two papers, both dealing with squamous cell esophageal carcinoma, the number of positive nodes and the lymph node ratio (i.e., the number of positive nodes as a function of the total number of nodes resected) were shown to be important prognostic factors [6, 9]. According to Kunisaki et al., the lymph node ratio can also be useful in determining the adequacy of lymphadenectomy [10]. Despite these results, the lymph node ratio is not included in the present staging system for esophageal cancer [1].

Stage Grouping Controversies

Hsu et al. compared the performance of the 6th and 7th editions of the AJCC staging classification of esophageal cancer. They analyzed 392 SCC patients receiving primary surgical resection through a three-incisional approach and found that in the 6th edition the Kaplan Meier plot showed overlapping curves among stages IIB, III, and IV. Most patients in stage IV had non-regional lymph node metastases while most in stage IIB and III had regional node metastases. The authors stated that identifying non-regional lymph node metastases (M1a) is unnecessary, because there is no difference in survival.

The 7th edition of the AJCC staging system has better homogeneity, discriminatory ability, and monotonicity of gradients compared with the previous edition. Survival curves are similar only between stages IIA and IIB and between stages IIIB and IIIC. Statistical analysis did not identify a significant prognostic value for tumor location and histologic grade, accounting for the worse discriminatory ability in stages IIA and IIB. There was also no statistical difference between N2 and N3 patients, which explains the lack of difference in survival between stages IIIB and IIIC [11].

These findings agree with data published by Hofstetter et al. and Rizk et al., even though in their patients there was a prevalence of adenocarcinoma [12, 13].

Non-anatomic factors are included in the present AJCC 7th edition, but not in the UICC staging system. These factors are histologic type, histologic grading, and tumor location (upper, middle, or lower third of the esophagus). As shown in the paper by Rice et al. [1], these factors have prognostic impact especially in groups with the best survival, i.e., N0 patients. Nevertheless, in the database used for the analysis, SCC histologic type constitutes less than half of the cases. In analyses of SCC-predominant databases, the role of non-anatomic factors is more controversial [11, 14]. The UICC classification does not consider non-anatomic factors, which is more in line with the results of the current literature than the AJCC classification, particularly for SCC.

2.2 Staging after Neoadjuvant Chemoradiotherapy

Preoperative chemoradiotherapy (CRT) is increasingly administered to patients with locally advanced esophageal carcinoma in order to achieve down-sizing and down-staging of the primary tumor and to sterilize nodal metastases, thus increasing the rate of complete tumor resection. The degree of regression produced by therapy (down-staging) is considered by some authors to be of prognostic importance [15].

So far, the esophageal specimen after treatment is still staged according to the TNM classification (ypTNM). However, preoperative CRT produces important changes—both in the tumor cells and in stromal tissues—that are not considered by the TNM classification. Moreover, neoadjuvant therapy causes many cytological changes in tumor cells such that preoperatively treated cancers are often upgraded to poorly differentiated cancers [16].

Since the TNM system is unsatisfactory in re-staging esophageal cancer after CRT, several classification systems have been proposed to assess the pathologic response of the primary tumor (T). The most widely used is Mandard classification, which estimates the degree of residual carcinoma in relation to the total tumor area. The authors distinguish five grades: TRG1: absence of residual tumor; TRG2: rare residual cancer cells scattered through fibrosis; TRG3: more residual tumor cells, but fibrosis still predominating; TRG4: residual cancer cells predominating in the fibrosis; TRG5: no signs of tumor regression [17]. Despite the widespread use of this classification several controversial issues remain. The Mandard system lacks quantitative measurements; hence, it is not easy to classify partial responders. Moreover, it is

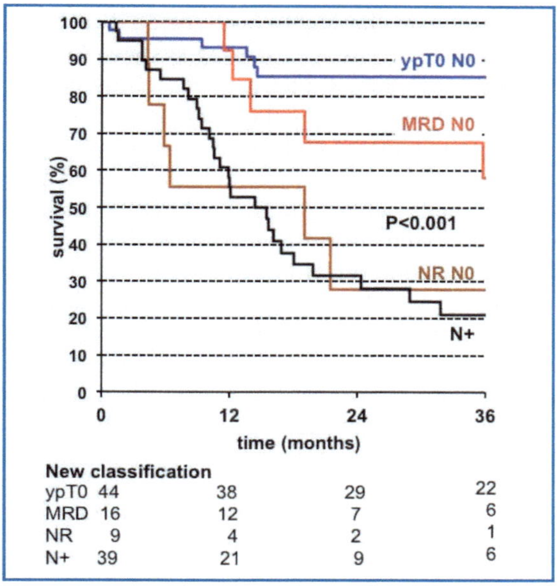

Fig. 2.2 Three-year disease-related survival curves for patients staged with SPR (size-based pathological response) classification of response ($p < 0.001$) [20]. *ypT0*, Pathological tumor category 0 after chemoradiotherapy (complete response); *N0*, no nodal involvement; *MRD*, minimal residual disease; *NR*, non response; *N+*, nodal involvement

focused on the primary tumor and does not take into account the relationship between T response and N stage. Other authors tried to create a response classification based on the percentage of residual cancer cells, but none of these systems has gained universal acceptance [18, 19].

In a paper published by our institution, we proposed a classification (SPR: size-based pathological response) based on the size of residual foci, with the aim of improving reproducibility. We identified, among partial responders, a group of patients with residual foci of ≤ 10 mm (minimal residual disease, MRD), whose survival was intermediate between pathologic complete responders and non-responders (residual cancer > 10 mm) (Fig. 2.2). We also demonstrated that adding the N category both to the Mandard and to our classification significantly increased the amount of prognostic information. In conclusion, we were able to demonstrate that the Mandard and SPR classifications are useful in the assessment of tumor response after CRT and in the evaluation of prognosis, with our system being less operator-dependent and considering the interplay between T and N [20].

2.3 Conclusions

Even though the 7th edition of the AJCC staging system is better than the previous one in terms of monotonicity, discriminatory, and homogeneity, controversial issues remain.

Lymph node classification according to the location of regional involved nodes is no longer included in the latest AJCC/UICC staging system. Also, in a recent paper, Tachimori and colleagues claimed that it is absolutely correct to consider the number of involved nodes, which is the strongest prognostic factor for esophageal cancer, whereas the site of metastasis is less important, not even if the positive nodes are located in the supraclavicular area. Those authors concluded by saying that supraclavicular nodes should be considered as regional nodes for esophageal cancer, thus being N and not M [21].

The analysis so far has been limited to surgical patients without neoadjuvant or post-operative therapy, both of which are now widely used also for SCC and probably have a prognostic impact. There are many classifications of pathologic response to neoadjuvant CRT, but none of them is universally accepted. Further investigation to create a universally accepted classification of response seems crucial to better define the prognosis of patients who undergo neoadjuvant treatments followed by surgery.

References

1. Rice TW, Rusch VW, Ishwaran H, Blackstone EH (2010) Cancer of the esophagus and esophagogastric junction: data-driven staging for the seventh edition of the American Joint Committee on Cancer/International Union Against Cancer Cancer Staging Manuals. Cancer 116:3763-3773
2. Clinical aspects (2008). In: Japanese Society for Esophageal Disease: Japanese classification of Esophageal Cancer, 10th edn. Kanehara & Co., Ltd., Tokyo
3. Edge SB, Byrd DR, Compton CC, eds. (2010) AJCC Cancer Staging Manual, 7th ed., Springer, New York, NY
4. Eguchi T, Nakanishi Y, Shimoda T et al (2006) Histopathological criteria for additional treatment after endoscopic mucosal resection for esophageal cancer: analysis of 464 surgically resected cases. Mod Pathol 19:475-480
5. Rice TW, Blackstone EH, Rybicki LA et al (2003) Refining esophageal cancer staging. J Thorac Cardiovasc Surg 125:1103-1113
6. Hsu WH, Hsu PK, Hsieh CC et al (2009) The metastatic lymph node number and ratio are independent prognostic factors in esophageal cancer. J Gastrointest Surg 13:1913-1920
7. Hu Y, Hu C, Zhang H et al (2010) How does the number of resected lymph nodes influence TNM staging and prognosis for esophageal carcinoma? Ann Surg Oncol 17:784-790
8. Altorki NK, Zhou XK, Stiles B et al (2008) Total number of resected lymph nodes predicts survival in esophageal cancer. Ann Surg 248:221-226
9. Liu YP, Ma L, Wang SJ et al (2010) Prognostic value of lymph node metastases and lymph node ratio in esophageal squamous cell carcinoma. Eur J Surg Oncol 36:155-159
10. Kunisaki C, Akiyama H, Nomura M et al (2005) Developing an appropriate staging system for esophageal carcinoma. J Am Coll Surg 201:884-890
11. Hsu PK, Wu YC, Chou TY et al (2010) Comparison of the 6th and 7th editions of the American Joint Committee on Cancer tumor-node-metastasis staging system in patients with resected esophageal carcinoma. Ann Thorac Surg 89:1024-1031
12. Hofstetter W, Correa AM, Bekele N et al (2007) Proposed modification of nodal status in AJCC esophageal cancer staging system. Ann Thorac Surg 84:365-373
13. Rizk N, Venkatraman E, Park B et al (2006) The prognostic importance of the number of involved lymph nodes in esophageal cancer: implications for revisions of the American Joint Committee on Cancer staging system. J Thorac Cardiovasc Surg 132:1374-1381

14. Wijnhoven BP, Tran KT, Esterman A (2007) An evaluation of prognostic factors and tumor staging of resected carcinoma of the esophagus. Ann Surg 245:717-725
15. Korst RJ, Kansler AL, Port JL et al (2006) Downstaging of T or N predicts long-term survival after preoperative chemotherapy and radical resection for esophageal carcinoma. Ann Thorac Surg 82:480-484
16. Chang F, Deere H, Mahadeva U, George S (2008) Histopathologic examination and reporting of esophageal carcinomas following preoperative neoadjuvant therapy: practical guidelines and current issues. Am J Clin Pathol 129:252-262
17. Mandard AM, Dalibard F, Mandard JC et al (1994) Pathologic assessment of tumor regression after preoperative chemoradiotherapy of esophageal carcinoma. Clinicopathologic correlations. Cancer 73:2680-2686
18. Schneider PM, Baldus SE, Metzger R et al (2005) Histomorphologic tumor regression and lymph node metastases determine prognosis following neoadjuvant radiochemotherapy for esophageal cancer: implications for response classification. Ann Surg 242:684-692
19. Swisher SG, Hofstetter W, Wu TT (2005) Proposed revision of the esophageal cancer staging system to accommodate pathologic response (pP) following preoperative chemoradiation (CRT). Ann Surg 241:810-817
20. Verlato G, Zanoni A, Tomezzoli A et al (2010) Response to induction therapy in oesophageal and cardia carcinoma using Mandard tumour regression grade or size of residual foci. Br J Surg 97:719-725
21. Tachimori Y, Nagai Y, Kanamori N et al (2011) Pattern of lymph node metastases of esophageal squamous cell carcinoma based on the anatomical lymphatic drainage system. Dis Esophagus 24:33-38

Preoperative Work-up: Conventional Radiology, Ultrasonography, CT Scan, and MRI

3

Stefania Montemezzi, Daniela Cenzi, Massimiliano Motton, and Thomas J. Re

3.1 Introduction

The optimal assessment and staging of esophageal cancer (EC) is crucial as it has an important impact on patient selection with respect to appropriate treatment (surgery, neo-adjuvant therapy with or without surgery, palliative treatment) [1]. Preoperative evaluation requires knowledge of the esophageal anatomy and of the patterns of tumor spread. As mentioned in Chap. 2, the staging criteria for esophageal cancer include depth of local invasion, nodal involvement, and presence or absence of distant metastases. The various imaging modalities have different strengths and weaknesses in evaluating each of these criteria such that a combined multimodality imaging approach is usually necessary for an optimal assessment [2].

3.2 Tumor Spread

3.2.1 Direct Extension of the Tumor

The lack of a serosa as a barrier between the esophagus and the surrounding structures facilitates tumor spread through the esophageal wall and thus extra-esophageal involvement. Consequently, it is quite common to find early direct infiltration of the thyroid gland, larynx, large airway, aorta, thoracic duct, lung, pericardium, and diaphragm [3-7].

S. Montemezzi (✉)
Radiology Unit, Borgo Trento Hospital,
Verona, Italy

G. de Manzoni (Ed.), *Treatment of Esophageal and Hypopharyngeal Squamous Cell Carcinoma*,

3.2.2 Lymphatic Spread

Between 74% and 88% of patients with EC have lymphatic spread [8]. The frequency of nodal metastases is related to the size and depth of tumor invasion. An experimental study showed that dye injected into the esophageal wall at one level drains to nodes at all other levels of the esophagus and frequently directly into the thoracic duct. This finding can explain the presence of mediastinal, supraclavicular, and celiac lymph node metastases in at least 75% of EC patients [9] and also the not negligible incidence of "skip metastases" [10]. However, it is difficult to definitively establish whether two separate lesions represent synchronous primary tumors or the same cancer with disseminated lymphatic metastases [11].

3.2.3 Hematogenous Metastasis

Patients with advanced disease usually also have hematogenous metastases. The organ most commonly involved is the liver, because the distal part of the esophagus is drained by the portal vein. Other sites of hematogenous spread include the lung, bone, adrenal gland, and brain. By contrast, cancers of the distal esophagus seldom develop peritoneal metastases [1].

3.3 Pre-treatment Imaging

The diagnosis of EC is usually made by endoscopy, with multiple biopsies. After detection of the disease, pre-treatment tumor staging is planned in order to select the appropriate therapy.

The most widely available imaging techniques for evaluating EC are: endoscopic ultrasonography (EUS), computed tomography (CT), and magnetic resonance imaging (MRI). All are commonly used to provide pre-operative staging. Conventional radiology and ultrasonography (US) play only a secondary role in disease assessment even though in some cases they reveal the disease as an incidental finding while the patient is undergoing an exam for other reasons.

Since all imaging techniques have their advantages and disadvantages, a multi-modality imaging approach is currently considered the best way to obtain the most accurate staging.

The following flow-chart (Fig. 3.1) is a suggestion for a routine work-up in the diagnosis and treatment of esophageal cancer (EC). In patients diagnosed with EC based on gastroscopy and biopsy findings, a computed tomography (CT) scan is performed as it plays a crucial role in the detection of involved lymph nodes, hematogenous metastases, and organ infiltration. In case of distant metastases, palliative care with best supportive care is chosen. Any patient without distant metastases, regardless of whether organ infiltration is suspected (T4a and T4b), should undergo complete disease staging by bronchoscopy

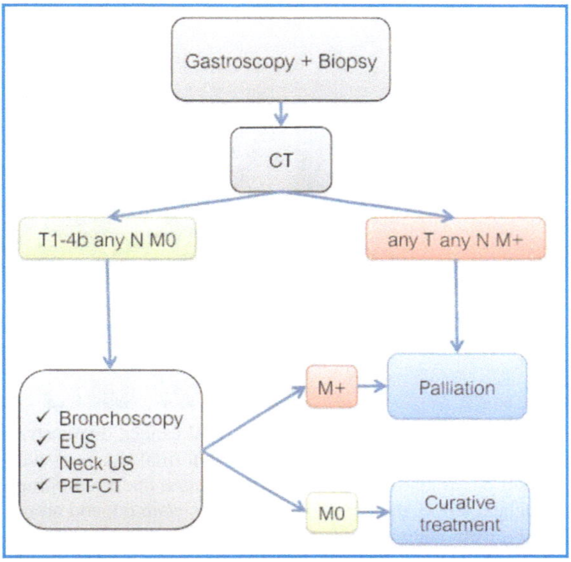

Fig. 3.1 Work-up guidelines in the diagnosis and treatment of esophageal cancer

(to exclude tracheal infiltration, vocal cord paralysis, or concomitant neoplasms in the airways), neck ultrasound (to detect nodes in the neck area, not easily visualized on CT), endoscopic ultrasound (EUS) with potential fine-needle aspiration (to study the depth of tumor invasion and exclude regional nodal metastases), and positron emission tomography PET-CT (to confirm staging, and especially to exclude distant metastases).

3.3.1 Conventional Radiology

As noted above, conventional radiological investigation plays a secondary role in EC imaging studies.

Plain radiographs have no primary application in EC although mediastinal abnormalities can be identified at chest radiograph in about 50% of patients with advanced cancer [12]. The most common signs of disease are: (a) enlargement of the mediastinal silhouette (due to the abnormal-appearance of right and/or left paratracheal stripes); (b) an opacity in the retrocardiac region; (c) an abnormal bulge in the aortopulmonary window; (d) tracheal displacement, with abnormal thickening of the posterior tracheal stripe; (e) dilatation of the esophagus, with an unusual air-fluid level (Fig. 3.2) [12-14]. Tracheal anterior convex displacement, as well as widening of the posterior tracheal stripe > 3 mm at the thoracic inlet and > 5.5 mm at the carina, might be related to direct invasion of the tumor or to lymphatic spread. Dilatation of the esophagus with the evidence of an intraluminal air-fluid level can be demonstrated in large tumors in the distal esophagus or at the esophagogastric junction (EGJ), even if such findings are also common in case of inflammatory stenosis, scleroderma, and achalasia.

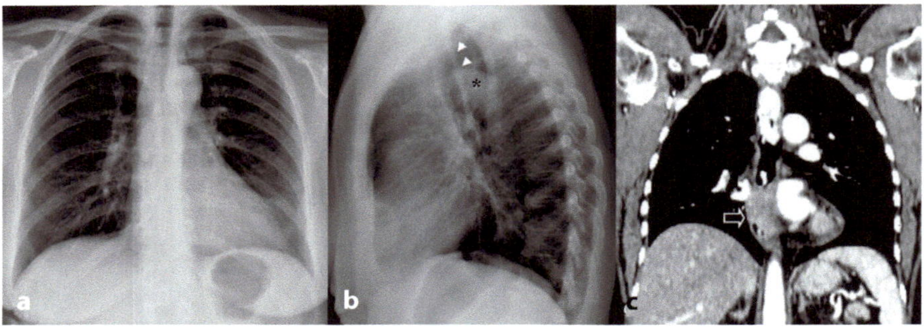

Fig. 3.2a-c Chest radiographs in a 62-year-old patient with lower esophageal cancer, demonstrated at CT coronal reconstruction (**c**). A frontal chest radiograph shows no abnormal signs (**a**), with the normal appearance of the right and left paratracheal stripes. However, lateral chest radiograph (**b**) shows widening of the posterior tracheal stripe, thickened > 5 mm (*arrowheads*), and an unusual dilation of the esophagus (*asterisk*). Both signs should raise suspicion of distal esophageal stenosis. Enhanced CT coronal scan (**c**) highlights an irregular stenotic tumor of the lower esophagus (*large arrow*). This mass causes dilation of the upper and middle esophagus, which is filled with contrast material

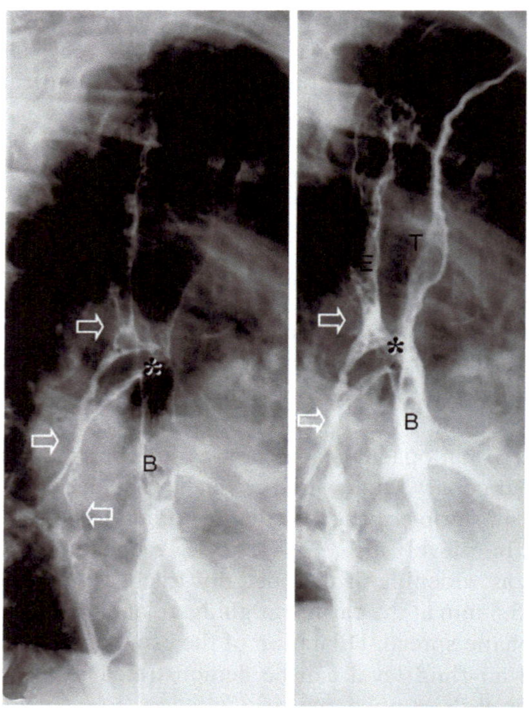

Fig. 3.3 Double-contrast esophagogram of a large cancer extending from the middle to the distal esophagus (*large arrows*), with evidence of tracheo-bronchial fistula (*asterisk*); two subsequent scans on oblique projection are shown. The tumor is demonstrated as an irregular stricture, with a very tight stenosis about 5 cm below the carina. The fistula is seen as a small leakage at the carina, with the passage of contrast medium from the esophagus (*E*) to the main left bronchus (*B*) and, consequently, to the trachea (*T*). It is a typical feature of direct airway invasion

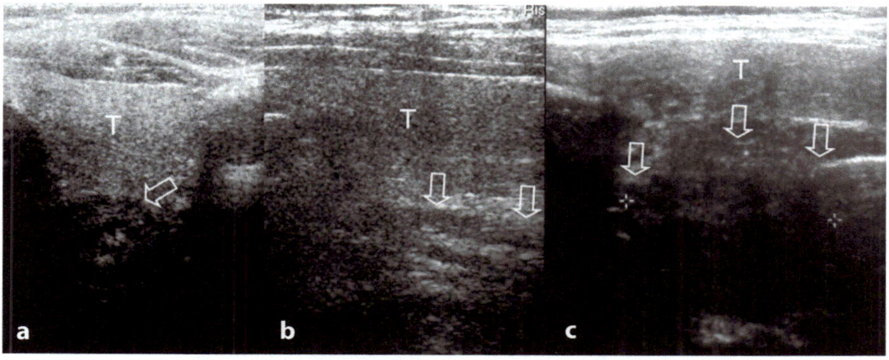

Fig. 3.4 Cervical esophagus as seen on axial (**a**) and longitudinal (**b, c**) ultrasound scans of the neck using a high-frequency linear transducer (10 MHz): two different patients, one with a normal esophagus (**a, b**), the other with cervical esophageal cancer (**c**). The esophagus (*large arrows*) is usually highlighted on the left side of the neck, just behind the left thyroid lobe (*T*). At axial scan (**a**), the normal esophagus is demonstrated as an oval structure with the typical target appearance of the bowel, while in the longitudinal plane (**b**) it has a tubular appearance, with different linear echoes corresponding to the different layers of the wall. Although difficult to demonstrate at ultrasound, a large hypoechoic ovoid mass with irregular borders behind the left thyroid lobe (**c**) should raise suspicion of esophageal cervical cancer. The linear echo appearance is completely disrupted and the esophageal walls are abnormally thickened

In patients with dysphagia, barium upper GI series are usually performed to exclude inflammatory disease or cancer. A double-contrast esophagogram can be used to assess the mucosal surface lesion of the esophagus but it provides little information about the extramucosal extent of the disease. For this reason, its usefulness is limited to local detection and staging.

The tumor may appear as a fungating polypoid mass, an ulcerating mass, or as an irregular stricture (Fig. 3.3). Malignant strictures are usually very tight and often prevent the passage of an endoscopy probe. Submucosal extension may produce the appearance of a "varicoid carcinoma." Unlike true varices, the filling defects of varicoid carcinoma will not change in appearance with Valsalva maneuvers or varying amounts of esophageal distension. The least common appearance is a "superficially spreading" carcinoma, in which subtle small filling defects can be seen only on a high-quality air contrast examination [15-18].

3.3.2 Ultrasound

General Principles and Technique

Transcutaneous US has no application in the routine evaluation of EC, since it provides access only to the cervical (Fig. 3.4) and distal abdominal portions of the esophagus. The thoracic esophagus is surrounded by the lungs and vertebral, sternal and rib bones, making it almost impossible to obtain an appropriate acoustic window for use in the study [19].

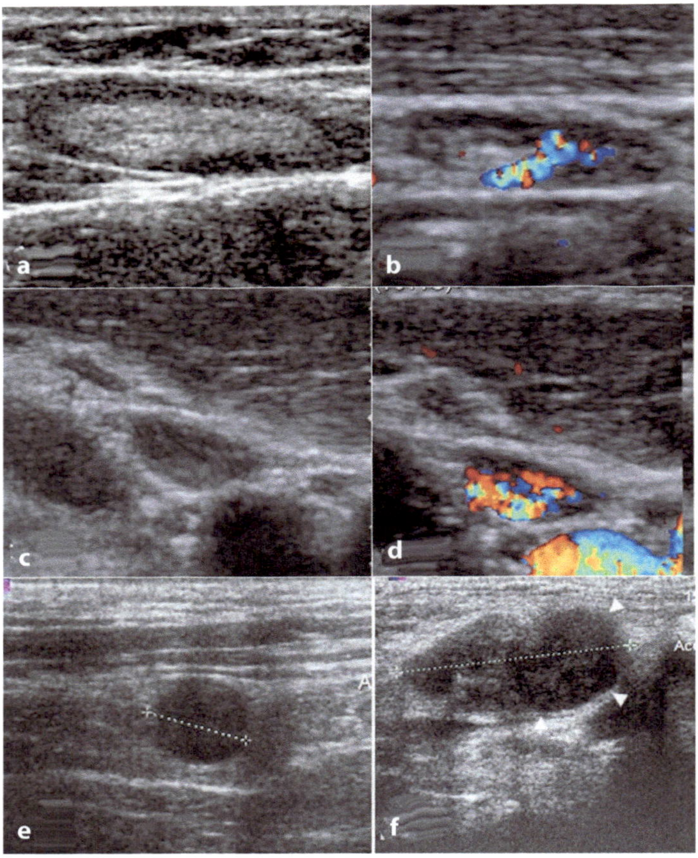

Fig. 3.5. Ultrasound (US) comparison of a reactive node (**a, b**), a node with suspicious characteristics (**c, d**), and metastatic nodes (**e, f**). A typical reactive lymph node of the lateral cervical chain appears is oval in shape, with smooth borders, a central hyperechoic hilum, and regular cortical contours (**a**). Doppler-US shows a radially branching hilar vessel (**b**). Diffuse cortical thickening, with no clear demonstration of the echoic hilum (**c**) and increased, chaotic hilar and transcapsular vasculature at Doppler-US (**d**) suggest nodal invasion: in such cases, fine-needle aspiration biopsy is mandatory to confirm the diagnosis. Finally, two different metastatic lymph nodes of the neck, one at the supraclavicular fossa (**e**), the other of the right internal jugular chain (**f**), are shown. A rounded hypoechoic lymph node with loss of the central hilum (**e**) or nodal enlargement with asymmetric thickening creating focal, hypoechoic, outward bulging, and lobulation in the outer contour (*arrowheads*) (**f**) are certain features of metastatic involvement

Although US may incidentally identify a cervical EC or one at the EGJ, it cannot be proposed for T staging. Nevertheless, it is well known that US is highly accurate and plays an important role in demonstrating lymph node malignancies of the neck (Fig. 3.5) [20, 21]. For this reason, it should be considered as the first choice examination in EC for N staging.

The cervical portion of the esophagus can be visualized during US studies of the neck by using high-frequency linear transducers (7.5–15 MHz). The examination should be performed thoroughly in both the transverse and longitudinal planes and should be extended laterally on both sides to identify enlarged jugular chain nodes, superiorly to visualize submandibular adenopathy, and inferiorly to detect any pathologic supra- and sub-clavicular nodes. The esophagus is usually found laterally, on the left side, just behind the left thyroid lobe, at 2–3 cm from the skin plane. It is clearly identified by its target-pattern appearance in the transverse plane (Fig. 3.4a) and by its peristaltic movement when the patient swallows [22].

The abdominal distal portion of the esophagus and the EGJ are visualized with the target-pattern appearance of the bowel in the transverse plane, behind the left hepatic lobe, lateral to the caudate lobe, above the vertebral body and the suprarenal aorta [19].

T Staging

Cervical EC can be demonstrated on US if the tumor is at least 5 mm in diameter, in which case it may appear as a hypoechoic nodule, round or oval, sometimes with irregular borders, just behind the left thyroid lobe (Fig. 3.3c). The target-sign appearance may be completely disrupted and the walls abnormally thickened [23]. No changes in morphology are observed during US compression of the lesion, whereas the normal esophagus can be compressed and gas bubbles displaced [23, 24].

Distal esophageal and EGJ cancers may appear as an exophytic mass, an asymmetric thickened segment of gut with or without ulceration, or as a sizable intraluminal mass [23, 25]. Eckardt et al., using these features as a reference, reported a high sensitivity (100%) and specificity (82%) for lesions > 8 mm [26].

Despite its capacity to identify lesions, conventional US cannot determine the exact depth of tumor infiltration of the esophageal wall, so that it is very difficult to define T staging.

N Staging

Ultrasound is largely and widely used in highlighting neck adenopathies (Fig. 3.5). In uncertain cases, it enables US-guided fine-needle aspiration biopsy (FNAB) [21].

Apart from size and shape criteria, US can evaluate six other different parameters to define whether nodes are benign or malignant: (1) echogenicity of the hilum, (2) level of echogenicity, (3) necrosis, (4) extracapsular spread, (5) vascularity characteristics, and (6) calcifications. Neoplastic infiltration occurs primarily in the cortex; therefore, malignant nodes have a tendency to a greater transverse diameter, with a round, asymmetric morphology (Fig. 3.5e, f). The long-to-short axis ratio (L\S ratio) can be employed to distinguish between benign (L\S > 2) and malignant (L\S < 2) nodes. The hilum may be thin, eccentric, or completely lacking (Fig. 3.5c, d), with associated eccentric

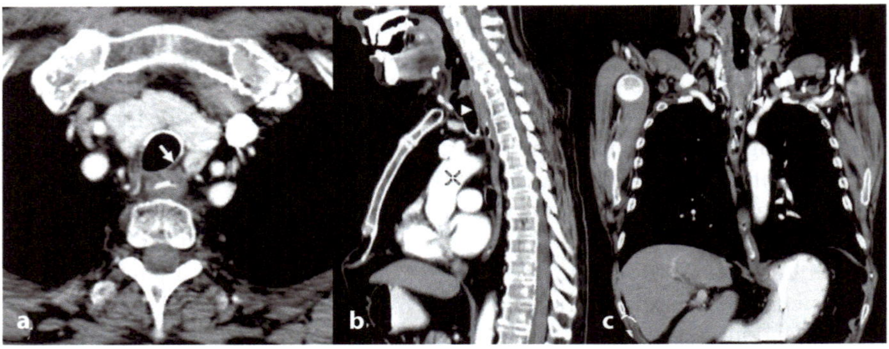

Fig. 3.6 T3 N0 M0 (stage III) carcinoma of the upper thoracic esophagus in a 55-year-old man. Diffuse esophageal wall thickening > 5 mm is demonstrated at axial CT (**a**), obtained at the level of the superior border of the sternum. The anterior outer contours are irregular, with a small spiculation extending into the periesophageal fat plane (*arrow*), suggestive of fat infiltration. Sagittal (**b**) and coronal (**c**) CT reconstructions show the extent of esophageal wall thickening (*arrowhead*), which involves the esophagus from the thoracic inlet to the level of D3. Evidence of the irregular stenotic lumen is better evaluated at coronal reformatted image (**c**), comparing the diameter with that of the middle esophagus by filling the lumen with contrast medium and gas

cortical widening. In patients with a known EC, the presence of necrosis in a lymph node is highly suggestive of malignancy. Margins may be rounded and well-defined, or less defined and sharp, due to possible extracapsular spread. Most malignant nodes show aberrant vessels and a chaotic capsular blood flow pattern. No single sonographic criterion is absolutely specific for a benign or malignant nature; however, rounded shape, absence of hilum, an irregular outline, coagulative or cystic necrosis, and chaotic capsular blood flow pattern are all signs highly suspicious of malignancy, especially when they are present in the same node [20, 27]. For uncertain cases, the most reliable diagnostic modality is US-guided FNAB, based on its high sensitivity (89–98%), specificity (95–100%), and accuracy (95–97%) [20, 21, 27].

3.3.3 Computed Tomography

The mainstay for preoperative staging is a computed tomography study, as it yields information on tumor size, location, extension, mediastinal involvement, nodal metastasis, and distant spread [4]. The development of multidetector CT (MDCT) has provided an extraordinary capacity for fast data acquisition and thin collimation, with significant gains in spatial resolution. MDCT allows isotropic, or near-isotropic voxel acquisition, permitting high-quality multiplanar reconstructions and 3D visualization, achieving a high level of anatomic detail (Fig. 3.6) [28]. MDCT scanners permit also a more accurate assessment of tumor length.

General Principles and Technique

A biphasic (arterial and venous phases) enhanced CT scan of the thorax and abdomen following intravenous injection of contrast medium is the standard technique used to evaluate the region of the primary esophageal tumor and to search for distant metastatic disease. Just before the exam, oral contrast medium or water is administered to the patient to obtain adequate distension of the esophagus, which is a prerequisite for a correct assessment of the esophageal walls, usually collapsed at conventional CT scans and therefore not evaluable. With enough esophageal lumen distension, it is possible to visualize any intraluminal and intramural pathology, as well as the shape, anatomic location, and size of the lesion; extraluminal planes, such as the fat layers between the tumor and the adjacent organs; or airway tree involvement. Due to the rapid transit of contrast medium in the esophagus, it is essential to perform the exam immediately after its oral administration in order to achieve an optimal distension at the moment of acquisition. It is better to use water or oral contrast medium diluted with water, since undiluted oral contrast medium could have the same density of the tumor, making image interpretation difficult [29]. Some authors have recently proposed the use of water and effervescent granulate as a negative contrast agent; alternatively, direct lumen distension can be achieved by instilling air through a 14 French Foley catheter placed transorally [3, 30-32]. The use of an antiperistaltic drug is not necessary, as the induction of pharmacological hypotonia has not been shown to produce a clear improvement in lumen distension.

Thoracic and abdominal CT scans must be acquired during a single breath-hold in full inspiration. Optimization of intravenous contrast material injection is particularly necessary when performing MDCT. Proper contrast enhancement offers improved differentiation of tumor tissue from normal mucosa [33] and increases the detection of liver metastases. Axial images, with a slice thickness of at least 3 mm and 1-mm reconstruction increments, together with multiplanar reformatting in the sagittal and coronal planes should be routinely evaluated. MDCT is especially valuable in T staging and in determining the actual tumor length, which is important in the evaluation of upper and lower resection margins. CT estimates of tumor length made with multiplanar reformatted images are more accurate than those made with axial scans alone, especially for EC at the EGJ (Fig. 3.7) [1, 3].

T Staging

The normal esophageal wall is usually < 3 mm thick when the esophagus is distended; thus, any wall thickness > 5 mm or asymmetric thickening of the esophageal wall should be considered abnormal. These anomalies are considered a primary but non-specific CT finding of EC [1].

CT can highlight wall thickening but it is not able to demonstrate the different layers of the esophageal wall. As a consequence, it is unable to adequately differentiate between T1, T2, and T3 disease. This drawback is mainly due to contrast resolution as the tumor's attenuation is similar to that of the

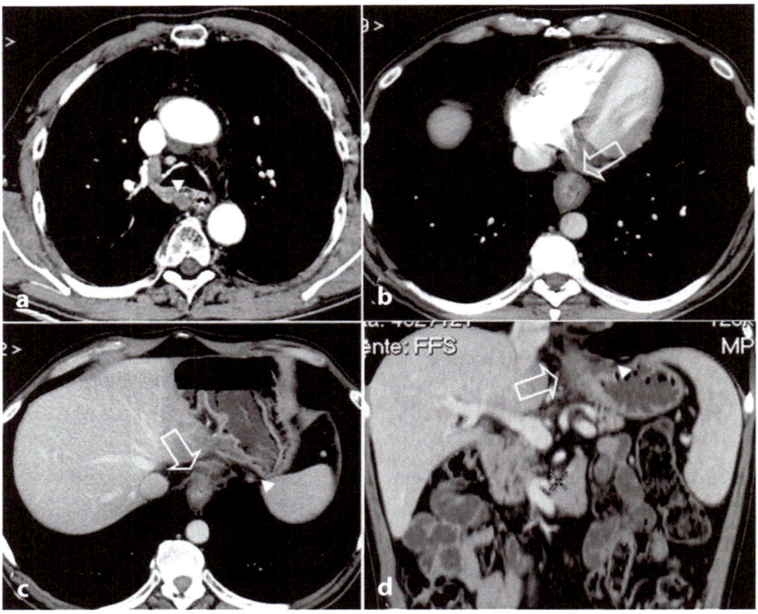

Fig. 3.7 T3N+M0 distal esophageal cancer in a 48-year-old man. **a** Axial CT scan obtained at the level of the carina shows a rounded hypodense lymph node (*arrowhead*) just behind the trachea and in the right para-esophageal space. The esophageal wall is not thickened at this site. **b** Axial CT scans obtained at the level of left ventricle and **c** diaphramatic hiatus demonstrate diffuse esophageal wall thickening (*large arrow*), with irregular borders and strand-like areas of increased attenuation extending into the peri-esophageal fat. Note the preserved fat plane between the mass and the heart, and the triangular fat space between the esophagus and the aorta. The tumor involves the gastro-esophageal junction, better seen at coronal CT reconstruction (**d**). A small perigastric lymph node (*arrowhead*) is highlighted, on the axial and coronal images, raising suspicion of metastatic involvement. However, the lymph node's location is better highlighted at coronal reconstruction, where it appears on the left side, next to the cardia, just below the distal margin of the tumor

esophageal wall, with only slight differences in contrast enhancement. Accordingly, the major role of CT is to detect the invasion of adjacent organs (cT4 disease). CT has a proven high negative predictive value for T4 disease as the preservation of fat planes between the EC and adjacent structures is a highly specific sign [34]. Unfortunately, fat planes are obscured in many patients with loss of body weight due to dysphagia or in those who have undergone radiation therapy; thus, whereas frank infiltration of adjacent structures is easily detected, it is usually difficult to exclude minimal invasion [35].

EC may manifest as a focal area of mural thickening with or without ulceration, as a flat or polypoid lesion, or as a generalized mural thickening. The probability of transmural extension of the tumor is directly correlated with mural thickness; fat invasion is shown when the outer contours become blurred

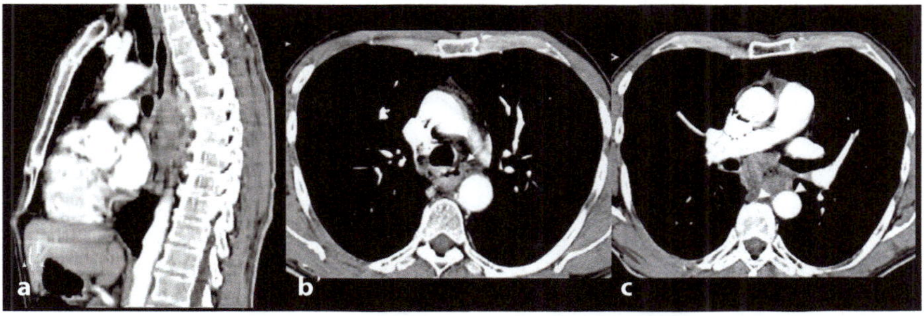

Fig. 3.8 T4 N+ M0 mid-esophageal cancer in a 45-year-old man. A large stenotic tumor of the middle esophagus is highlighted at CT sagittal reconstruction (**a**). The walls are irregularly thickened on axial imaging, obtained at the level of the carina (**b**); there is complete stenosis of the esophageal lumen, as seen on axial CT obtained at the level of the right pulmonary artery (**c**). Note a small left para-esophageal lymph node (*arrow*) (**b**) and the absent fat plane between the esophagus and the aorta (*arrowheads*) (**c**), with 80–90° direct contact between the tumor and the circumference of the aorta. This is pathognomonic of aortic invasion

and strand-like areas of increased attenuation are seen extending into the periesophageal fat plane (Fig. 3.8) [3].

The CT criteria for local infiltration of adjacent structure include the loss of fat planes between the tumor and other structures in the mediastinum, and the displacement or indentation of other mediastinal structures due to a mass effect [1]. Aortic invasion is a very rare finding. It is suggested on imaging if there is at least 90° of direct contact between the tumor and the circumference of the aorta (accuracy around 80%) or if there is obliteration of the triangular fat space between the esophagus, aorta, and spine adjacent to the primary tumor (sensitivity 100%; specificity 82%) (Fig. 3.8c) [36, 37]. Unfortunately, according to other studies, these criteria are unreliable [38] and the suspicion of aortic invasion is difficult to prove preoperatively; in most cases, this determination is a surgical one [2].

Unlike aortic invasion, tumor spread into the central airways is not rare. Flattening and indentation of the membranous portion of the trachea or main bronchus have proved to be accurate predictors of tracheobronchial invasion, although this finding may be caused by simple mass effect upon the membranous portion of the airway, without invasion. Tracheobronchial fistula and frank abnormal soft-tissue extension into the airway lumen are typical features of tracheobronchial invasion (Fig. 3.9) [2, 35]. Overall, the reported sensitivity for tracheobronchial involvement ranges from 31 to 100%, specificity from 68 to 98%, and accuracies from 74 to 97% [39]. Imaging features suggesting invasion should be further evaluated and confirmed with bronchoscopy + biopsy [2].

Pericardial invasion is suspected if pericardial thickening, pericardial effusion, or indentation of the heart with loss of the pericardial fat plane is visualized. Extensive invasion is unresectable, while minimal invasion may be resectable [1, 35].

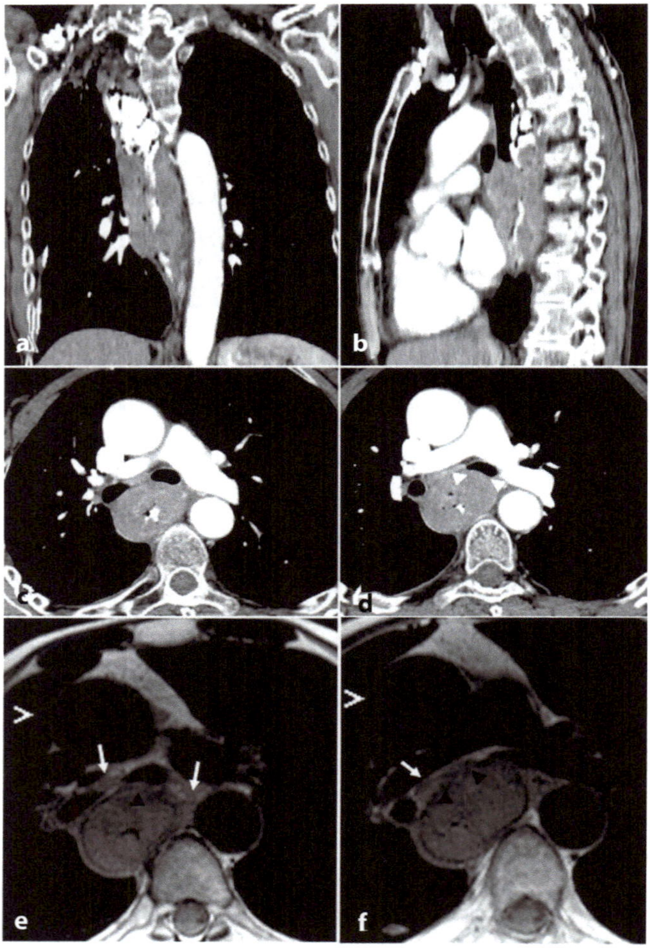

Fig. 3.9 T4 N+ M0 upper and middle esophageal cancer in a 64-year-old female. Sagittal (**a**) and coronal (**b**) reformatted CT images demonstrate a large stenotic mass of the mid-esophagus that involves the esophageal wall from the level of the aortic arch to that of the mid-left atrium. The lumen upstream is enlarged and filled with air and contrast medium. Tumor length is better evaluated on multiplanar coronal and sagittal reconstructions. Contrast-enhanced CT scans obtained at the level of the tracheal carina (**c**) and pulmonary artery (**d**) highlight diffuse wall thickening and define the relationship with the adjacent anatomic structures: a broad interface between the esophageal mass and the left main bronchus (*arrowheads*) is seen, as is subsequent flattening and narrowing of the left main bronchus. This is suspicious of airway infiltration. The normal fat plane between the thoracic aorta and esophagus is seen on sagittal and axial images, with no evidence of aortic invasion. T2-weighted axial MRI (**e, f**) can be helpful in determining trachea-bronchial invasion vs. a simple mass effect upon the membranous portion of the airway. The outer low-signal-intensity muscularis propria is focally disrupted anteriorly, with tumor spread at the site of the membranous portion of the left main bronchus, which is flattened (*arrowhead*) (**e**); this is a definite sign of tumor infiltration. Also worth noting is the loss of a high-signal fat plane and the nodular irregularity into the peri-esophageal fat just below the tracheal carina (**f**) along with small peri-esophageal lymph nodes (*white arrows*), which are not always demonstrated on CT images

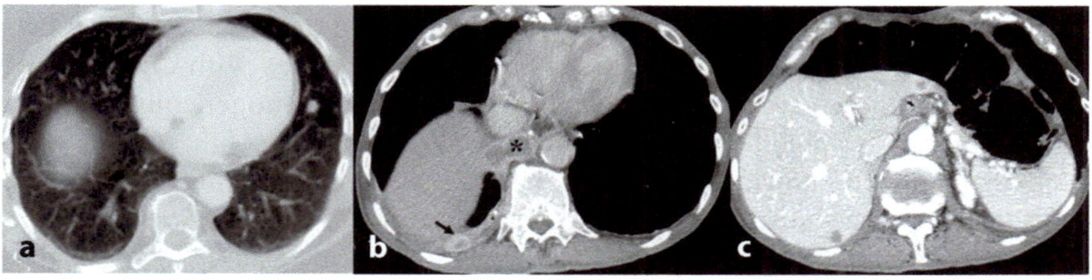

Fig. 3.10 Metastatic spread of esophageal cancer: three different cases. **a** CT axial image at lung window demonstrates a 1-cm metastatic nodule on the left side; this is common evidence of esophageal cancer with metastatic disease; **b** the demonstration of pleural effusion with small metastatic nodules (*arrow*) showing pleural attachment is rare. In this patient, this finding was associated with evidence of enlarged necrotic lymph nodes (*asterisk*) in the right diaphragmatic crus space; **c** hypodense nodules extending into the liver on the left side and at segment VII are typical features of metastatic liver disease

The reported sensitivity and specificity of CT for detecting mediastinal invasion in patients with esophageal cancer are 88–100% and 85–100%, respectively [36, 40]. CT accuracy for overall pre-operative T staging was traditionally low, between 49% and 59% [1]; it has undoubtedly improved with the development MDCT technology [28, 30], but further studies are needed before its true accuracy can be confirmed. However, most comparative studies have demonstrated that endoscopic US (EUS) is more accurate than CT in the assessment of preoperative T, so that EUS is considered the method of choice in T staging [34, 41]. In a recent international multicenter study, EUS staging was compared with staging by CT alone and the additional information obtained by EUS was shown to change patient management in one-third of the reported cases [42].

N Staging

Lymph node assessment remains a challenge even with MDCT and the diagnosis of regional nodal metastasis is complex for two main reasons: (1) a bulky primary tumor may obscure adjacent involved nodes (Fig. 3.9d, f) [43] and (2) the diagnosis of lymph node disease is based exclusively on size criteria. Indeed, enlarged nodes may be reactive and benign, whereas small nodes may harbor microscopic metastases. In addition, a significant correlation between lymph node size and the frequency of nodal metastases has not been established [44]. As the detection of metastatic nodes depends primarily on size criteria, the sensitivity and specificity of CT are strictly dependent on the definition of an abnormally enlarged node. In general, intrathoracic and abdominal lymph nodes > 1 cm and supraclavicular nodes with a short axis > 5 mm are considered to be pathologic [45, 46]. Most studies that use the common size criterion of 1 cm to define an enlarged node report a sensitivity of CT of 30–60%, whereas specificity tends to be somewhat higher (60–80%) (Fig. 3.10b) [47, 48]. Ba-Ssalamah et al. recently suggested that both morphologic and enhancement criteria be evaluated to increase the diagnostic accuracy: better results can be achieved if peri-esophageal lymph nodes with diameters of at least 6 mm, rounded shape, and marked or inhomogeneous contrast enhancement are judged as positive (Fig. 3.8b) [3].

EUS has been shown to be superior to CT even in detecting lymph node metastases, with accuracy for N staging ranging from 72 to 80% [49]. However, its sensitivity and specificity in detecting lymph node metastases vary depending on location, with better results in the assessment of celiac lymph nodes than mediastinal lymph nodes. Importantly, EUS can only visualize lymph nodes close to the esophageal wall, as the probe has a limited field of view of approximately 5 cm, whereas CT can demonstrate both regional and distant lymph nodes. According to a recent meta-analysis, EUS was significantly more sensitive but less specific than CT for the detection of regional lymph node metastases, and EUS and CT studies are to be combined in N staging [50].

M Staging

Computed tomography has a crucial role in the identification of distant metastases, which are typically localized in the liver and lungs (Fig. 3.10) and, more rarely, in the adrenal glands or in the bones. Contrast-enhanced MDCT is currently the preferred method for liver evaluation: liver metastases are highlighted as hypodense lesions. Most metastases are best visualized during the portal venous phase of liver enhancement.

The sensitivity of spiral CT for the detection of masses $\geq$ 1 cm is approximately 90% [51]; however, in patients with known malignancy, only 50% of lesions < 1.5 cm and 12% of lesions < 1 cm are metastatic [52, 53]. No recent data regarding the accuracy of MDCT have been reported in the literature, even if an improvement in the detection of small lesions ($\leq$ 5 mm) is expected.

CT is very sensitive in the detection of pulmonary nodules. Pulmonary metastases are usually rounded, smooth bordered, and non-calcified. Given the high prevalence of incidentally detected nodules at screening CT, suspect pulmonary lesions should be confirmed by further examinations, especially when the presence of pulmonary metastases has an influence on therapeutic planning. A synchronous primary lung cancer should be considered in patients with EC when the pulmonary lesion is solitary, as smoking is related to carcinogenesis of both esophageal and lung cancer [1].

It is important to realize that both CT and positron emission tomography with 2-[fluorine-18]-fluoro-2-deoxy-D-glucose (FDG-PET) can be used to detect distant metastases. In a recent meta-analysis, the pooled sensitivity of CT for the detection of distant metastases was lower than that of FDG-PET, whereas specificity was equivalent [50]. Furthermore, several publications have reported the additional value of FDG-PET in the detection of distant metastases, in 5–28% of patients with EC [54], and suggested that an FDG-PET exam be performed in case of equivocal CT-findings.

3.3.4 Magnetic Resonance Imaging

The role of MRI in the diagnosis and staging of esophageal tumors has not been thoroughly evaluated and evidence of a distinct advantage over traditional imaging modalities has not been established [55-57]. At most institutions, MRI is rarely performed for EC staging, probably because it is more difficult to perform, requiring respiratory and cardiac gating to optimize images and to avoid motion artifacts. Recent advances in MRI technology have improved the achievable signal to-noise ratio, thus improving performance in terms of spatial and temporal resolution. This has opened new possibilities in the local staging of EC. It is well known that MRI, like CT, can successfully be used in the evaluation of wall thickness, mediastinal involvement, adjacent lymphadenopathy, and distant spread, with contrast resolution higher than CT (Fig. 3.9e, f) [4]. Recent studies have developed imaging criteria for the local staging of EC using high-resolution T2-weighted imaging and have suggested the potential of this technique as an alternative non-invasive method to CT and EUS for local staging (Fig. 3.11) [58, 59].

Compared to MRI, EUS remains the imaging modality of choice for local staging, but several of its limitations may be overcome by MRI, at least in selected cases. For example, the accuracy of EUS remains highly operator dependent and in up to 17–24% of cases EUS is unable to stage tumor T and N due to the presence of unsurpassable stenosis.

General Principles and Technique

Until recently, the conventional MRI approach consisted of T1-weighted and T2-weighted spin-echo or turbo spin-echo sequences, in axial and sagittal planes with respiratory and cardiac triggering [55]; unfortunately, this approach did not provide useful information about the separate layers of the esophageal wall.

Recent studies have demonstrated the potential of MRI to depict the different esophageal wall layers. Some authors proposed the use of an endoluminal surface coil attached to the tip of a modified endoscope, with encouraging preliminary results. This technique has some limitations: the inability of the coil to traverse strictures; a short radius for receiving signal (3–4 cm), which necessitates repositioning of the endoscope for evaluation of long tumors; and motion artifacts due to peristalsis [60-62]. Other authors have focused on the development of high-spatial-resolution T2-weighted imaging techniques using external surface coils. They were encouraged by the technique's non-invasiveness and by the success that high-resolution MRI has already achieved in imaging of the pelvis. These authors demonstrated that T2-weighted high resolution MRI is able to produce detailed images of the different layers of the esophageal wall [58, 59, 63, 64].

The standard protocol of high-resolution T2-weighted MRI starts with an initial sagittal sequence for localizing the esophagus and to guarantee optimum coil placement. Subsequently, axial images are acquired perpendicular to

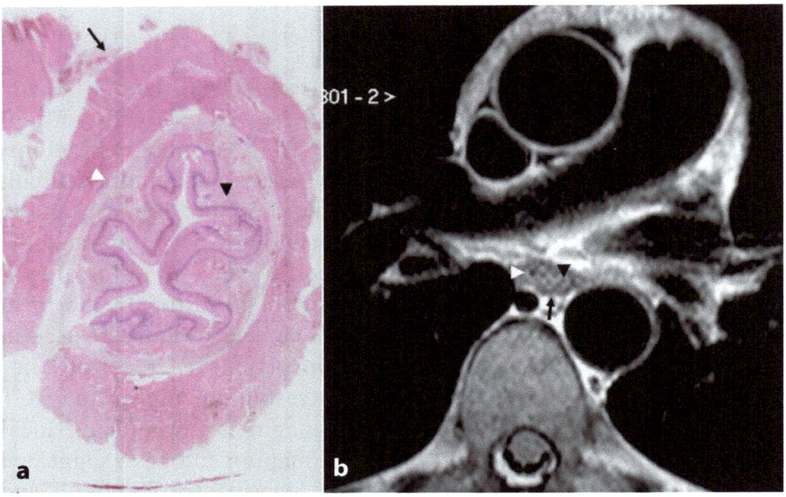

Fig. 3.11 Correlation between a histological anatomic section of the esophagus, (**a**) and high-resolution T2-weighted axial MRI at 3 Tesla in a healthy 33-year-old man (**b**). Images show the different layers of the esophageal wall: mucosa (*black arrowhead*), submucosa (*white arrowhead*), and muscularis propria (*arrow*). High-resolution T2-weighted axial MRI can demonstrate all layers of the wall. The mucosa appears as a fine, intermediate-signal-intensity, corrugated layer surrounded by the high-signal-intensity submucosa and the outer low-signal-intensity muscularis propria. (Images courtesy of Dr. A. Tomezzoli)

the long axis of the esophagus using a standard fast spin-echo T2-weighted sequence similar to that used for pelvic imaging but modifying baseline sequence parameters by using cardiac gating, a reduction in the field of view, and an increased signal to noise ratio [58, 59].

T Staging

Preliminary results reported by Riddell et al. using high-resolution T2 weighted MRI are very encouraging [58, 59, 65]. The normal esophageal wall is usually only 3 mm thick but with this technique the different sub-layers of the wall are clearly visible: normal mucosa is characterized by a fine intermediate signal layer, which is often corrugated. This layer is surrounded by high-signal-intensity submucosa and the outer low-signal-intensity muscularis propria; the esophagus is surrounded by high-signal peri-esophageal fat (Fig. 3.11) [59]

These authors also demonstrated that the degree of wall infiltration on MRI correlates with the pathological T stage in the majority of cases, with a tendency to overstage T1 tumors, which due to their minimal mass effect on the esophageal wall are difficult to differentiate from normal wall [59]. Thickening of the esophageal wall and an alteration in the cross-sectional appearance of the esophagus from the normal elliptical shape to a circular one may help to identify tumor location. Riddell et al. proposed several MRI criteria for the local staging of esophageal cancer: T2 cancer has intermediate sig-

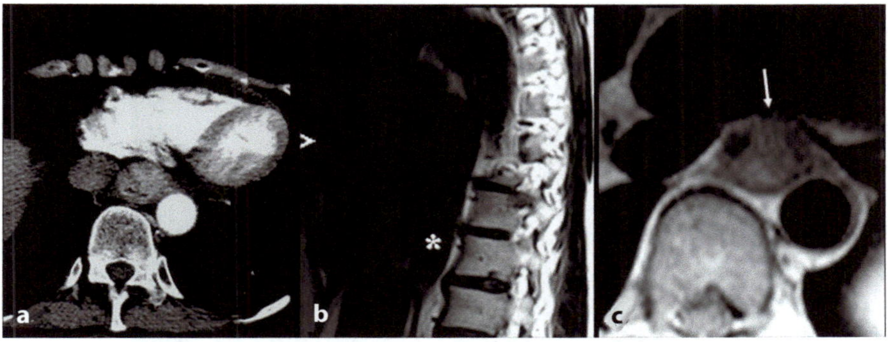

Fig. 3.12 Comparison between local staging by CT and MRI. The CT axial image obtained at the level of the right ventricle (**a**) demonstrates an eccentric polypoid esophageal mass of the lower esophagus. The fat plane evident between the mass and the heart and the preserved triangular fat space between the esophagus, aorta, and spine are consistent with T2 or T3 disease. In this case, it is quite difficult to distinguish tumor from the normal esophageal wall, as there are only slight differences in contrast enhancement. Sagittal and axial MRI (**b**, **c**) shows higher contrast resolution. Focal thickening of the distal esophageal wall is seen on the sagittal image (**b**), with evidence of a polypoid mass of intermediate signal filling the lumen (*asterisk*). At axial T2-weighted MRI (**c**) the tumor is seen to involve the anterior and left anterolateral walls, with irregular loss of the outer low-signal-intensity muscularis propria, which corresponds to focal peri-esophageal fat invasion in a T3 tumor. Posteriorly, the low signal intensity of the muscularis propria is well demonstrated

nal intensity within the high-signal submucosa and low-signal muscularis propria, without any disruption of the outer margin, which remains clearly defined. Nodular irregularity of the outer margin of the muscularis propria with intermediate signal intensity into the peri-esophageal tissues should be considered a typical feature of a T3 carcinoma (Fig. 3.12), whereas T4 tumors are demonstrated as masses of intermediate signal intensity extending into adjacent structures (Fig. 3.13) [65]. As in the case of CT, MRI criteria for the local infiltration of adjacent structures are the loss of fat planes between the tumor and other structures in the mediastinum, and the mass effect over other mediastinal structures. However, spatial and contrast resolution are superior in MRI compared to CT, so that the relationship of extramural tumor to its surrounding structures is more clearly defined [65].

Despite the relevance of all these initial findings, further studies with larger numbers of cases are needed to define the real clinical impact of high-resolution T2 MRI in the local staging of EC.

N Staging

Like CT, conventional MRI is inaccurate in preoperative nodal staging because it relies on insensitive and nonspecific nodal size criteria. Conventional MRI is mainly limited because signal intensity evaluation does not reliably differentiate benign from malignant lymph nodes. The sensitivity of conventional MRI in depicting N metastases is 36%, specificity 86%, accuracy 77%, positive predictive value 38%, and negative predictive value 85% [66].

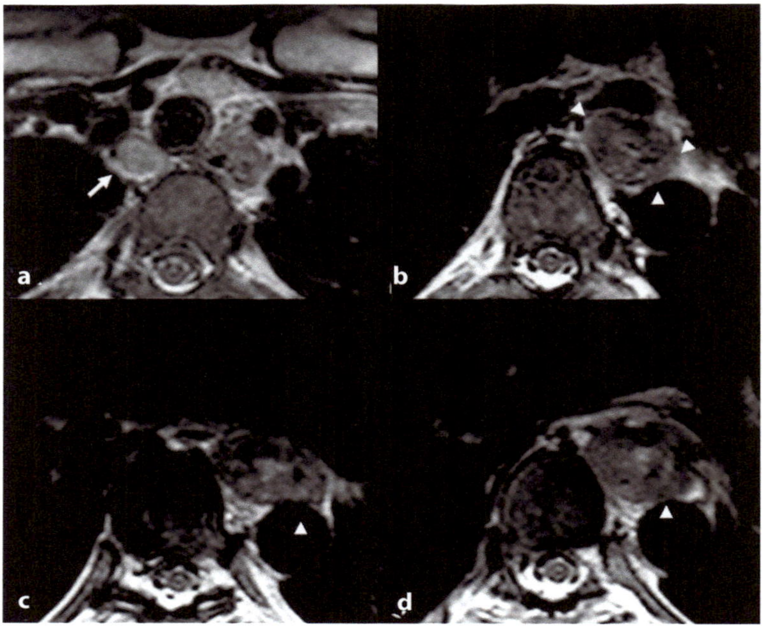

Fig. 3.13 Local staging by high-resolution T2-weighted MRI in a T4N+M0 upper and middle esophageal cancer in a 51-year-old female. Axial MRI demonstrates a bulky esophageal tumor, with irregular thickening of the cervical and middle esophageal walls, extending from the suprasternal notch (**a**) to the left atrium (**d**). A thoracic outlet tumor involves the anterior and left anterolateral walls, with local spreading into the peri-esophageal fat (**a**). An enlarged necrotic lymphadenopathy is seen on the right para-tracheal side (*arrow*). Inferiorly, the circumferential tumor shows evidence of multiple sites of focally disrupted, low-signal-intensity outer muscularis propria. At axial MRI at the level of the left main bronchus (**b**), there is focal disruption of the right anterolateral and left posterolateral walls (*arrowheads*). A slight direct contact between tumor and aortic adventitia is highlighted, suggesting focal infiltration. Axial image obtained 1 cm below, at the level of the left hilum (**c**), demonstrates the close relationship between the esophageal posterior wall and the aortic adventitia (*arrowhead*). At this site, there is no evidence of disruption of the low-signal-intensity muscularis propria, thus excluding tumor infiltration. Finally, the axial image obtained at the level of the pulmonary artery (**d**) shows irregular thickening mainly involving the posterior walls, which are irregular and less well defined, with direct contact and infiltration of the aortic adventitia (*arrowhead*)

Multiple efforts to increase MRI accuracy in N staging have been attempted, with contradictory results. Nanoparticle-enhanced MRI has proven to be very useful for the characterization of lymph nodes [67-69] but its use in clinical practice is still under evaluation. The development of high-resolution MRI has suggested that the likelihood of node-positive disease might be increased in the presence of nodular densities > 2 mm in size within the peri-esophageal tissues, but histopathologic studies to confirm this finding are missing [59]. Sakurada et al. have tried to assess the value of diffusion-weighted magnetic resonance imaging (DWI) in detecting EC and assessing lymph node status. However, although DWI is an excellent non-invasive imaging technique that also provides functional information, it has only a restricted role in T and N staging [70].

Finally, Alper et al. recently observed that the characteristics of lymph nodes with turbo-spin-echo (TSE) sequence with short-term inversion recovery (STIR) are much more feasible than with CT and conventional MRI. According to their experience, the signal intensity value of the lymph nodes enabled the differentiation between metastatic and non- metastatic lymph nodes. Mean signal intensities values were found to be higher in metastatic than in non-metastatic nodes and metastatic intensity values were equal to or greater than those for the pathologic esophagus. With TSE-STIR, they achieved a sensitivity of 81.3%, a specificity of 98.3%, a positive predictive value of 92.9%, and a negative predictive value of 95.2% in detecting nodal metastases, even for lymph nodes < 1 cm in diameter [71].

3.4 Re-staging after Neoadjuvant Therapy

The identification after neoadjuvant chemoradiation therapy (CRT) of patients who had a good response and thus may benefit from surgery is an important objective, with a strong impact on treatment choices [72-74].

Imaging is divided into two main stages. In the "early-response assessment" stage, a short time after the start of treatment, tumor responsiveness is evaluated and non-responding patients are identified. In the "late-response assessment" stage, several weeks after the completion of induction therapy, the extent of down-staging of the primary tumor is determined.

Assessment of therapeutic response has traditionally been performed with CT, endoscopic gastroduodenoscopy, and EUS [75]. However, the extent of tumor necrosis, inflammation, and fibrosis that follow CRT decrease the accuracy of these methods in the evaluation of the extent of residual malignancy [1, 74, 75].

CT has been widely used for monitoring non-surgical therapy in patients with various solid tumors but in EC it is not considered sufficiently accurate for the assessment of treatment response [1]. The sensitivity of response assessment in CT reportedly range from 27% to 55%, and the specificity from 50 to 91% [76, 77]. These poor results are most likely related to the fact that the only feature suggesting treatment response is a change in the size of the mass (Fig. 3.14). It is extremely difficult using CT to differentiate between viable tumor and reactive change, such as inflammation or scar tissue (Fig. 3.15) [1], and no specific MDCT studies have been reported thus far.

Perfusion CT is a recent development that seems to be useful in predicting the response to CRT [78-81]. Tumor angiogenesis is regarded as a prerequisite for tumor progression and blood supply may be one of the tumor's biological characteristics that influence the effect of adjuvant therapies. CT perfusion is a non-invasive, objective, and reproducible technique to assess microvascular density within the tumor in vivo, through the quantitative analysis of hemody-

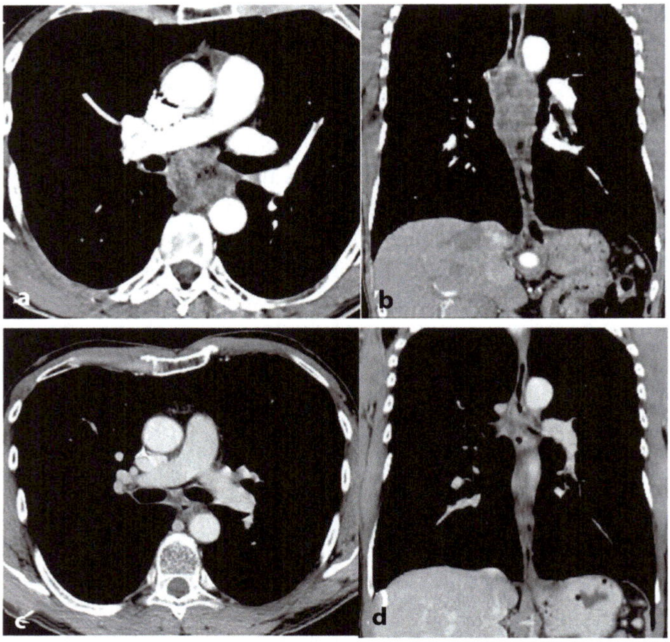

Fig. 3.14 Initial (a, b) and re-staging (c, d) evaluation of a middle esophageal cancer (same patient as in Fig. 3.6) after neoadjuvant chemoradiation therapy. a, b Axial and coronal reformatted CT images obtained at initial staging show a large stenotic mass in the middle esophagus; c, d post-therapy CT scan obtained at the same levels shows a significant decrease in the size of the esophageal mass, and in peri-esophageal infiltration, both of which suggest a good response to inductive therapy and confirm the high positive predictive value of CT

namic parameters. Chen et al. showed a higher blood value and longer time to peak in esophageal squamous cell carcinoma than in normal esophagus [80], while Hayano et al. demonstrated that esophageal tumor with a higher blood flow, higher blood volume, or shortened mean transit time at pre-CRT might have a better clinical response to CRT, with an accuracy of 90.3% for the detection of clinical responders [78]. Also, Makari et al. found a significant correlation between blood flow and tumor size reduction by CRT [79]. Therefore, perfusion CT to assess the early response to neoadjuvant treatment appears promising, but further, large cohort studies are needed before its clinical usefulness can be fully exploited.

3.5 Conclusions

Currently, a multi-modality imaging approach is recommended to achieve the most accurate staging in EC (tumor wall invasion, lymphatic involvement, and

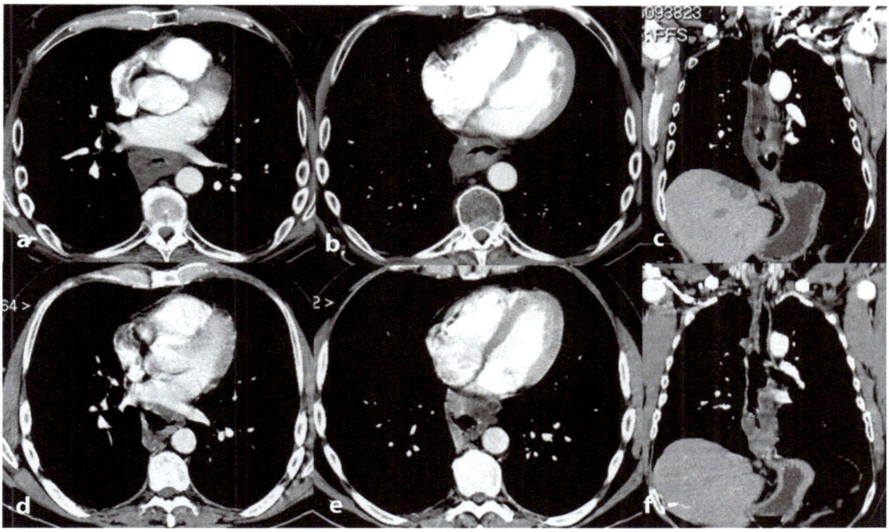

Fig. 3.15 Initial (**a-c**) and re-staging (**d-f**) evaluation of a mid-lower esophageal cancer in a 39-year-old man who underwent neoadjuvant therapy. Axial (**a, b**) and coronal reformatted images (**c**) obtained at initial staging show a large mass in the middle and lower esophagus that has caused irregular thickening of the esophageal walls. Follow-up axial and coronal CT images obtained at the same levels (**d-f**) after completion of neoadjuvant radiation therapy show no significant changes in the size of the mass, suggesting no response. Actually, there was a partial response to chemoradiation therapy, demonstrated at CT-PET and at histopathological examination after surgical resection. The persistence of wall thickening was mainly due to fibrotic tissue changes related to radiation therapy. At CT scan, it is impossible to distinguish between residual tumor mass and fibrotic tissue

metastatic spread). CT, EUS, and PET/PET-CT all play important roles in disease staging, while conventional radiology, US, and MRI are not currently used in the routine study of EC (see Fig. 3.1). However, imaging techniques continue to evolve, especially regarding the staging of advanced cases. According to the literature, the most promising emerging imaging techniques are high-resolution T2-weighted MRI and perfusion-CT. In EC, the former may become a non-invasive alternative to EUS in the initial staging of the disease, while perfusion CT may soon play a role in assessing tumor response to neoadjuvant therapy.

References

1. Kim TJ, Kim HY, Lee KW, Kim MS (2009) Multimodality assessment of esophageal cancer: preoperative staging and monitoring of response to therapy. RadioGraphics 29:403-421
2. Quint LE and Bogot NR (2008) Staging esophageal cancer. Cancer Imaging 8: S33-S42
3. Ba-Ssalamah A, Zacherl J, Noebauer-Huhmann IM et al (2009) Dedicated multi-detector CT of the esophagus: spectrum of diseases. Abdom Imaging 34:3-18

4. Jang MK, Lee KS, Lee KS et al (2002) The spectrum of benign esophageal lesions: Imaging findings. Korean J Radiol 3:199-210
5. Yamada A (1979) Radiologic assessment of respectability and prognosis in esophageal cancer. Gastrointestinal Radiol 4:213-218
6. Mannell A (1982) Carcinoma of the esophagus. Curr Probl Surg 19:553-647
7. Levine MS and Halvorsen RA (2002) Carcinoma esofageo. In: Gore, Levine Eds. Trattato di Radiologia Gastro-intestinale Vol.1. Verduci Ed., Roma, pp 409-438
8. Siewert JR (2007) Esophageal carcinoma. Chirurg 78:475-484
9. Suga K, Shimizu K, Kawakami Y et al (2005) Lymphatic drainage from esophagogastric tract: feasibility of endoscopic CT lymphography for direct visualization of pathways. Radiology 237:952-960
10. Mandard AM, Chasle J, Marnay J et al (1981) Autopsy findings in 111 cases of esophageal cancer. Cancer 48:329-335
11. Glickman JN. II (2003) Pathology and pathologic staging of esophageal cancer. Semin Thorac Cardiovasc Surg 15:167-179
12. Lindell MM, Hill CA, Libshitz HI (1979) Esophageal cancer: radiographic chest findings and their prognostic significance. AJR 133:461-465
13. Gibbs JM, Chandrasekhar CA, Ferguson EC, Oldham SAA (2007) Lines and stripes: where did they go? From conventional radiography to CT. RadioGraphics 27:33-48
14. Whitten CR, Khan S, Munneke GJ, Grubnic S (2007) A Diagnostic Approach to Mediastinal Abnormalities. RadioGraphics 27:657-671
15. Gloyna RE, Zornoza J, Goldstein HM (1977) Primary ulcerative carcinoma of the esophagus. AJR 129:599-600
16. Yates CW Jr, Le Vene MA, Jensen KM (1977) Varicoid carcinoma of the esophagus. Radiology 122:605-608
17. Mori M, Mimori K, Sadanaga N et al (1994) Polypoid carcinoma of th esophagus. Jpn J Cancer Res 85:1131-1136
18. Buck JL (2001) Neoplastic and non-neoplastic tumors of the esophagus. Eur Radiol 11:S97-S103
19. Martinoli C, Givagnorio F, Derchi LE (2006) Anatomia ecografia normale del tratto gastroenterico. In: Arienti V (ed) Ecografia clinica del tratto gastroenterico. Unimedia srl- Athena srl, Modena, pp 75-84
20. Esen G (2006) Ultrasound of superficial lymph nodes. Eur J Radiol 58:345-359
21. de Bondt RBJ, Nelemans PJ, Hofmana PAM et al (2007) Detection of lymph node metastases in head and neck cancer: A meta-analysis comparing US, USgFNAC, CT and MR imaging. Eur J Radiol 64:266-272
22. Solbiati L, Charboneau JW, Osti V et al (2005) The thyroid gland. In: Rumack CM, Wilson SR, Charboneau JW (eds) Diagnostic ultrasound, 3rd edn. Mosby, St. Louis, pp 735-770
23. Vitale F, Arienti V (2006) Semeiotica ecografica. In: Arienti V (ed) Ecografia clinica del tratto gastroenterico. Unimedia srl- Athena srl Modena, pp 109-118
24. Doldi SB, Lattuada E, Zappa MA et al (1997) Ultrasonographic imaging of neoplasms of the cervical esophagus. Hepatogastroenterology 44:724-726
25. Tanomkiat W, Chongchitnan P (1999) Transabdominal sonography of gastroesophageal junctions. J Clin Ultrasound 27:505-512
26. Eckardt VF, Schmitt T, Kanzler G (2004) Transabdominal ultrasonography in achalasia. Scan J Gastroenterol 39:634:637
27. Solbiati L, Osti V, Cova L, Tonolini M (2002) Ultrasound of thyroid, parathyroid glands and neck lymph nodes. In: Ultrasound Categorial Course ECR 2002 Beart LA Ed, Eur Radiol Supplement Springer-Verlag, pp 320-333
28. Onbas O, Eroglu A, Kantarci M et al (2006) Preoperative staging of esophageal carcinoma with multidetector CT and virtual endoscopy. Eur J Radiol 57:90-95
29. Mazzeo S, Caramella D, Gennai A et al (2004) Multidetector CT and virtual endoscopy in the evaluation of the esophagus. Abdom Imaging 29:2-8
30. Panebianco V, Grazhdani H, Iafrate F et al (2006) 3D CT protocol in the assessment of the

esophageal neoplastic lesions: can it improve TNM staging? Eur Radiol 16:414-421
31. Carrascosa P, Capun˜ay C, Lòpez EM et al (2009) Esophageal stenosis: three dimensional multidetector CT and virtual endoscopy. Abdom Imaging 34:19-25
32. Ulla M, Cavadas D, Mun˜oz I et al (2010) Esophageal cancer: pneumo-64-MDCT. Abdom Imaging 35:383-389
33. Kumano S, Tsuda T, Tanaka H et al (2007) Preoperative evaluation of perigastric vascular anatomy by 3-dimensional computed tomographic angiography using 16-channel multidetector-row computed tomography for laparoscopic gastrectomy in patients with early gastric cancer. J Comput Assist Tomogr 31:93-97
34. Rice TW (2000) Clinical staging of esophageal carcinoma. CT, EUS, and PET. Chest Surg Clin N Am 10:471-485
35. Diederich S (2007) Staging of oesophageal cancer. Cancer Imaging 7:S63-S66
36. Picus D, Balfe DM, Koehler RE et al (1983) Computed tomography in the staging of esophageal carcinoma. Radiology 146:433-438
37. Takashima S, Takeuchi N, Shiozaki H et al (1991) Carcinoma of the esophagus: CT vs MR imaging in determining resectability. AJR Am J Roentgenol 156:297-302
38. Lehr L, Rupp N, Siewert JR (1988) Assessment of resectability of esophageal cancer by computed tomography and magnetic resonance imaging. Surgery 103:344-350
39. Rankin S (1990) The role of computerized tomography in the staging of oesophageal cancer. Clin Radiol 42:152-153
40. Daffner RH, Halber MD, Postlethwait RW et al (1979) CT of the esophagus. II. Carcinoma. AJR Am J Roentgenol 133:1051-1055
41. Marzola MC, de Manzoni G, Grassetto G et al (2010) Extended staging of oesophageal cancer using FDG-PET. A critical appraisal. Eur J Radiol, doi: 10.1016/j.ejrad2010.10.018
42. Mortensen MB, Edwin B, Hunerbein M et al (2007) Impact of endoscopic ultasonography (EUS) on surgical decision-making in upper gastrointestinal tract cancer: an international multicenter study. Surg Endosc 21:431-438
43. Kumbasar B (2002) Carcinoma of esophagus: radiologic diagnosis and staging. Eur J Radiol 42:170-180
44. Schroder W, Baldus SE, Monig SP et al (2002) Limph node staging of esophageal squamous cell carcinoma in patients with and without neoadjuvant radiochemotherapy: histo-morphologic analysis. World J Surg 26:584-587
45. Dorfman RE, Alpern MB, Gross BH, Sandler MA (1991) Upper abdominal lymph nodes: criteria for normal size determined with CT. Radiology 180:319-322
46. Fultz PJ, Feins RH, Strang JG, et al (2002) Detection and diagnosis of nonpalpable supraclavicular lymphnodes in lung cancer at CT and US. Radiology 222:245-251
47. Block MI, Patterson GA, Sundaresan RS et al(1997) Improvement in staging of esophageal cancer with the addition of positron emission tomography. Ann Thorac Surg 64:770-777
48. Kato H, Kuwano H, Nakajima M et al (2002) Comparison between positron emission tomography and computed tomography in the use of the assessment of esophageal carcinoma. Cancer 94:921-928
49. Souquet JC, Napoleon B, Pujol B et al (1994) Endoscopic ultrasonography in the preoperative staging of esophageal cancer. Endoscopy 26:764-766
50. van Vliet EPM, Heijenbrok-Kal MH, Hunink MGM et al (2008) Staging investigations for oesophageal cancer: a meta-analysis. British J Cancer 98: 547-557
51. Kuszyk BS, Bluemke DA, Urban BA et al (1996) Portalphase contrast-enhanced helical CT for the detection of malignant hepatic tumors: sensitivity based on comparison with intraoperative and pathologic findings. AJR Am J Roentgenol 166:91-95
52. Jones EC, Chezmar JL, Nelson RC, Bernardino ME (1992) The frequency and significance of small (less than or equal to 15 mm) hepatic lesions detected by CT. AJR Am J Roentgenol 158:535-539
53. Schwartz LH, Gandras EJ, Colangelo SM et al (1999) Prevalence and importance of small hepatic lesions found at CT in patients with cancer. Radiology 210:71-74
54. Kato H, Miyazaki T, Nakajima M et al (2005) The incremental effect of positron emission to-

mography on diagnostic accuracy in the initial staging of esophageal carcinoma. Cancer 103:148-156
55. Giovagnoni A, Valeri G, Ferrara C (2002) MRI of esophageal cancer. Abdom Imaging 27:361-366
56. Wu LF, Wang BZ, Feng JL et al (2003) Preoperative TN staging of esophageal cancer: Compaison of miniprobe ultrasonography, spial CT and MRI. Wordl J Gastroenterol 9:219-224
57. Jamil LH, Gill KRS and Wallace MB (2008) Staging and restaging of advanced esophageal cancer. Current Opinion in Gastroenterology 24:530-534
58. Riddell AM, Richardson C, Scurr E, Brown G (2006) The development and optimization of high spatial resolution MRI for imaging the oesophagus using an external surface coil. Br J Radiol 79: 873-879
59. Riddell AM, Allum WH, Thompson JN et al (2007) The appearances of oesophageal cancinoma demonstrated oh high-resolution T2-weighted MRI, with histopathological correlation. Eur Radiol 17:391-399
60. Inui K, Nakazawa S, Yoshino J et al (1995) Endoscopic MRI: preliminary results of a new technique for visualization and staging of gastrointestinal tumors. Endoscopy 27:480-485
61. Kulling D, Feldman DR, Kay CL et al (1998) Local staging of esophageal cancer using endoscopic magnetic resonance imaging: prospective comparison with endoscopic ultrasound. Endoscopy 30:745-749
62. Dave UR, Williams AD, Wilson JA et al (2004) Esophageal cancer staging with endoscopic MR imaging: pilot study. Radiology 230:281-286
63. Yamada I, Murata Y, Izumi Y et al (1997) Staging of esophageal carcinoma in vitro with 4.7-T MR imaging. Radiology 204:521-526
64. Yamada I, Izumi Y, Kawano T et al (2001) Superficial esophageal carcinoma: an in vitro study of high-resolution MR imaging at 1.5 T. J Magn Reson Imaging 13:225-231
65. Riddell AM, Davies DC, Allum WH et al (2007) High-resolution MRI in evaluation of surgical anatomy of the esophagus and posterior mediastinum. AJR Am J Roentgenol 188:W37-W43
66. Nishimura H, Tanigawa N, Hiramatsu M et al (2006) Preoperative esophageal cancer staging: magnetic resonance imaging of lymph node with ferumoxtran-10, an ultrasmallsuperparamagnetic iron oxide. J Am Coll Surg 202:604-611
67. Sigal R, Vogl T, Casselman J et al (2002) Lymph node metastases from head and neck squamous cell carcinoma: MR i1aging with ultrasmall superparamagnetic iron oxide particles (Sinerem MR) – results of a phase-III multicenter clinical trial. Eur Radiol 12:1104-1113
68. Harisinghani M, Saksena M, Hahn P et al (2006) Ferumoxtran-10-enhanced mr lymphangiography: does contrast-enhanced imaging alone suffice for accurate lymph node characterization? AJR Am J Roentgenol 186:144-148
69. Saksena M, Harisinghani M, Hahn P et al (2006) Comparison of lymphotropic nanoparticle-enhanced MRI sequences in patients with various primary cancers. AJR Am J Roentgenol 187:W582-W588
70. Sakurada A, Takahara T, Kwee TC et al (2009) Diagnostic performance of diffusion-weighted magnetic resonance imaging in esophageal cancer. Eur Radiol 19:1461-1469
71. Alper F, Turkyilmaz A, Kurtcan S et al (2010) Effectiveness of the STIR turbo spin–echo sequence MR imaging in evaluation of lymphadenopathy in esophageal cancer. Eur J Radiol. doi:10.1016/j.ejrad.2010.08.003
72. Kelsen DP, Ginsberg R, Pajak TF et al (1998) Chemotherapy followed by surgery compared with surgery alone for localized esophageal cancer. N Engl J Med 339:1979-1984
73. Ancona E, Ruol A, Santi S et al (2001) Only pathologic complete response to neoadjuvant chemotherapy improves significantly the long term survival of patients with resectable esophageal squamous cell carcinoma: final report of a randomized, controlled trial of preoperative chemotherapy versus surgery alone. Cancer 91:2165-2174
74. Bruzzi JF, Munden RF, Truong MT et al (2007) PET-CTof esophageal cancer: its role in clinical management. RadioGraphics 27:1635-1652
75. Westerterp M, van Westreenen HL, Reitsma JB et al (2005) Esophageal cancer: CT, endoscop-

ic US, and FDG PET for assessment of response to neoadjuvant therapy–systematic review. Radiology 236:841-851
76. Swisher SG, Maish M, Erasmus JJ et al (2004) Utility of PET, CT, and EUS to identify pathologic responders in esophageal cancer. Ann Thorac Surg 78:1152-1160
77. Cerfolio RJ, Bryant AS, Ohja B et al (2005) The accuracy of endoscopic ultrasonography with fine-needle aspiration, integrated positron emission tomography with computed tomography, and computed tomography in restaging patients with esophageal cancer after neoadjuvant chemoradiotherapy. J Thorac Cardiovasc Surg 129:1232-1241
78. Hayano K, Okazumi S, Shuto K et al (2007) Perfusion CT can predict the response to chemoradiation therapy and survival in esophageal squamous cell carcinoma: initial clinical results. Oncol Rep 18:901-908
79. Makari Y, Takushi Y, Yuichiro D et al (2007) Correlation between tumor blood flow assessed by perfusion CT and effect of neoadjuvant therapy in advanced esophageal cancers. J Surg Oncol 96:220-229
80. Chen TW, Yang ZG, Li Y et al (2009) Quantitative assessment of first-pass perfusion of oesophageal squamous cell carcinoma using 64-section MDCT: initial observation. Clinical Radiology 64:38-45
81. Chen TW, Yang ZG, Li Y et al (2010) Whole tumour first-pass perfusion using a low-dose method with 64-section multidetector row computed tomography in oesophageal squamous cell carcinoma. Eur J Radiol. doi:10.1016/j.ejrad.2010.07.006

Preoperative Work-up: EsophagoGastroDuodenoScopy, Tracheobronchoscopy, and Endoscopic Ultrasonography

4

Luca Rodella, Angelo Cerofolini, Francesco Lombardo,
Filippo Catalano, Walid El Kheir, and Giovanni de Manzoni

4.1 Endoscopy

Patients with esophageal squamous cell carcinoma (ESCC) frequently describe "alarm" symptoms, such as as dysphagia, bleeding, and weight loss. In these cases, endoscopy of the upper gastrointestinal (GI) tract is the first diagnostic examination usually performed. In a series of 4018 patients, Bowrey et al. [1] identified 123 cases of esophagogastric carcinoma (3%), and in 85% of these patients "alarm" symptoms were present. A comparison of this subgroup with the entire series showed that in the former the tumors were significantly more advanced (47% vs. 11%); there were fewer indications for surgery (50% vs. 95%) and a worse survival (median 11 vs. 39 months).

4.1.1 Early Cancer

The extensive use of new endoscopic methodologies (discussed below) has enabled the detection of a higher number of non-invasive neoplastic lesions defined as "in situ cancer" or invasive "superficial" tumors that correspond to the T1 stage of the TNM classification, in which invasion is limited to the mucosa and submucosa. The macroscopic classification of superficial esophageal cancer recognizes:
Type 0: Superficial
Type 0-I: Superficial and protruding (Ip: protruding; Is: sessile)
Type 0-II: Superficial and flat (IIa: slightly elevated; IIb: flat; IIc: slightly depressed)

L. Rodella(✉)
Surgical Endoscopy Unit, Borgo Trento Hospital,
Verona, Italy

G. de Manzoni (Ed.), *Treatment of Esophageal and Hypopharyngeal Squamous Cell Carcinoma*,

Type 0-III: Superficial and distinctly depressed (Japanese Society of Esophageal Disease [2, 3]

In the esophagus, protruding lesions are infrequent and have a sessile morphology (0-Is). The elevation or depression of superficial lesions may be measured using a single jaw of a biopsy forceps (1.2-mm) as a calibrating gauge.

The endoscopic detection of superficial neoplastic lesions can be supplemented by other endoscopic methodologies such as:

High-definition (HD) and high-magnification (HM) endoscopy. Standard video-endoscopes produce an image signal of 100,000–300,000 pixels. The advent of HD endoscopes has resulted in the production of signal images with resolutions ranging from 850,000 to more than 1 million pixels. This modality is different from HM endoscopy, which simply moves the image closer on the display, while maintaining the image display resolution [4]. Nonetheless, the role of HD or HM in the identification of superficial, early ESCC is still questionable.

Chromoendoscopy. The endoscopic morphology of superficial lesions can be assessed after spraying them with an iodine-potassium solution (Lugol solution 1.5–2.0%) that stains normal epithelium dark brown, while the neoplastic areas remain discolored. It is safe and quick to perform, with a very high sensitivity (90–100%) but low specificity (60–70%), allowing more precise biopsy samples. An endoscopic screening conducted in 62 French endoscopy centers using Lugol staining (1095 patients) showed a 9.9% prevalence of ESCC in high-risk patients, i.e., with a history of head, neck, or tracheobronchial carcinoma [5]. Indigo carmine, a contrast solution that accumulates in the spaces between mucosal folds, may serve as a diagnostic alternative, improving evaluation of the mucosal pattern on HD endoscopy [6].

Narrow-band imaging (NBI). This is a new contrast-enhancing technique that, instead of staining agents, uses optical narrow-bandwidth filters in a red-green-blue sequential illumination system. NBI may disclose the irregular surface architecture of the epithelium (pit pattern) and abnormal vascular networks. In ESCC, the intrapapillary capillary loops undergo changes in caliber and shape or show dilatation and weaving [7]. NBI is more suitable for the targeted meticulous inspection of suspicious areas previously detected with HD or autofluorescence endoscopy. Goda et al. compared HM with NBI and EUS in 72 patients. The sensitivity rates of the three techniques in diagnosing superficial ESCC were 72, 78, and 83%, respectively, with specificity rates of 92, 95, and 89%. The authors concluded that the clinical utility of HM endoscopy with NBI does not seem to be significantly different from that of non-HM endoscopy or endoscopic ultrasonography (EUS) [8] .

Endoscopic mucosal resection (EMR)/endoscopic submucosal dissection (ESD). In case of suspected superficial cancer, endoscopic resection (ER) may provide a precise diagnosis, with the entire specimen submitted for histological inspection (depth of invasion, grading, lymph/vascular invasion, margins of resection). All visible lesions should be removed by ER, which has been shown to influence patient management in up to 30% of the cases. The indications for

EMR, as defined by the Japanese Esophagus Association, are restricted to m1 or m2 cancer, while for m3 or sm1 invasion the local recurrence rate is reportedly 7.8–20%, and 23–57%, respectively [9-11]. Compared to EMR, ESD allows better study of the lateral and vertical margins of the tumor [12]. Oyama performed ESD with the hook knife, obtaining en bloc resection in 95% of the cases and without any local recurrence. The median size of the resected specimen was 32 mm (range: 8-76 mm) [13]. However, ESD is more time-consuming than EMR and correlates with a higher risk of complications (perforation, hemorrhage). In Western countries, ESD series are still limited; a recent European survey reported that ESD was performed in ex vivo models in only 12 endoscopic centers [14].

4.1.2 Advanced Cancer

Advanced cancer of the thoracic esophagus has been macroscopically classified in five types by the Japanese Society of Esophageal Disease [15]:
Type 1: Protruding
Type 2: Ulcerative and localized
Type 3: Ulcerative and infiltrating
Type_4: Diffusely infiltrating
Type 5: Unclassified

An accurate description, according to Savary and Miller [16], also includes: location of the proximal and distal margins, longitudinal and circumferential extent and location, degree of mobility and fixation, diameter of the lumen, appearance of the mucosa proximal to the cancer, histological type, and status of the larynx and vocal cords to evaluate recurrent laryngeal nerve function.

A particular diagnostic approach is needed in case of tumors located in the cervical esophagus, extending from the lower border of the cricopharyngeal muscle (upper esophageal sphincter) to the thoracic inlet. These tumors must be distinguished from those of the hypopharynx or larynx, best appreciated by an ear-nose-throat specialist, who should perform a laryngoscopy to evaluate the need for a total laryngectomy associated with an esophagectomy

In high-risk patients, HM endoscopy and NBI offer a new approach to pharyngeal squamous cell cancer screening [17]. At present, the double-contrast esophagogram is the preferred diagnostic approach only if an esophagorespiratory fistula is suspected.

4.2 Endoscopic Ultrasonography

4.2.1 Clinical Staging

T Staging

Endoscopic ultrasonography is essential to identify those patients who are unlikely to benefit from surgery and in whom a conservative palliative treatment is indicated, or patients with early cancer for whom endoscopic treatment may be ideal. When any distant metastasis has been excluded, EUS should be the next step in locoregional staging. Radial or linear scanners with high-frequency probes (7.5-20 MHz) and 3-D interrogation are currently used, with an overall diagnostic accuracy of approximately 80% [18]. EUS can detect wall layer thickening and disruption (T) and node involvement (N). The highest accuracy is obtained for T3-T4 cancers and the lowest for intraesophageal tumors (T1-T2).

In case of high-grade stenosis, a dilatation may be necessary to enable EUS staging; indeed, evaluation limited to the proximal site of the stenosis has a poor accuracy (< 50%) [19]. By using a guide-wire, it is possible to pass an 8-mm/12-MHz probe (Olympus MH-908) through the stenosis, with a reported accuracy in T staging of 89% [20]. An alternative is the use of miniprobes, which are available with 1.8- to 2.6-mm diameters and frequencies of 12, 15, 20, and 30 MHz. These instruments distinguish nine layers within the wall in contrast to the five layers seen with conventional EUS and have been proposed in the differentiation between cancers limited to the mucosa and those with submucosal infiltration, with an accuracy ranging of 67–94% [21]. Unfortunately, these miniprobes do not accurately study the external margins of infiltrating tumors and adjacent lymph nodes [22].

According to many authors, the role of EUS in the staging of high-grade dysplasia and early esophageal cancer is inadequate and its clinical impact on the workup is disappointing [23, 24]. EMR or ESD, as discussed before, can be performed in a diagnostic setting, overcoming the limitations of EUS. The "non-lifting sign" (no elevation of the lesion), due to submucosal infiltration, has 100% sensitivity, 99% specificity, and 83% positive predictive value, as shown in studies involving colonic polyps [25].

N Staging

The EUS features suggestive of lymph node metastasis are: size (> 10 mm), shape (round), echogenicity (hypoechoic pattern), and borders (smooth). No single criterion is diagnostic, while the presence of all four criteria has an accuracy of 80–100% [23]. Additional criteria are node location (i.e., celiac region), number of lymph nodes identified (> 5), and advanced T staging (T3, T4) [24]. In case of positivity of less than five criteria, EUS-guided fine-needle aspiration for cytological examination increases the accuracy to 87–100% [25]. EUS-guided fine-needle aspiration is indicated only if the lymph node status will change the therapeutic approach. During this procedure, it is important to keep the needle away from the primary tumor, in order to avoid false-positive results. The combined approach of computed tomography (CT), positron emission tomography (PET), and EUS was reported to change the treatment plan of patients with ESCC, reducing the number of unnecessary operations to 21% from 44% when CT alone was used [26, 27].

4.2.2 Staging after Neoadjuvant Treatment

A common observation in neoadjuvant trials is that patients with good clinical response have a very good prognosis. This has pointed out the need for an objective method to evaluate this response [28]. Clinical response has been evaluated by endoscopy with biopsies and by EUS. Endoscopic response evaluation is easy to perform; however, the false negative rate of results compared to the final pathologic examination is around 40–50% among all clinical experiences [28-30], and the technique is therefore too inaccurate to predict major pathologic tumor regression or complete response. Also, re-biopsies in the area of cancer after treatment are not useful in clinical decision-making. Indeed, while a positive re-biopsy was shown to secure proof of residual tumor, in half of the cases in which there was a negative result histopathologic examination of the resected specimen revealed residual tumor [28-30]. In conclusion, all patients with negative endoscopy or negative re-biopsies after neoadjuvant treatment should undergo esophagectomy. Endoscopy with re-biopsy is not suggested if performed only to stage treatment response.

The first study on the accuracy of EUS after neoadjuvant treatment was published in 1999 by our group [31]. We analyzed 87 patients who underwent EUS after completion of a chemo/radiotherapy protocol and then esophagectomy after 4–6 weeks. The overall accuracy of EUS in T staging was 48%, and 71% in N staging. These poor results were confirmed by other studies [30, 32] and in some the results were even worse. For example, Agarval [33] reported correct T staging in 29% of 97 patients analyzed, with the majority of cases (55%) overstaged. Also, the sensitivity of EUS in N staging was worse (48% for N0 and 52% for N1). Therefore, according to the most of the published results, there is no benefit in response evaluation by EUS as it is inaccurate in differentiating residual tumor from tissue reaction after chemo/radiotherapy (inflammation, necrosis, fibrosis) [31, 32].

4.3 Tracheobronchoscopy (TBS)

Tracheobroncoscopy (TBS) has an important role in ESCC staging in the evaluation of direct airway invasion, involvement of the recurrent laryngeal nerves, and the presence of synchronous cancer in the respiratory tract.

ESCC has a high risk of local spread to surrounding tissues, with involvement of the tracheobronchial tree in 6–46% of cases and fistula development in 1–13%. TBS may show compression or infiltration from the adjacent cancer and helps to choose the appropriate palliative treatment (laser, stent, or brachytherapy). Choi et al. [34] proposed what has become the most often used classification of airway infiltration:

Grade I: No abnormalities

Grade IIa: Slight compression of the trachea or bronchus; normal mobility of the wall; parallel and regular longitudinal folds of the pars membranacea

Grade IIb: Impingement or deviation of the trachea or bronchus or widening of the carina, associated with reduction of the mobility during coughing and breathing

Grade III: Frank mucosal invasion [34, 35]

Impingement alone is not considered as a T4 lesion and is therefore still considered resectable. A standardized classification scheme has been proposed for central airway stenosis, considering degree (code 0: non stenosis – code 1:< 25% - code 2: 26-50% - code 3: 51-75% - code 4: 76-90% - code 5: 90-complete ostruction), type (functional or structural: exophytic, extrinsic distortion, scar) and location of stenoses in order to provide universally accepted informations for the operators, avoiding repeated examinations [36]. When the tumor is located in the middle or the upper part of the esophagus, TBS with biopsy and brushing has an accuracy of more than 95%. A comparison of TBS and CT scan showed a discordance in 40% of the cases, with higher specificity and positive predictive values for TBS [37]. Careful inspection of the larynx also evaluates the function of the vocal cords: the impairment of one or both of them is indicative of infiltration of the recurrent laryngeal nerves (T4).

Recently, autofluorescence bronchoscopy (AF) was shown to have a higher sensitivity in detecting early tracheobronchial lesions and the growth process from adjacent ESCC. The technique makes use of fluorescence light produced by a xenon lamp and recognizes different degrees of abnormal fluorescence in suspected areas due to differences in the amount of fluorophores or to angiogenesis, thus permitting a more accurate analysis of the depth of infiltration [38].

References

1. Bowrey DJ, Griffin SM, Wayman J et al (2006)Use of alarm symptoms to select dyspeptics for endoscopy causes patients with curable esophagogastric cancer to be overlooked. Surg Endosc 20:1725-1728
2. Japanese Society for Esophageal Disease (1992) Guidelines for clinical and pathologic studies on carcinoma of the esophagus, 8th edn. Kanehara, Tokyo, pp 31-58
3. The Paris endoscopic classification of superficial neoplastic lesions: esophagus, stomach and colon (2003) Gastrointest Endosc 58: S3-S43
4. ASGE Technology Committee (2009) High-resolution and high-magnification endoscopes. Gastrointest Endosc 69: 399-407
5. Dubuc J, Legoux JL, Winnock M et al (2006) Endoscopic screening for esophageal squamous-cell carcinoma in high-risk patients: a prospective study conducted in 62 French endoscopy centers. Endoscopy 38: 690-695
6. Inohue H, Rey JF, Lightdale C (2001) Lugol chromoendoscopy for esophageal squamous cell cancer. Endoscopy 33:75-79
7. Yoshida T, Inohue H, Usui S et al (2004) Narrow-band imaging system with magnifying endoscopy for superficial esophageal lesions. Gastrointest Endosc 59:288-295
8. Goda K, Tajiri H, Ikegami M et al (2009) Magnifying endoscopy with narrow band imaging for predicting the invasion depth of superficial esophageal squamous cell carcinoma. Dis Esoph 22:453-460
9. Takeo Y, Yoshida T, Shigemitu T et al (2001) Endoscopic mucosal resection for early esophageal

cancer and esophageal dysplasia. Hepatogastroenterology 48:453-457
10. May A, Gossner L, Beherens A et al (2003) A prospective randomized trial of two different endoscopic resection techniques for early stage cancer of the esophagus. Gastrointest Endosc 58:167-175
11. Japanese Society of Esophageal Disease (1999) Guidelines for clinical and pathologic studies on carcinoma of the esophagus. 9th Ed. Kanehara Shuppan
12. Catalano F, Trecca A, Rodella L et al (2009) The modern treatment of early gastric cancer: our experience in an Italian cohort. Surg Endosc 23:1581-1586
13. Oyama T, Tomori A, Hotta K et al (2005) Endoscopic submucosal dissection of early esophageal cancer. Clin Gastroenterol Hepatol 3:S67-S70
14. Neuhaus H (2009) Endoscopic submucosal dissection in the upper gastrointestinal tract: present and future view of Europe. Digest Endosc 21: S4-S6
15. Kumagai Y, Makuuchi H, Mitomi T, Ohmori T (1993) A new classification system for early carcinoma of the esophagus. Dig Endosc 5:139-150
16. Savary M, Miller G (1978) The esophagus. Handbook and atlas of endoscopy. Gassman, Solothurn, Switzerland
17. Muto M, Minashi K, Yano T et al (2010) Early detection of superficial squamous cell carcinoma in the head and neck region and esophagus by narrow band imaging: a multicenter randomized controlled trial. J Clin Oncol 28:1566-1572
18. Plukker JTM, van Westreenen HL (2006) Staging in oesophageal cancer. Best Practice Research Clin Gastroenterol 20: 877-891
19. Catalano MF, Van Dam J, Sivak Jr MV (1995) Malignant esophageal strictures: staging accuracy of endoscopic ultrasonography. Gastrointest Endosc 41:535-539
20. Binmoeller KF, Seifert H, Seitz U et al (1995) Ultrasonic esophago-probe for TNM staging of highly stenosing oesophageal carcinoma. Gastrointest Endosc 41:547-552
21. Waxman I (2006) EUS and EMR/ESD: is EUS in patients with Barrett's esophagus with high-grade dysplasia or intramucosal adenocarcinoma necessary prior to endoscopic mucosal resection? Endoscopy 38:S2-S4
22. Scotiniotis IA, Kochman ML, Lewis JD et al (2001) Accuracy of EUS in the evaluation of Barrett's esophagus and high-grade dyspla-sia or intramucosal carcinoma. Gastrointest Endosc 54:689-696
23. Pouw RE, Heldoorn N, Alvarez Herrero L et al (2011) Do we still need EUS in the workup of patients with early esophageal neoplasia? A retrospective analysis of 131 cases. Gastrointest Endosc (in press)
24. Young PE, Gentry AB, Acosta RD et al.(2010) Endoscopic ultrasound does not accurately stage early adenocarcinoma or high-grade dysplasia of the esophagus. Clin Gastroenterol Hepatol 8:1037-42
25. Kato H, Haga S, Endo S et al (2001) Lifting of lesions during endoscopic mucosal resection (EMR) of early colorectal cancer: implication for the assessment of respectability. Endoscopy 33:568-573
26. Bhutani MS, Hawes RH, Hoffman BJ (1997) A comparison of the accuracy of echo features during endoscopic ultrasound (EUS) and EUS-guided fine needle aspiration for diagnosis of malignant lymph node invasion. Gastrointest Endosc 45:474-479
27. Vazquez-Sequeiros E, Levy MJ, Clain JE et al (2006) Routine vs. selective EUS-guided FNA approach for preoperative nodal staging of esophageal carcinoma. Gastrointest Endosc 63:204-211
28. Vogel SB, Mendenhall WM, Sombeck MD et al (1995) Downstaging of esophageal cancer after preoperative radiation and chemotherapy. Ann Surg 221:685-693
29. Bates BA, Detterbeck FC, Bernard SA et al (1996) Concurrent radiation therapy and chemotherapy followed by esophagectomy for localized esophageal carcinoma. J Clin Oncol 14:156-163
30. Schneider PM, Metzger R, Schaefer H et al (2008) Response evaluation by endoscopy, rebiopsy, and endoscopic ultrasound does not accurately predict histopathologic regression after neoadjuvant chemoradiation for esophageal cancer. Ann Surg 248:902-908

31. Laterza E, de Manzoni G, Guglielmi A et al (1999) Endoscopic ultrasonography in the staging of esophageal carcinoma after preoperative radiotherapy and chemiotherapy. Ann Thorac Surg 67:1466-69
32. Kahla I, Kaw M, Fukami N et al (2004)The accuracy of endoscopic ultrasound for restaging oesophageal carcinoma after chemoradiation therapy. Cancer 101:940-947
33. Agarwal B, Swisher S, Ajani G et al (2004) Endoscopic ultrasound after preopetative chemoradiation can help identify patients who benefit maximally after surgical esophageal resection. Am J Gastroenterol 99:1258-1266
34. Choi TK, Siu KF, Lam KH, Wong J (1984) Bronchoscopy and carcinoma of the esophagus I. Findings of bronchoscopy in carcinoma of the esophagus. Am J Surg 147:757-759
35. Baisi A, Bonavina L, Peracchia A (1999) Bronchoscopic staging of squamous cell carcinoma of the upper thoracic esophagus. Arch Surg 134:140-143
36. Freitag L, Ernst A, Unger M et al (2007) A proposed classification of central airway stenosis. Eur Rest J 30:7-12
37. Riedel M, Hauck RW, Stein HJ et al (1998) Preoperative bronchoscopic assessment of airway invasion by esophageal cancer: a prospective study. Chest 113:687-695
38. Wagner M, Ficker JH (2007) Autofluorescence bronchoscopy. UNI-MED Verlag, Bremen, Germany

Preoperative Work-up: PET and PET-CT

5

Valentina Ambrosini, Maria Cristina Marzola, Paola Caroli, Stefano Fanti, and Domenico Rubello

5.1 Introduction

Esophageal cancer is characterized by an overall poor prognosis. Due to late onset of symptoms and early metastatic spread, only about 15–20% of patients undergo curative resection [1]. Accurate staging in esophageal squamous cell carcinoma (SCC) is essential to decide the correct therapeutic strategy. Currently, a limited number of patients are candidates for curative resection while in those with advanced-stage disease a combination of neoadjuvant chemotherapy and/or radiotherapy followed by surgery is recommended.

There are several different and complementary diagnostic tools that should be used to stage SCC disease, especially endoscopic ultrasound (EUS) and computed tomography (CT).

Recently, the use of positron emission tomography (PET) in the preoperative diagnostic flow chart and staging of SCC has been increasing with further diagnostic benefits obtained with 18F-fluorodeoxyglucose (18F-FDG) based on the high glucose uptake of SCC (Fig. 5.1) [2, 3].

The major advantage of PET in the diagnostic work-up is related to its ability to detect otherwise unsuspected metastatic disease (Figs. 5.2, 5.3) [4-6]. Several studies have investigated the role of PET with 18F-FDG, comparing it to other imaging modalities (mainly CT and EUS) for SCC staging; however, a unanimous consensus was not reached [7-10].

D. Rubello (✉)
Dept. of Nuclear Medicine, "Santa Maria della Misericordia" Hospital, Rovigo, Italy

G. de Manzoni (Ed.), *Treatment of Esophageal and Hypopharyngeal Squamous Cell Carcinoma*,

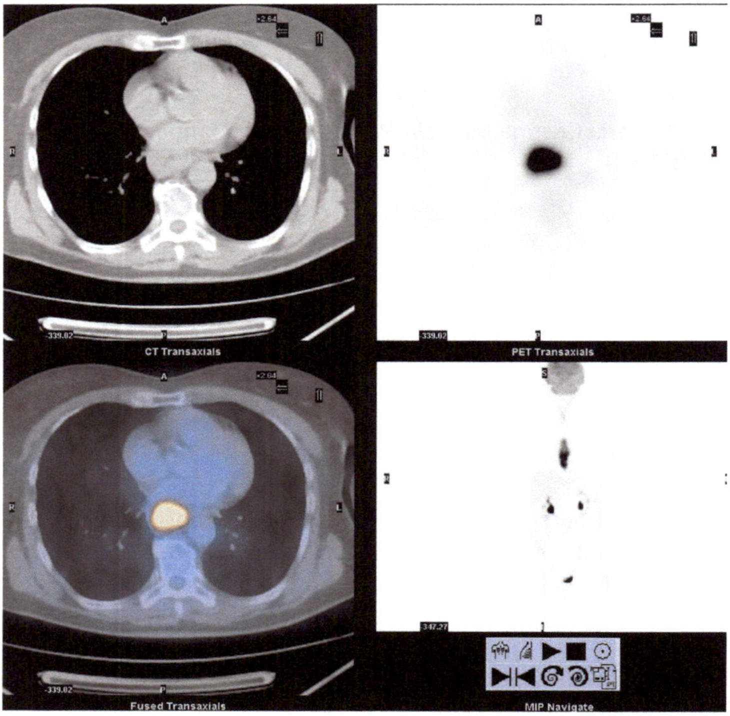

Fig. 5.1 Esophageal cancer at diagnosis: only the primary lesion, not metastatic deposits, is visualized. *Top left*, Axial CT image; *top right,* 18F-FDG PET image; *bottom left,* axial fused image; *bottom right*, MIP (maximum intensity projection) image

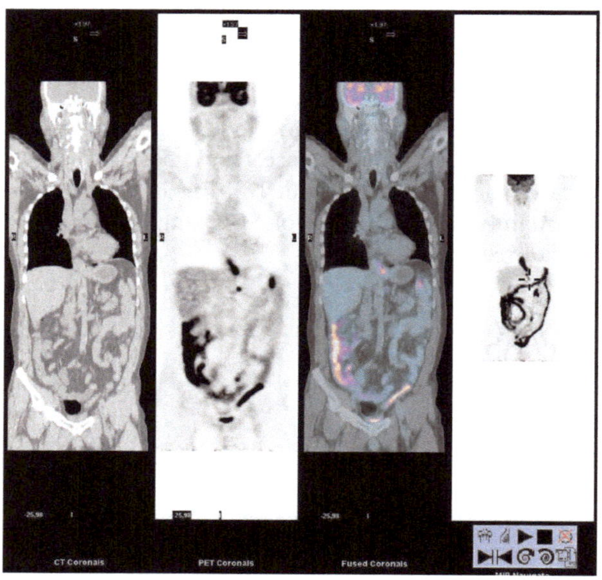

Fig. 5.2 Esophageal cancer at diagnosis; an inferior phrenic metastatic lymph node was detected. *Left*, CT coronal image; *middle*, 18F-FDG PET coronal image; *right*, fused coronal image

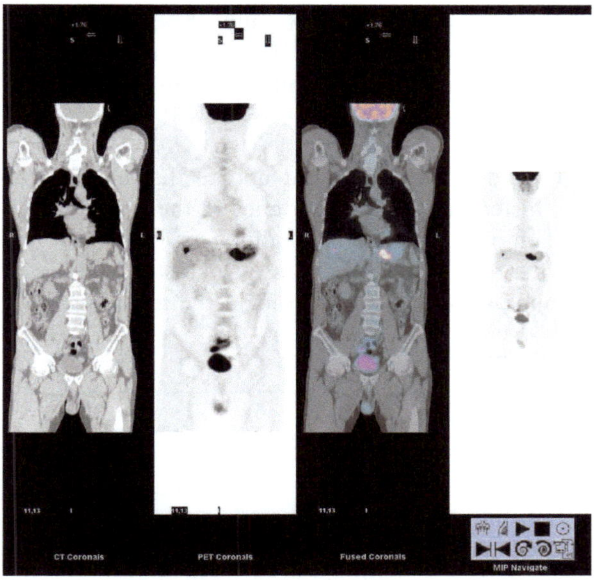

Fig. 5.3 Esophageal cancer at diagnosis, with liver metastasis at segments VII-VIII. *Left,* CT coronal image; *middle*, 18F-FDG PET image; *right*, fused image

5.2 T Staging

In a meta-analysis comprising 12 studies and 490 patients with esophageal cancer who were studied for pre-operative staging by PET, CT, and EUS, the reported sensitivity of PET alone (51%) was significantly lower than that of CT, but when PET and EUS were combined the sensitivity was higher than that obtained with EUS alone, with a relatively high specificity in both procedures (84% for PET) [11]. The main limitation of PET in T stage evaluation is the impossibility to define tumor infiltration, which prevents the distinction between superficial and advanced cancers and especially the identification of T4 carcinomas. Moreover, as reported by Kato et al. [12], PET-CT has a low sensitivity (43%) for the detection of small and superficial tumors (T1).

Hence, the impossibility to define the exact T stage and the inability to obtain more information than provided by EUS and CT limit the role of PET-CT in T staging.

5.3 N Staging

A recent meta-analysis reported a sensitivity and specificity for locoregional N staging of 57% and 85%, respectively [13]. In a prospective study performed on 75 ESCC patients [14], similar performance in nodal staging was shown for

PET, CT, and EUS, with sensitivities of 82%, 84%, and 85%, respectively. However, there are important limitations for PET-CT: intense uptake by the primary tumor could hide nodal uptake, inflammation could mimic a metastasis, and a spatial resolution of 5 mm is not sufficient to allow the detection of small metastatic nodes.

The possibility to identify nodes with sufficient uptake that are not too close to the primary tumor is instead of great importance in therapeutic decision-making and is the main aim of PET-CT in N staging.

In summary, PET-CT plays a role in the detection of metastatic nodes far from the primary tumor, although important limitations of the technique have been described.

5.4 M Staging

Computed tomography remains the first imaging tool in the detection of metastatic disease, even though more recent studies are in favor of the preoperative use of PET-CT, based on the possibility to obtain more accurate whole-body staging [15] with equal specificity but higher sensitivity.

In one large study (191 cases), PET-CT showed distant metastases in 9% of patients, resulting in a change in the clinical management of 26% of these patients [16].

Additionally, a recent paper, in which a large population (200 patients) was studied, investigated the change in SCC clinical management based on information provided by PET-CT [17]. PET-CT was able to identify unsuspected distant metastases, including systemic or non-regional node metastases, in 11% of the patients. These patients with subsequently up-staged disease were treated with palliation and were therefore spared useless surgical procedures. Moreover, in 7.5% of the patients the disease was down-staged, such that 12/15 were candidates for radical treatment. Overall, the treatment strategy was modified in 34 out of 200 patients (17%).

The lack of glucose uptake by the metastasis and the presence of abundant necrosis, in which the neoplastic foci are too small to be detected (< 5 mm), are the most important drawbacks of PET-CT in M staging.

In summary, PET-CT, despite its limitations, plays a prominent role in M staging and results in changes in the management of patients with ESCC in 10–25% of the cases. It is of particular value in detecting unsuspected metastases, which rules out resection, but of less use in disease downstaging, due both to the impossibility of effectively defining the pathological absence of disease and to the lack of data in the current literature.

Finally, the use of PET-CT before and during/after neoadjuvant treatments has been reported to provide prognostic information [18-20], an application that its described in detail in Chapter 6.

5.5 Conclusions

PET-CT with 18F-FDG provides additional advantages to currently used diagnostic tools, mainly because it allows more accurate staging of distant otherwise unsuspected metastases. The importance of PET-CT in SCC staging is increasing and its use in clinical practice seems justified.

References

1. Falk GW (2009) Risk factors for esophageal cancer development. Surg Oncol Clin N Am 18:469-85
2. Harewood GC, Wiersema MJ (2002) A cost analysis of endoscopic ultrasound in the evaluation of esophageal cancer. Am J Gastroenterol 97:452-458
3. van Westreenen HL, Westerterp M, Bossuyt PM et al (2004) Systematic review of the staging performance of 18F-fluorodeoxyglucose positron emission tomography in esophageal cancer. J Clin Oncol 22:3805-3812
4. Flamen P (2004) Positron emission tomography in gastric and esophageal cancer. Curr Opin Oncol 16:359-363
5. Heeren PA, Jager PL, Bongaerts F et al (2004) Detection of distant metastases in esophageal cancer with (18)F-FDG PET. J Nucl Med 45:980-987
6. Gananadha S, Hazebroek EJ, Leibman S et al (2008) The utility of FDG-PET in the preoperative staging of esophageal cancer. Dis Esoph 21:389-394
7. Salahudeen HM, Balan A, Naik K et al (2008) Impact of the introduction of integrated PET-CT into the preoperative staging pathway of patients with potentially operable oesophageal carcinoma Clinical Radiol 63:765-773
8. Walker AJ, Spier BJ, Perlman SB et al (2011) Integrated PET-CT fusion imaging and endoscopic ultrasound in the pre-operative staging and evaluation of esophageal cancer. Mol Imaging Biol 13:166-171
9. Chuang HH, Macapinlac HA (2009) The evolving role of PET-CT in the management of esophageal cancer. Q J Nucl Med Mol Imaging 53:201-209
10. Schreurs LM, Janssens AC, Groen H et al (2011) Value of EUS in determining curative resectability in reference to CT and FDG-PET: the optimal sequence in preoperative staging of esophageal cancer? Ann Surg Oncol. Epub ahead of print
11. van Westreenen HL, Westerterp M, Bossuyt PM et al (2004) Systematic review of the staging performance of 18F-fuorodeoxyglucose positron emission tomography in esophageal cancer. J Clin Oncol 22:3805-3812
12. Kato H, Miyazaki T, NakajimaM et al (2005) The incremental effect of positron emission tomography on diagnostic accuracy in the initial staging of esophageal carcinoma. Cancer 103:148-156
13. van Vliet EP, Heijenbrok-Kal MH, Hunink MG et al (2008) Staging investigations for oesophageal cancer: a meta-analysis Br J Cancer 98:547-557
14. Lowe VJ, Booya F, Fletcher JG et al (2005) Comparison of positron emission tomography, computed tomography and endoscopic ultrasound in the initial staging of patients with esophageal cancer. Mol Imaging Biol 7:422-430
15. Thurau K, Palmes D, Franzius C (2011) Impact of PET-CT on primary staging and response control on multimodal treatment of esophageal cancer. World J Surg 35:608-616
16. Noble F, Bailey D, Tung K, Byrne JP (2009) Impact of integrated PET-CT in the staging of oesophageal cancer: a UK population based cohort study. Clin Radiol 64:699-705

17. Gillies RS, Middleton MR, Maynard ND et al (2011) Additional benefit of a-F-fluorodeoxyglucose integrated positron emission tomography/computed tomography in the staging of oesophageal cancer. Eur Radiol 21:274-280
18. van Westreenen HL, Plukker JT, Cobben DC et al (2005) Prognostic value of the standardized uptake value in esophageal cancer. AJR Am J Roentgenol 185:436-440
19. Hong D, Lunagomez S, Kim EE et al (2005) Value of baseline positron emission tomography for predicting overall survival in patient with nonmetastatic esophageal or gastroesophageal junction carcinoma. Cancer 104:1620-1626
20. Cerfolio RJ, Bryant AS (2006) Maximum standardized uptake values on positron emission tomography of esophageal cancer predicts stage, tumor biology, and survival. Ann Thorac Surg 82:391-394

Role of PET-CT in the Prediction of Response to Neoadjuvant Treatment

6

David Fuster, Maria Cristina Marzola, Francesca Pons, Giovanni de Manzoni, and Domenico Rubello

6.1 Introduction

Even if surgery is still the main therapeutic option in patients with esophageal squamous cell carcinoma (SCC), recent studies have shown that neoadjuvant chemoradiotherapy (CRT) can reduce the incidence of local recurrence and improve the overall survival rate [1-3].

Once esophageal cancer has been diagnosed, correct disease staging is essential to decide the best therapeutic approach. Currently, computed tomography (CT) and endoscopic ultrasonography (EUS) are the first-line modalities used for staging. However, for many malignant tumors, PET-CT has proved to be more useful than other image diagnostic modalities in the examination of tumor spread or treatment response. The role of PET-CT in routine clinical practice for the staging of esophageal SCC is well-established, since a whole-body search can be conducted with a single study, thus allowing the detection of previously unknown distant metastases.

Even though several published studies have suggested the use of PET-CT in tumor response evaluation following CRT, their results remain to be confirmed by well-designed clinical trials [4-6].

6.2 Evaluation of Treatment Response

For different types of malignant tumors, PET-CT reportedly provides an accurate evaluation of response to both radiation therapy and chemotherapy, often before any change is seen on a CT scan. The timing and reliability of PET-CT

M. C. Marzola (✉)
Dept. of Nuclear Medicine, "Santa Maria della Misericordia" Hospital,
Rovigo, Italy

G. de Manzoni (Ed.), *Treatment of Esophageal and Hypopharyngeal Squamous Cell Carcinoma*,

studies in predicting tumor response have been the subject of numerous prospective studies. The implications of this approach are significant in terms of optimizing treatments, minimizing unnecessary morbidity, and reducing costs.

In patients with locally advanced esophageal SCC without distant metastases, esophagectomy is a treatment option after neoadjuvant CRT. Consequently, accurate staging at initial presentation and clear assessment of the therapeutic response after neoadjuvant therapy are essential in optimal management. In esophageal SCC, there are as yet no biological predictive markers of response. Instead, the response to neoadjuvant CRT is monitored using CT; however, this approach is unable to distinguish between radiochemically induced fibrosis and cancer tissue.

Earlier studies on the use of PET-CT after neoadjuvant CRT in patients with esophageal SCC did not clearly support its use as a predictor of pathological response and survival [1]. Vallbohmer et al. [2] found that PET-CT failed to effectively characterize major and minor response groups, neither did it predict survival, although other trials reported encouraging results [3, 4]. A quantitative variable, the standardized uptake value (SUV), is the most common index used to quantify uptake in diagnosed lesions. However, systemic treatment and especially radiotherapy generally cause local inflammatory reactions in normal tissue, which often manifest as glucose uptake in PET-CT scans, thus limiting the use of this modality for metabolic measurement soon after or during neoadjuvant treatment for esophageal SCC. Consequently, to accurately assess tumor response, it may be better to perform PET-CT several weeks or even months after the patient has completed radiotherapy.

6.2.1 Predicting Response

The early detection of response to neoadjuvant CRT might point out the need to change the therapeutic strategy, that is, either to continue CRT or to recommend that the patient proceed to surgery. Early-response evaluation is defined as the assessment of response during treatment, whereas late evaluation is performed after the completion of induction therapy. Early-response assessment could allow the identification of non-responding patients, i.e., those who will not benefit from further CRT and could be better treated with surgical resection. Based on this distinction, only responding patients would complete treatment, while non-responders would avoid potentially harmful treatments. Late-response assessment is limited to a prognostic appraisal, as a change in therapeutic strategy is no longer an option. CT is currently the most widely used imaging modality in assessing the early and late treatment responses of most solid tumors. Nevertheless, the images obtained do not clearly differentiate between treatment-induced morphological changes and persistent tumor presence [7]. Some studies that have assessed the use of FDG-PET in a variety of solid tumors concluded that it is a trustworthy technique in the differential diagnosis between residual tumoral tissue and fibrotic or scar tissue [8, 9].

Recent studies suggested that the quantitative decrease in FDG uptake seen after neoadjuvant therapy correlates with pathologic response to therapy and patient survival [10]. Moreover, PET-CT has an important role in detecting distant metastases, especially new interval metastases, after CRT.

Nonetheless, some relevant problems remain regarding the utilization of PET-CT in the detection of response to treatment. First, no study used PET-CT to change the therapeutic strategy of patients undergoing CRT; the only study in which the strategy was changed was the MUNICON trial (discussed below), but the patients had adenocarcinoma and were being treated with chemotherapy, not CRT. Second, on PET-CT, the inflammation that characteristically occurs during radiation therapy may be misinterpreted. Third, the correct timing for a PET-CT scan in early treatment response has yet to be determined, and an appropriate marker of response as well as the threshold value of that marker are still highly debated.

As there are still no established guidelines for the optimal timing of PET-CT in response assessment, in most studies PET-CT was performed after patients had completed neoadjuvant therapy. In patients with esophageal cancer, a PET-CT scan may show inflammation or ulceration within the esophagus, resulting in a false-positive interpretation [11]. The problem of timing is then particularly relevant: indeed, if throughout the chemoradiation period the resulting inflammation masks the uptake by residual tumor, the chance of detecting an early response would be minimal, reducing the impact of PET-CT in decision-making. So far, no study has been able to establish the correct timing to perform an early-response evaluation during CRT.

When treatment consists only of chemotherapy, the problem of timing is reduced, since the inflammation is less pronounced and early detection is thus more accurate.

Ott et al. [12] assessed tumor glucose uptake using PET in 65 patients with locally advanced esophageal adenocarcinoma (AC) both before chemotherapy and 14 days after the beginning of therapy. Patients were classified as metabolic responders when the metabolic activity of the primary tumor had decreased by more than 35% at the time of the second PET. Metabolic responders showed a high pathologic response rate (44%), with a 3-year survival rate of 70%. In contrast, prognosis was poor for metabolic non-responders, with a pathologic response rate of 5% and a 3-year survival rate of 35%. These results were largely confirmed in a prospective study of 119 patients subsequently published by the same group. The MUNICON trial was the first published study to document a change in treatment strategy during chemotherapy, using the percentage decrease between time-0 PET and PET performed 2 weeks after treatment begin (ΔSUV) [13]. However, the results of the MUNICON trial have yet to be reproduced by other groups. Thus, further investigation is essential to discover the marker that best defines response. As reported in a recent meta-analysis [10], different markers of response and different threshold values have been proposed. ΔSUV is a very well-accepted marker, but the threshold value is strongly debated. We questioned its role and proposed the use of final SUV as a marker of response. In a cohort of 27 patients studied with PET-CT after completion of treatment, we found that non-responders had a median final SUV of 7, while in responders the median value was 4. Unfortunately, the spatial resolution could not distinguish pathological complete responders from partial responders and was unable to identify small nodal metastases.

In a study by Malik et al. [14], PET-CT was found to be a non-reliable early predictor of pathologic response to neoadjuvant CRT. Thirty-seven patients with locally advanced AC of the esophagus underwent pre-treatment and an intra-treatment PET-CT scan in the second week of a 6-week regimen of neoadjuvant CRT. Indeed, responders had an increased ΔSUV, but the groups overlapped considerably and a threshold value could not be identified. Moreover, there was no detectable survival benefit for responders identified with PET-CT, based on two different ΔSUV cutoffs (26% and 35%). Hence, even though histopathologic responders had a grater reduction in ΔSUV than histopathologic non-responders, the overlapping values made ΔSUV a non-reliable marker of the early detection of response in this trial.

Taken together, these findings suggest the potential of PET-CT to predict response early in the course of treatment, but further studies are essential to define timing, marker, and threshold values. So far, restaging with PET-CT early during CRT is only investigational and a change in strategy due to the results of a PET-CT scan might be hazardous. However, late PET-CT scans, obtained after the completion of treatment, could be used to identify the correct timing of the scan, the most appropriate marker, its threshold value, and particularly disease progression.

6.3 Tumor Recurrence

Recurrent esophageal cancer is relatively common after curative surgical removal and the prognosis of these patients is poor. Two-thirds of patients with relapse have a recurrence within 1 year and nearly all within 2 years after the primary operation. Since treatment options are limited, routine surveillance in asymptomatic patients remains controversial. Tumor recurrences usually appear as metastatic disease, can be clinically occult, and occur in unpredicted sites. However, the early detection of relapse could help in the selection of effective palliative treatment.

Siersema et al. [15] demonstrated that metabolic response was the only factor predicting recurrence in patients after R0 resection. Roedl et al. [16] showed that the reduction of tumor length, as demonstrated by PET-CT before and after CRT, was a better predictor of time to recurrence than the decrease in SUV.

PET-CT achieved a sensitivity of 91% and a specificity of 81% in identifying sites of tumor recurrence. Overstaging of the disease, with 20% false-positive PET-CT-detected lesions, could be corrected by comparing the PET-CT findings with clinical data and conventional CT images, thus avoiding the negative impact of these equivocal lesions.

6.4 Conclusions

The current literature on treatment monitoring and response prediction of esophageal cancer is still quite limited. Neither defined markers nor threshold values nor the correct timing of response assessment have been identified yet. The only study that documented a changed therapeutic strategy during treatment (MUNICON trial) considered only chemotherapy in patients with AC and could not be reproduced for CRT. Even though FDG uptake seems to be reduced in metabolic responders and a correlation between reduced SUV and pathological response is more than hypothetical, PET-CT cannot be deemed safe for decision-making during preoperative CRT. Nevertheless, its potential role deservers further in-depth evaluation and investigation, as in non-responding patients it would avoid useless and potentially harmful CRT and a delay in surgery. Currently, however, PET-CT already has a definite and standardized utility in assessing the absence of response and disease progression after CRT.

Furthermore, there is some evidence that PET-CT provides additional valuable information for the diagnosis of recurrent disease. It was shown to be more specific than CT in the detection of local recurrences at the anatomic site and more sensitive than CT in the detection of metastatic disease [17]. However, the usefulness of PET-CT in the follow-up of SCC patients who have undergone R0 resection has not been established yet.

References

1. Schmidt M, Bollschweiler E, Dietlein M et al (2009) Mean and maximum standardized uptake values in [18F]FDG-PET for assessment of histopathological response in oesophageal squamous cell carcinoma or adenocarcinoma after radiochemotherapy. Eur J Nucl Med Mol Imaging 36:735-744
2. Vallböhmer D, Hölscher AH, Schneider PM et al (2010) 18F]-fluorodeoxyglucose-positron emission tomography for the assessment of histopathologic response and prognosis after completion of neoadjuvant chemotherapy in gastric cancer. J Surg Oncol 102:135-140
3. Shields AF, Mankoff DA, Link JM et al (1998) Carbon-11-thymidine and FDG to measure therapy response. J Nucl Med 39:1757-1762
4. Kluge R, Schmidt F, Caca K et al (2001) Positron emission tomography with [(18)F]fluoro-2-deoxy-D-glucose for diagnosis and staging of bile duct cancer. Hepatology 33:1029-1035
5. Westerterp M, Van Westreenen HL, Reitsma JB et al (2005) Esophageal cancer: CT, endoscopic US, and FDG PET for assessment of response to neoadjuvant therapy–systematic review. Radiology 236:841- 851
6. Rebollo AC, Ramos-Font C, Villegas R et al (2009) 18F-fluorodeoxiglucose positron emission tomography for the evaluation of neoadjuvant therapy response in esophageal cancer: systematic review of the literature. Ann Surg 250:247-254
7. Jones DR, Parker LA Jr, Detterbeck FC, Egan TM (1999) Inadequacy of computed tomography in assessing patients with esophageal carcinoma after induction chemoradiotherapy. Can-

cer 85:1026-32
8. Weber WA, Ott K, Becker K et al (2001) Prediction of response to preoperative chemotherapy in adenocarcinomas of the esophagogastric junction by metabolic imaging. J Clin Oncol 19:3058-3065
9. Ott K, Fink U, Becker K et al (2003) Prediction of response to preoperative chemotherapy in gastric carcinoma by metabolic imaging: results of a prospective trial. J Clin Oncol 21: 4604-4610
10. Krause B, Herrmann K, Wieder H, Meyer zum Buschenfelde C (2009) 18F-FDG PET and 18F-FDG PET-CTfor Assessing Response to Therapy in Esophageal Cancer. J Nucl Med 50:89S-96S
11. Kim TJ, Kim HY, Lee KW, Kim MS (2009) Multimodality assessment of esophageal cancer: preoperative staging and monitoring of response to therapy. Radiographics 29:403-421
12. Ott K, Weber WA, Lordick F et al (2006) Metabolic imaging predicts response, survival and recurrence in adenocarcinomas of the oesophagogastric junction. J Clin Oncol 24:4692-4698
13. Lordick F, Ott K, Krause BJ et al (2007) PET to assess early metabolic response and to guide treatment of adenocarcinoma of the oesophagogastric junction: the MUNICON phase II trial. Lancet Oncol 8:797-805
14. Malik V, Lucey JA, Duffy GJ et al (2010) Early repeated 18F-FDG PET scans during neoadjuvant chemoradiation fail to predict histopathologic response or survival benefit in adenocarcinoma of the esophagus. J Nucl Med 51:1863-1869
15. Siersema PD (2007) Pathogenesis, diagnosis and therapeutic possibilities of esophageal cancer. Curr Opin Gastroenterol 23:456-461
16. Roedl JB, Harisinghani MG, Colen RR et al (2008) Assessment of treatment response and recurrence in esophageal carcinoma based on tumor length and standardized uptake value on positron emission tomography-computed tomography. Ann Thorac Surg 86:1131-1138
17. Flamen P, Lerut A, Van Cutsem E et al (2000) The utility of positron emission tomography for the diagnosis and staging of recurrent esophageal cancer. J Thorac Cardiovasc Surg 120:1085-1092

Role of Molecular Biology in the Prediction of Response to Neoadjuvant Treatment

7

Milena Gusella, Felice Pasini, and Giovanni de Manzoni

In esophageal cancer, molecular markers representing tumor biological properties or patient features could provide significant determinants for predicting therapeutic response. To date, however, there is no sufficient evidence that current diagnostic methods can be used to improve the efficacy of multimodality neoadjuvant therapies. Molecular research in esophageal cancer has focused on two principal categories: (1) mRNA from cancer biopsies, searching for a relationship between outcome and the different gene expression levels; (2) DNA from healthy tissues, searching for associations between outcome and constitutive inter-individual genetic variations. This second option is a very attractive one, in that a small volume of peripheral blood is sufficient to obtain genomic DNA from lymphocytes-monocytes.

A variety of potentially predictive markers with respect to radiation and chemotherapy sensitivity has been published for different tumors but only a limited number of molecular markers have been studied specifically for esophageal squamous cell carcinoma (ESCC).

7.1 Studies on Gene Expression Levels

Messenger RNA levels influence biological responses through the control of protein synthesis and, consequently, various enzyme activities. The development of high-density cDNA microarrays has given this field a huge technical opportunity in that the analysis of an entire human genome is now possible. The goal is to identify genes, as yet unknown, that are associated with therapy response.

Recent studies, mostly published in the last year, have correlated more or

M. Gusella (✉)
Dept. of Medical Oncology, "Santa Maria della Misericordia" Hospital,
Rovigo, Italy

G. de Manzoni (Ed.), *Treatment of Esophageal and Hypopharyngeal Squamous Cell Carcinoma*,

Table 7.1 Studies on the association between gene expression profile and outcome in esophageal cancer patients treated with neoadjuvant chemoradiotherapy

Author (year)	Genes	Patients (N.)	Positive results	Gene function/pathway
Luthra (2006) [1]	14,593	19	*PERP* *S100A2* *SPRR3*	involved in apoptosis tumor suppressor gene component of cell envelope
Duong (2007) [3]	9,389	46	*SIAH2*	degradation of specific proteins
Maher (2009) [4]	28,000	53	*CCL28* *EPB41L3* *IRF8* *NOV* *RNPC1* *RTKN* *STAT5B* *NMES1*	mucosae-associated epithelial chemokine tumor suppressor transcription factor extracellular protein involved in cell migration rna RNA binding protein involved in cell cycle control involved in cell growth and transformation transcription factor onco-suppressor
Warnecke-Eberz (2010) [5]	17	41	*DPYD* *ERCC1* *c-erbB-2*	5fu 5 FU metabolism DNA repair epidermal growth factor receptor
Metzger (2010) [6]	29,000	66	*STK11* *CUL2*	tumor suppressor protein degradation
Kim (2010) [7]	48,702	64	*SPARK* *SPP1*	extracellular matrix protein secreted glycoprotein

less broad gene-expression profiles with outcome in ESCC patients treated with neoadjuvant chemoradiotherapy (CRT) (Table 7.1). The number of patients studied was generally small, in the dozens, because of several common drawbacks in array analysis, such as the need for relatively large, very high quality, possibly frozen samples; the delicate and time-consuming procedures; and the high costs of the necessary materials and reagents.

The general study design consisted in a first-phase in which the expression levels of thousand of unselected genes were tested in parallel. An analysis of the association between expression profiles and outcome generally identified a group of several genes differentially expressed in the different prognostic classes. Among these genes, some were chosen for validation according to their higher level of significance, since array results are considered as not conclusive.

In a second phase of the study another methodology, based on gene amplification, was applied in order to directly quantify gene expression and verify its up- or down-regulation; this resulted in the individuation of a smaller number of genes with potential predictive value. Unfortunately, results from different studies have never reported the same genes.

Luthra et al. [1] profiled pretreatment endoscopic cancer biopsies from 19 esophageal carcinomas for response to neoadjuvant chemoradiotherapy with fluorouracil (5-FU), irinotecan, and docetaxel. A gene combination of *PERP* (apoptosis effector), *S100A2* (tumor suppressor gene), and *SPRR3* (cell envelope component) discriminated between pathologic complete response (higher expression of the three genes) from less than complete response (significantly lower expression of the three genes) with high sensitivity and specificity (85%). Two of these genes are located in the same genomic region, the so-called highly conserved epidermal differentiation complex (EDC, chr:1q21), implicated in the maturation and maintenance of the stratified esophageal mucosa. Both loci and the flanking segments were re-analyzed in a second work by the same group [2] on the same samples: all EDC genes were expressed at high levels in responders but at low levels in resistant tumors.

Duong et al. [3] identified a 32-gene profile that could predict clinical response to neoadjuvant CRT in squamous carcinoma (21 patients), but not in adenocarcinoma (25 patients). Among them *SIAH2* (protein degradation) was a potential marker of interest.

Maher et al. [4] identified a 103-gene pattern associated with response: genes related to apoptosis, oncogenesis, cell proliferation, and differentiation were down-regulated in responders compared to non-responders, whereas genes associated with signal transduction and cell adhesion were up-regulated in responders compared to non-responders. Among these genes, eight that were differentially expressed were found to predict response with high sensitivity and specificity.

Very recently, Warnecke-Eberz et al. [5] published expression data on 17 genes, related to apoptosis, angiogenesis, cell cycle, DNA repair, and growth factors and their receptors, as profiled in pretreatment biopsies from 20 patients with responding and 21 patients with non-responding esophageal cancer. *DPYD* mRNA (5-FU metabolism) was associated with histopathologic response; in addition, a combination of *DPYD* with *ERCC1* (DNA repair effector) and *c-erbB-2* (epidermal growth factor receptor), known to be predictive as determined in previous studies by the same group, provided better predictive values. Multivariate analysis including all 17 genes further improved the prediction potential (75% sensitivity and 81% specificity).

The same group [6] found that the expression of 3052 genes was statistically different in cancer samples obtained from responding vs. non-responding patients. Among those genes, *STK11* (tumor suppressor) and *CUL2* (protein degradation) were validated to be down-regulated in non-responders compared with responders. *STK11* showed a significant association with response to treatment in the adenocarcinoma subset, while the association of *CUL2* involved all histotypes.

Finally, Kim et al. [7] detected 452 genes with specific deregulation in the group of patients with worst survival; in addition, genes whose expression levels strongly differed in magnitude (≥ 4-fold) between the prognostic groups were further explored, validating two genes *SPARK* (extracellular matrix protein) and *SPP1* (secreted glycoprotein) whose expression was associated with overall survival.

7.2 Studies on Gene Structure Variations

Variations in DNA nucleotide sequence that are present in the population with a frequency of at least 1% are called polymorphisms. The most common are single-nucleotide polymorphisms (SNPs), which consist of a change in only one nucleotide in the same position of the gene between individuals. SNPs have biological consequences because they may alter protein structures and activities; over the last 10 years, they have been the most widely studied molecular markers.

The association of SNPs and treatment outcome in esophageal cancer has been evaluated in at least 16 papers, mostly published in the last few years (Table 7.2) [8–24]. The size of the study population varied widely, from 31 to 370 patients, and overall survival was generally the primary endpoint. Of note, all of these studies were retrospective, non-randomized, and often comprised patients treated with different drug regimens. Specific data on the neoadjuvant setting were included in eight of these studies.

Overall 65 polymorphic genes were evaluated, but only two genes, *XRCC1* and *GSTP1*, had a consistently positive association in at least two independent studies.

Eleven other genes had a single un-replicated reported association (*MDM2*, *PTEN/AKT1/AKT2/FRAP*, *VEGF*, *EGF*, *MPO*, *XPA*, *ECRG1*, *GNAS1*), while conflicting data were reported for seven other genes (*p53*, *MTHFR*, *MTR*, *TYMS*, *MDR1*, *XPD*, *ERCC1*); no association was reported for the other 45 genes.

The strategy of these studies was based on a gene-candidate approach; that is, the genes to be investigated were chosen on the basis of their plausible relevant role in cell physiology and drug action.

For example, the cytotoxic effects of platinating agents and ionizing radiation are principally due to the ability of these agents to induce DNA damage, with resistance or sensitivity to treatment thought to depend on the activation of DNA repair enzymes. Polymorphisms involved in this setting are among the best studied in relation to prognosis.

XRCC1 is a repair protein involved in removing small DNA lesions. The gene presents two SNPs. The first is a polymorphism in position 194 of the protein that causes an amino acid change (Arg194Trp). None of the patients with one copy of the altered gene (Trp) responded to treatment with cisplatin and 5FU [8]. The second polymorphism, at position 399, also causes an amino acid change (Arg399Gln). In these patients, pathological complete response and survival were significantly lower than in patients with the wild-type gene [9].

The SNP of *XPA*, encoding another DNA repair protein, is located in the promoter area, such that gene expression is modified (*XPA* G23A). Wu et al. [9] demonstrated that the GG genotype was associated with a lower risk of death than the AA genotype. In our series, the XPA AA genotype was significantly associated with worse disease-free survival and overall survival compared to the other XPA genotypes [10].

Table 7.2 Studies on the association between genolymorphisms and outcome in esophageal cancer patients treated with chemoradiotherapy

Author (year)	N. patients	N. of genes (SNPs)#	Treatment homogeneity	Positive results*	Gene function/pathway
Liao (2006) [12]	146	1 (1)	Neoadjuvant	0	
Sarbia (2006) [13]	68	3 (3)	Neoadjuvant	MTR	Folate metabolism
Wu (2006) [9]	210	22 (30)	mix	MTHFR MDR1 XRCC1 GSTP1 MPO XPA	Folate metabolism Drug efflux transporter DNA repair detoxification myeloperoxidase DNA repair
Jain (2007) [14]	79	5 (5)	mix	EGF	Grow factor
Jatoi (2007) [15]	54	3 (6)	Neoadjuvant	0	
Okuno (2007) [11]	31	5 (8)	mix	TYMS GSTP1	5FU- target detoxification
Lanuti (2008) [16]	312	1 (1)	mix	0	
Alakus (2009) [17]	51	1 (1)	Neoadjuvant	GNAS1	G-protein
Bachmann (2009) [18]	107	1 (1)	mix		1
Bradbury (2009) [19]	361	1 (3)	mix	VEGF	Growth factor
Bradbury (2009) [20]	370	2 (4)	mix (70% neoadjuvant)	XPD ERCC1	DNA repair DNA repair
Bradbury (2009) [21]	313	3 (4)	mix	0	
Cescon (2009) [22]	371	2 (2)	mix (50% neoadjuvant)	p53 MDM2 AKT1 AKT2	Pro-apoptosis Anti-apoptosis Protein kinasi, involved in anti-apoptosis Protein kinasi, involved in glucose metabolism

(cont.) →

Table 7.2 (*continued*)

Hildebrand (2009) [23]	186	5 (16)	mix	PTEN FRAP	Tumor suppressor Tumor suppressor
Warnecke (2009) [8]	52	12 (17)	Neoadjuvant	ERCC1 XRCC1	DNA repair DNA repair
Narumiya (2011) [24]	262	1 (1)	Neoadjuvant	MDR1	Drug efflux transporter

#Number of genes (and SNPs) investigated.
*Genes demonstrated to have an association with outcome.

Detoxification pathways are important in chemotherapy effects and glutathione S transferase P is known to be associated with cisplatin resistance. Two independent studies found an association with survival for two different SNPs on the same gene: Ile105Val [11] and Ala 114 Val [9].

Other genes that were investigated were selected based on their role in drug metabolism (activation, deactivation) and kinetics (absorption, distribution, elimination), the drug's mechanism of action (target enzymes), or because of their involvement in cell proliferation and apoptosis. In all cases, the results were negative or inconclusive. It should be noted that practically all of the papers on SNPs caution that the studies were exploratory and in need of validation or replication.

7.3 Conclusions

Currently, there is no molecular marker for the prediction of tumor response to neoadjuvant CRT. There is evidence that gene expression or polymorphisms may predict response or survival in CRT; however, since existing data are conflicting, firm conclusions cannot be drawn. Molecular studies should be embedded into large prospective randomized controlled trials to provide convincing evidence that their application is appropriate in routine clinical practice.

References

1. Luthra R, Wu T, Luthra MG et al (2006) Gene expression profiling of localized esophageal carcinomas: association with pathologic response to preoperative chemoradiation. J Clin Oncol 24:259-267
2. Luthra MG, Ajani JA, Izzo J et al (2007) Decreased expression of gene cluster at chromosome 1q21 defines molecular subgroups of chemoradiotherapy response in esophageal cancers. Clin Cancer Res 13:912-919
3. Duong C, Greenawalt DM, Kowalczyk A et al (2007) Pretreatment gene expression profiles can be used to predict response to neoadjuvant chemoradiotherapy in esophageal cancer. Ann Surg Oncol 14:3602-3609
4. Maher SG, Gillham CM, Duggan SP et al (2009) Gene expression analysis of diagnostic biopsies predicts pathological response to neoadjuvant chemoradiotherapy of esophageal cancer. Ann Surg 250:729-737
5. Warnecke-Eberz U, Metzger R, Bollschweiler E et al (2010) TaqMan low-density arrays and analysis by artificial neuronal networks predict response to neoadjuvant chemoradiation in esophageal cancer. Pharmacogenomics 11:55-64
6. Metzger R, Heukamp L, Drebber U et al (2010) CUL2 and STK11 as novel response-predictive genes for neoadjuvant radiochemotherapy in esophageal cancer. Pharmacogenomics 11:1105-1113
7. Kim SM, Park YY, Park ES et al (2010) Prognostic biomarkers for esophageal adenocarcinoma identified by analysis of tumor transcriptome. PLoS One 5:e15074
8. Warnecke-Eberz U, Vallböhmer D, Alakus H et al (2009) ERCC1 and XRCC1 gene polymorphisms predict response to neoadjuvant radiochemotherapy in esophageal cancer. J Gastrointest Surg 13:1411-1421

9. Wu X, Gu J, Wu TT et al (2006) Genetic variations in radiation and chemotherapy drug action pathways predict clinical outcomes in esophageal cancer. J Clin Oncol 24:3789-3798
10. Gusella M, de Manzoni G, Marinelli R et al (2009) XPA and XRCC3 gene polymorphisms predict survival in esophageal cancer patients receiving neo-adjuvant radio-chemotherapy with cisplatin (CDDP), docetaxel (DTX) and 5-fluorouracil (FU). J Clin Oncol 27:e14571
11. Okuno T, Tamura T, Yamamori M et al (2007) Favorable genetic polymorphisms predictive of clinical outcome of chemoradiotherapy for stage II/III esophageal squamous cell carcinoma in Japanese. Am J Clin Oncol 30:252-257
12. Liao Z, Liu H, Swisher SG et al (2006) Polymorphism at the 3'-UTR of the thymidylate synthase gene: a potential predictor for outcomes in Caucasian patients with esophageal adenocarcinoma treated with preoperative chemoradiation. Int J Radiat Oncol Biol Phys 64:700-708
13. Sarbia M, Stahl M, von Weyhern C et al (2006) The prognostic significance of genetic polymorphisms (Methylenetetrahydrofolate Reductase C677T, Methionine Synthase A2756G, Thymidilate Synthase tandem repeat polymorphism) in multimodally treated oesophageal squamous cell carcinoma. Br J Cancer 94:203-207
14. Jain M, Kumar S, Upadhyay R et al (2007) Influence of apoptosis (BCL2, FAS), cell cycle (CCND1) and growth factor (EGF, EGFR) genetic polymorphisms on survival outcome: an exploratory study in squamous cell esophageal cancer. Cancer Biol Ther 6:1553-1558
15. Jatoi A, Martenson JA, Foster NR et al (2007) Paclitaxel, carboplatin, 5-fluorouracil, and radiation for locally advanced esophageal cancer: phase II results of preliminary pharmacologic and molecular efforts to mitigate toxicity and predict outcomes: North Central Cancer Treatment Group (N0044). Am J Clin Oncol. 30:507-513
16. Lanuti M, Liu G, Goodwin JM et al (2008) A functional epidermal growth factor (EGF) polymorphism, EGF serum levels, and esophageal adenocarcinoma risk and outcome. Clin Cancer Res 14:3216-3222
17. Alakus H, Warnecke-Eberz U, Bollschweiler E et al (2009) GNAS1 T393C polymorphism is associated with histopathological response to neoadjuvant radiochemotherapy in esophageal cancer. Pharmacogenomics J 9:202-207
18. Bachmann K, Shahmiri S, Kaifi J et al (2009) Polymorphism Arg290Arg in esophageal-cancer-related gene 1 (ECRG1) is a prognostic factor for survival in esophageal cancer. J Gastrointest Surg 13:181-187
19. Bradbury PA, Zhai R, Ma C et al (2009) Vascular endothelial growth factor polymorphisms and esophageal cancer prognosis. Clin Cancer Res 15:4680-4685
20. Bradbury PA, Kulke MH, Heist RS et al (2009) Cisplatin pharmacogenetics, DNA repair polymorphisms, and esophageal cancer outcomes. Pharmacogenet Genomics 19:613-625
21. Bradbury PA, Zhai R, Hopkins J et al (2009) Matrix metalloproteinase 1, 3 and 12 polymorphisms and esophageal adenocarcinoma risk and prognosis. Carcinogenesis. 30:793-798
22. Cescon DW, Bradbury PA, Asomaning K et al (2009) p53 Arg72Pro and MDM2 T309G polymorphisms, histology, and esophageal cancer prognosis. Clin Cancer Res 15:3103-109
23. Hildebrandt MA, Yang H, Hung MC et al (2009) Genetic variations in the PI3K/PTEN/AKT/mTOR pathway are associated with clinical outcomes in esophageal cancer patients treated with chemoradiotherapy. J Clin Oncol. 27:857-871
24. Narumiya K, Metzger R, Bollschweiler E et al (2011) Impact of ABCB1 C3435T polymorphism on lymph node regression in multimodality treatment of locally advanced esophageal cancer. Pharmacogenomics 12:205-214

Patient Selection according to General Condition and Associated Disease

8

Giovanni de Manzoni, Corrado Pedrazzani, Andrea Zanoni,
and Jacopo Weindelmayer

8.1 Introduction

Esophagectomy and the complete spectrum of treatment of esophageal cancer are unanimously considered to be complex, with very high risks of treatment-related complications. Esophageal squamous cell carcinoma (ESCC) is a highly aggressive disease that is usually diagnosed at an advanced stage. Malnutrition, low performance status, and cachexia are frequently seen in these patients at diagnosis.

ESCC is characteristically diagnosed during the sixth and seventh decades of life, but sometimes even later. These patients frequently present with associated severe co-morbidities, are usually of low economic status, and are heavy smokers and drinkers. Furthermore, despite the complexity and quality of treatment, a considerable number of patients suffer early tumor relapse, resulting in poor survival and an inadequate quality of life.

Patient selection is one of the key factors that greatly influence the quality of care in esophageal cancer. Accordingly, numerous variables play an important role in selecting patients for the various treatment options, which makes it difficult to draw conclusions from a literature analysis.

Indeed, a definite advantage accorded by the use of neoadjuvant chemoradiotherapy (CRT) has not been demonstrated; rather, several approaches have been used in the treatment ESCC (i.e., primary surgery, neoadjuvant chemotherapy, neoadjuvant CRT, etc.), depending on the center and its experience. Different surgical approaches are employed with none clearly superior to the others. In ESCC, the most common procedures are Ivor-Lewis and McKeown esophagectomy, although trans-hiatal esophagectomy is often pro-

G. de Manzoni (✉)
Dept. of Surgery, Upper G.I. Surgery Division, University of Verona,
Verona, Italy

G. de Manzoni (Ed.), *Treatment of Esophageal and Hypopharyngeal Squamous Cell Carcinoma*,

posed. Moreover, minimally invasive techniques are being employed with increasing frequency. Notably, there are many differences among the various centers regarding postoperative patient care and management. Another consideration is the fact that most of the experiences reported in the literature come from the United States and Western Europe, where the majority of esophageal cancers involve the esophago-gastric junction or the distal esophagus and are adenocarcinoma, with fewer cases of ESCC.

8.2 Patient Predictors of Morbidity and Mortality

Esophagectomy remains the mainstay of therapy for ESCC. Despite technical advances and improvements in peri-operative care, this procedure is still associated with protracted recovery periods, high morbidity, and significant mortality. Consequently, there has been considerable interest in identifying specific factors that contribute to complications or death after surgical resection for esophageal cancer. Accurate, individualized operative risk stratification can help to guide patients in choosing the proper extent of surgery and to identify high-risk patients who should be referred to a high-volume center.

Dhungel et al. [1] investigated the association between specific patient variables and postoperative morbidity and mortality based on data collected by the American College of Surgeons National Surgical Quality Improvement Program (ACS-NSQIP) database. Data were available for 1,032 cases of esophageal cancer operated on between the years 2005 and 2008. Among the patient variables, age and diabetes had an impact on both morbidity and mortality; dyspnea was associated with mortality alone whilst, smoking within a year preoperatively, high alcohol consumption, history of peripheral vascular disease, history of cerebrovascular accident with neurological deficit, steroid use, preoperative WBC count, preoperative INR, and ASA class III were significantly associated with morbidity. Some patient factors, such as BMI, history of severe chronic obstructive pulmonary disease (COPD), steroid use, hypertension, history of cardiac surgery, and > 10% loss of body weight in the last 6 months were statistically significant in the univariate analysis but insignificant in the multivariate models. These results were probably due to the low rate of occurrence of these factors as reported in the ACS-NSQIP database.

Wright et al. [2] similarly analyzed data from 2315 esophagectomy cases, accrued by the Society of Thoracic Surgeons from January 2002 to December 2007, in order to create a risk model for postoperative mortality and major morbidity. Age, history of congestive heart failure, coronary artery disease, peripheral artery disease, hypertension, insulin-dependent diabetes, ASA class III, smoking habit, forced expiratory volume in 1 s (FEV1) < 60%, and chronic steroid use were predictors of major morbidity.

Several studies have focused on the predisposing factors for complications after esophagectomy, in order to construct a reliable predictive model. In general, these multivariate analyses identified advanced age, pulmonary dysfunction, and poor preoperative performance status as pronounced risk factors [3-6]. However there is as yet no scoring system that can be used to consistently predict morbidity and mortality after esophagectomy.

Importantly, in analyzing these findings, the epidemiological differences between esophageal SCC and adenocarcinoma patients as well as the respective differences in the prevalence of co-morbidities should be considered.

8.3 Patient Characteristics

The occurrence of postoperative complications with respect to patient characteristics has been addressed in several studies, as reviewed below. However, few studies have examined the effect of specific patient factors on postoperative morbidity and mortality after esophagectomy for cancer.

8.3.1 Age

The effect of age on the short- and long-term results of esophagectomy has been examined, with the great majority of studies setting age 70 years as the cut-off. As expected, the number of patients with co-morbidities increases with increasing patient age. However, the overall number of postoperative complications is not significantly different between patients < 70 and > 70 years. Interestingly, there were also no differences in terms of surgical morbidity [7-9], whereas medical complications are seen significantly more often in elderly patients [7]. Similarly, mortality rates were double for patients age 70 years or older, implying that postoperative complications are poorly tolerated by elderly patients, particularly those suffering from multiple associated co-morbidities [7]. Nonetheless, in selected patients, mortality after esophagectomy is reported to be within 10%, also for patients age 70 years and older. Based on these short-term results and the substantial long-term survival that can still be achieved, elderly patients should not be denied esophagectomy [10, 11].

Zehetner et al. [12] recently reported the results of 47 octogenarians who underwent esophagectomy for cancer. The authors concluded that esophagectomy can be performed safely in this group of patients by selecting those with good cardiac and pulmonary function. It is important to note that the cohort under study represented 8% of the total number of patients operated on during the study period. Other reports from Japan confirmed the feasibility of esophagectomy in selected cases [13]. The percentage of patients > 80 years in the majority of the series is around 5% and 20–30% of these patients were eligible for surgery.

In our current practice, neoadjuvant CRT usually precedes surgery in fit patients age 75 or less, whilst primary surgery is proposed for older patients with potentially curable disease and good performance status. The percentage of patients over age 80 undergoing esophagectomy in our series was around 4%.

Definitive CRT should be considered as an alternative for patients with advanced disease or those not eligible for surgical resection [14].

8.3.2 Body Mass Index

It is well demonstrated that obesity is associated with several medical co-morbidities, such as diabetes, hypertension, and coronary artery disease. Likewise, obesity is a recognized risk factor for adenocarcinoma of the distal esophagus and esophago-gastric junction [15]. In the USA, there is a strong association between esophageal adenocarcinoma and obesity, as seen in clinical practice, whereas this association occurs less frequently in Italy. By contrast, there is little association between obesity and ESCC.

Grotenhuis et al. [16] analyzed the prognostic value of BMI on short- and long-term outcome in patients who had undergone resection for esophageal cancer. Overall morbidity, mortality, and re-operation rates did not differ among under-weight and obese patients. However, obese patients more frequently experienced severe complications and the rate of anastomotic leak was double that seen in normal-weight and under-weight patients. By contrast, complete (R0) surgical resection was less frequently observed in underweight patients. However, an association between weight loss and R0 resection rate has been demonstrated in SCC of the esophagus. Grotenhuis et al. [16] concluded that BMI is not of prognostic value with respect to short- and long-term outcome in patients undergoing esophagectomy for cancer and is not an independent predictor of radical (R0) resection. Thus, patients eligible for esophagectomy should not be denied surgery on the basis of their BMI class. Similar findings were reported by Healy et al. [17] and Scipione et al. [18]. Interestingly, trans-hiatal esophagectomy is mostly performed in obese patients in order to reduce pulmonary complications.

8.3.3 Chronic Obstructive Pulmonary Disease

A decrease in pulmonary function has been shown to influence the short-term results after lung resection surgery [19]. FEV1 is a readily available and frequently adopted measure used to investigate pulmonary function. Indeed, several studies have demonstrated that a decrease in FEV1 is an independent predictor of postoperative complications after esophagectomy [1, 2, 20]. FEV1 $< 60\%$ seems to represent the threshold at which overall and pulmonary complication rates increase such that a surgical procedure must be ruled out [1].

Respiratory co-morbidity is of particular importance in elderly patients. Cijs et al. [7] and Elsayed et al. [21] showed COPD to be an independent predictor of postoperative mortality in patients age 70 years or older. In patients with severe respiratory co-morbidity, the use of induction CRT should be carefully evaluated due to the potentially adverse effect of radiotherapy on patients with postoperative pulmonary complications. Similarly, a trans-hiatal approach rather than a trans-thoracic approach should be considered. Several studies have suggested that any operation that includes a thoracotomy increases the risk of such complications, whereas the risk is reduced by adopting a trans-hiatal approach [22, 23]. Moreover it seems that preservation of the right bronchial artery and of the bronchial branches of the vagus nerve during mediastinal lymphadenectomy results in improved lung function, a reduced risk of tracheal ischemia, and thus a decrease in postoperative pulmonary complications. The benefits of this conservative surgery were proposed by Fujita and colleagues in 1988 [24] and were confirmed by Pramesh in 2004 [25] but only sparse data are available in the current literature.

Perioperative respiratory physiotherapy might be useful in patients with functional tests indicating an area of increased risk for developing pulmonary complications: in the experience of Nakamura and colleagues [26], respiratory physiotherapy was determined to be a protective factor for respiratory complications according to both univariate and multivariate analysis.

In summary, patients with FEV1 < 60% are probably not fit for surgery, while those with FEV1 > 70% are good candidates for radical surgery. In patients in whom the FEV1 is between 60% and 70%, surgery poses an increased risk and careful preventative measures should be taken to avoid respiratory complications, e.g., perioperative respiratory physiotherapy, vascular and nerve sparing surgery, and perhaps a minimally invasive approach.

Elimination of both thoracotomy and laparotomy, as achieved with minimally invasive esophagectomy, could minimize the impact of associated pulmonary co-morbidity, although no clear benefit has been demonstrated to date [27].

8.3.4 Cardiovascular Diseases

In several studies that analyzed the risk factors for postoperative complications, the presence of cardiovascular co-morbidities did not seem to significantly influence postoperative mortality rates [1, 2, 7]. The reported incidence of myocardial infarction after esophagectomy is low (1–2%) while peri-operative cardiac arrhythmias, especially atrial fibrillation, occur in about 20% of these patients. However, these data should be considered carefully, since there may have been selection bias in the respective studies, i.e., many patients with severe cardiovascular co-morbidity may have been excluded from surgical resection and neoadjuvant treatments.

At present, there is no evidence for routine preoperative cardiac stress testing in patients undergoing esophagectomy. However, in the presence of high cardiac risk (ischemic heart disease, history of congestive heart failure or cerebrovascular disease, insulin therapy for diabetes), routine and stress echocardiography is mandatory in order to assess the need for revascularization prior to esophagectomy.

Statin administration has been associated with decreased mortality in patients undergoing non-cardiac surgery and should thus be restarted as soon as possible postoperatively. By contrast, the role of beta-blocker therapy is controversial, with no clear benefits demonstrated for its routine use in the prevention of cardiovascular complications.

Regarding neoadjuvant treatments, radiotherapy as well as some chemotherapeutic agents, such as 5-FU, may induce short- and long-term complications involving the cardiovascular system. The most common symptom associated with 5-FU cardiotoxicity is angina-like chest pain. Myocardial infarction, arrhythmias, heart failure, cardiogenic shock, and sudden death also have been reported. The incidence of cardiotoxicity associated with 5-FU varies in the literature, ranging from 1% to 68%. Risk factors have not been firmly established, but high doses (800 mg/m^2) and continuous infusions of 5-FU have been linked to higher rates of cardiotoxicity (7.6%) as compared with bolus injections (2%). Other commonly cited risk factors include a history of pre-existing cardiovascular disease, prior mediastinal radiation, and the concurrent use of chemotherapy [28].

Patients with cardiovascular co-morbidities have not been shown to benefit from a trans-hiatal approach.

8.3.5 Cirrhosis and Portal Hypertension

Liver cirrhosis increases importantly the risk of postoperative complications in patients undergoing major surgical procedures. This is especially true of esophagectomy, due to both the intrinsic technical difficulty of the operation and the high surgical stress on the patient. The main cause of liver disease in patients with SCC is alcohol abuse, followed by HCV infection.

There is a paucity of data in the current literature evaluating esophagectomy in cirrhotic patients. A recent review by Mariette [29] reported a morbidity rate of 83–87% and a mortality rate of 17–30%. Pulmonary complications and anastomotic leaks are not more frequent in cirrhotic than in non-cirrhotic patients, but they strongly impact survival. The most common specific complication is ascitic effusion, which is related to interruption of the peri-esophageal vascular collaterals and extensive lymphadenectomy. This condition is responsible for the death of about one-third of the patients. Another important cause of morbidity and mortality is bleeding, which occurs with a higher frequency in cirrhotic patients. Fatal specific complications are acute liver failure, portal thrombosis, and hepatorenal syndrome.

In the peri-operative period, accurate hemostasis, nutritional support, water and sodium restriction, and the use of albumin and fresh frozen plasma infusions are considered essential.

The degree of liver disease correlates with the risk of peri-operative complications. The most commonly used classification in clinical practice is the Child-Pugh score [30]. However, if portal hypertension is present, the risk of peri-operative morbidity is increased, even in patients with Child class A cirrhosis [31]. In a Taiwanese trial [32], 16 patients with cirrhosis underwent esophagectomy. The surgical mortality was 10% for patients with Child A cirrhosis, increasing to 50% in those with Child B and 100% for the two Child C patients. These results are consistent with those reported in the current literature [29, 33, 34]. Low albumin level, prolonged INR, and the presence of ascites seem to be the strongest predictors of increased mortality risk.

In terms of survival, the prognosis of cirrhotic patients after the peri-operative period is similar to that of non-cirrhotic patients. Indeed, if well managed, these patients have a comparable long-term survival [29, 33]. The risk of frequently fatal complications contraindicates any surgical procedure in Child B and C patients; instead, they should be treated with palliative therapies such as radiotherapy. The role of chemotherapy in patients with liver disease is debated but in most cases chemotherapy is not indicated.

A particular case is the Child A patient with portal hypertension, in which there is a high likelihood of venous flow congestion in the gastric tube, with increased risk of anastomotic leaks. A shunt procedure during esophagectomy has been proposed [35], but the preoperative use of transjugular intrahepatic portosystemic shunt (TIPSS), as a bridge to esophagectomy, has been shown to achieve better results, allowing the patient to overcome the surgical procedure [31, 36, 37]. In three patients with ESCC and Child A cirrhosis, we used a combined approach consisting of TIPSS followed one month later by esophagectomy, without posoperative mortality.

Superficial SCC in patients with esophageal varices may pose a challenge. Some case reports in the literature claim that endoscopic mucosal resection can be safely performed in these patients after previous variceal eradication or synchronous sclerotherapy [38-40].

In summary, cirrhotic patients requiring esophagectomy must be carefully selected as the procedure is feasible and should be carried out in those meeting the selection criteria, with long-term survival after radical surgery similar to that of non-cirrhotic patients. Nevertheless, upfront surgery is the mainstay, also in Child A cases, since chemotherapy is rarely possible in patients with liver disease. Surgery is not appropriate in Child B and C patients, who should be treated instead with radiotherapy alone. If portal hypertension is present in Child A patients, a TIPSS approximately one month before esophagectomy can reduce the hypertension, thus allowing the surgical procedure. Careful attention in the peri-operative period is always deemed essential to achieve a good survival probability in these fragile patients.

References

1. Dhungel B, Diggs BS, Hunter JG (2010) Patient and peri-operative predictors of morbidity and mortality after esophagectomy: American College of Surgeons National Surgical Quality Improvement Program (ACS-NSQIP), 2005-2008. J Gastrointest Surg 14:1492-1501
2. Wright CD, Kucharczuk JC, O'Brien SM et al (2009) Society of Thoracic Surgeons Gener-

al Thoracic Surgery Database. Predictors of major morbidity and mortality after esophagectomy for esophageal cancer: a Society of Thoracic Surgeons General Thoracic Surgery Database risk adjustment model. J Thorac Cardiovasc Surg 137:587-595
3. Avendano CE, Flume PA, Silvestri GA et al (2002) Pulmonary complications after esophagectomy. Ann Thorac Surg 73:922-926
4. Law S, Wong KH, Kwok KF (2004) Predictive factors for postoperative pulmonary complications and mortality after esophagectomy for cancer. Ann Surg 240:791-800
5. Atkins BZ, D'Amico TA (2006) Respiratory complications after esophagectomy. Thorac Surg Clin 16:35-48
6. Grotenhuis BA, Wijnhoven BP, Grüne F (2010) Preoperative risk assessment and prevention of complications in patients with esophageal cancer. J Surg Oncol 101:270-278
7. Cijs TM, Verhoef C, Steyerberg EW (2010) Outcome of esophagectomy for cancer in elderly patients. Ann Thorac Surg 90:900-907
8. Alexiou C, Beggs D, Salama FD (1998) Surgery for esophageal cancer in elderly patients: the view from Nottingham. J Thorac Cardiovasc Surg 116:545-553
9. Ellis FH Jr, Williamson WA, Heatley GJ (1998) Cancer of the esophagus and cardia: does age influence treatment selection and surgical outcomes? J Am Coll Surg 187:345-551
10. Yang HX, Ling L, Zhang X et al (2010) Outcome of elderly patients with oesophageal squamous cell carcinoma after surgery. Br J Surg 97:862-867
11. Ruol A, Portale G, Zaninotto G et al (2007) Results of esophagectomy for esophageal cancer in elderly patients: age has little influence on outcome and survival. J Thorac Cardiovasc Surg 33:1186-1192
12. Zehetner J, Lipham JC, Ayazi S (2010) Esophagectomy for cancer in octogenarians. Dis Esophagus 23:666-669
13. Takeno S, Takahashi Y, Watanabe S (2008) Esophagectomy in patients aged over 80 years with esophageal cancer. Hepatogastroenterology 55:453-456
14. Davies L, Lewis WG, Arnold DT et al (2010) Prognostic significance of age in the radical treatment of oesophageal cancer with surgery or chemoradiotherapy: a prospective observational cohort study. Clin Oncol (R Coll Radiol) 22:578-585
15. Enzinger PC, Mayer RJ (2003) Esophageal cancer. N Engl J Med 349:2241-2252
16. Grotenhuis BA, Wijnhoven BP, Hötte GJ et al (2010) Prognostic value of body mass index on short-term and long-term outcome after resection of esophageal cancer. World J Surg 34:2621-2627
17. Healy LA, Ryan AM, Gopinath B (2007) Impact of obesity on outcomes in the management of localized adenocarcinoma of the esophagus and esophagogastric junction. J Thorac Cardiovasc Surg 134:1284-1291
18. Scipione CN, Chang AC, Pickens A et al (2007) Transhiatal esophagectomy in the profoundly obese: implications and experience. Ann Thorac Surg 84:376-382
19. Shapiro M, Swanson SJ, Wright CD (2010) Predictors of major morbidity and mortality after pneumonectomy utilizing the Society for Thoracic Surgeons General Thoracic Surgery Database. Ann Thorac Surg 90:927-934
20. Abunasra H, Lewis S, Beggs L (2005) Predictors of operative death after oesophagectomy for carcinoma. Br J Surg 92:1029-1033
21. Elsayed H , Whittle I, McShane J et al (2010) The influence of age on mortality and survival in patients undergoing esophagogastrectomies. A seven years experience in a tertiary center. Interact Cardiovasc Thorac Surg 11:65-69
22. Hulscher JB, Tijssen JG, Obertop H, van Lanschot JJ (2001) Transthoracic versus transhiatal resection for carcinoma of the esophagus: a meta-analysis.Ann Thorac Surg 72:306-313
23. Hulscher JB, van Sandick JW, de Boer AG et al (2002) Extended transthoracic resection compared with limited transhiatal resection for adenocarcinoma of the esophagus. N Engl J Med 347:1662-1629
24. Fujita H, Hawahara H, Yamana H, et al (1988) Mediastinal lymphnode dissection procedure during esophageal cancer operation—Carefully considered for preserving respiratory function. Jpn J Surg 18:31-34

25. Pramesh CS, Mistry RC, Sharma S et al (2004) Bronchial artery preservation during transthoracic esophagectomy. J Surg Oncol 85:202-203
26. Nakamura M, Iwahashi M, Nakamoni M et al (2008) An analysis of the factors contributing to a reduction in the incidence of pulmonary complications following an esophagectomy for esophageal cancer. Langenbecks Arch Surg 393:127-133
27. Decker G, Coosemans W, De Leyn P et al (2009) Minimally invasive esophagectomy for cancer.Eur J Cardiothorac Surg 35:13-20
28. Gayed I, Gohar S, Liao Z (2009) The clinical implications of myocardial perfusion abnormalities in patients with esophageal or lung cancer after chemoradiation therapy. Int J Cardiovasc Imaging 25:487-495
29. Mariette C (2008) Is there a place for esogastric cancer surgery in cirrhotic patients? Ann Surg Oncol 15:680-682
30. Pugh R, Murray-Lyon I (1973) Transection of the esophagus in bleeding esophageal varices. Br J Surg 60:646-652
31. Friedman LS (2010) Surgery in the patient with liver disease. Trans Am Clin Climatol Assoc 121:192-204
32. Lu MS, Liu YH, Wu YC et al (2005) Is it safe to perform esophagectomy in esophageal cancer patients combined with liver cirrhosis? Interact Cardiovasc Thorac Surg 4:423-425
33. Tachibana M, Kotoh T, Kinugasa S et al (2000) Esophageal cancer with cirrhosis of the liver: results of esophagectomy in 18 consecutive patients. Ann Surg Oncol 7:758-763
34. Belghiti J, Cherqui D, Langonnet F, Fékété F (1990) Esophagogastrectomy for carcinoma in cirrhotic patients. Hepatogastroenterology 37:388-391
35. Kato T, Motohara T, Kaneko Y et al (2001) Two cases of esophageal cancer with portal hypertension: esophagectomy with venous shunt procedure. Hepatogastroenterology 48:1656-1658
36. Azoulay D, Buabse F, Damiano I (2001) Neoadjuvant transjugular intrahepatic portosystemic shunt: a solution for extrahepatic abdominal operation in cirrhotic patients with severe portal hypertension. J Am Coll Surg 193:46-51
37. Kim JJ, Dasika NL, Yu E, Fontana RJ (2009) Cirrhotic patients with a transjugular intrahepatic portosystemic shunt undergoing major extrahepatic surgery. J Clin Gastroenterol 43:574-579
38. Iwase H, Kusugami K, Suzuki M et al (2000) Endoscopic resection of early-stage esophageal cancer accompanied by esophageal varices. Gastrointest Endosc 51:749-552
39. Inoue H, Endo M, Takeshita K et al (1991) Endoscopic resection of carcinoma in situ of the esophagus accompanied by esophageal varices. Surg Endosc 5:182-184
40. Ciocîrlan M, Chemali M, Lapalus MG (2008) Esophageal varices and early esophageal cancer: can we perform endoscopic mucosal resection (EMR)? Endoscopy 40:E91

9 Esophageal Cancer Surgery: the Importance of Hospital Volume

Giovanni de Manzoni and Alberto Di Leo

9.1 The Hospital Volume-outcome Relationship

Esophagectomy for esophageal carcinoma is one of most demanding and traumatic surgical procedures undertaken in general surgery. Postoperative morbidity and mortality are usually high; nevertheless better outcomes have been noted in some high-volume specialized centers [1-4], with reported death rates of 1–3%. A recent analysis showed an improvement in outcome after the process of centralization of esophageal resections for cancer. Hospitals with the highest operative volume had the largest improvement in terms of outcome [5]. As a consequence, it was speculated that the skill, knowledge, and experience not only of the surgical team but of the entire hospital staff (anesthesiologists, intensivists, nurses, and dieticians) could influence the quality of care for patients with esophageal cancer. In addition, in a hospital with a higher surgical workload, post-operative complications can be better managed, since the hospital staff is better trained in their early recognition and is able to treat them more effectively [4]. The definition of low- and high-volume centers remains to be definitively established. Indeed, a clear volume cut-off point at which a center is justified to perform esophageal resections has yet to be determined.

At present, most of the information regarding hospital volume is obtained from studies based on state or national hospital discharge databases whereas clinical data for risk adjustment, such as cancer stage and/or coexisting diseases, are often not analyzed. Moreover, information on the surgical technique adopted and number and skill level of the involved surgeons are often missing.

G. de Manzoni (✉)
Dept. of Surgery, Upper G.I. Surgery Division, University of Verona,
Verona, Italy

G. de Manzoni (Ed.), *Treatment of Esophageal and Hypopharyngeal Squamous Cell Carcinoma*,

The majority of reports concern the relationship between surgical volume and operative mortality, which is a valid and objective outcome measure. In some studies, operative morbidity and long-term survival also have been investigated.

9.2 Outcome Measures

9.2.1 Morbidity

Postoperative complications after esophagectomy, such as pulmonary problems and anastomotic leak, have not only been associated with higher postoperative mortality rates and increased use of hospital and other healthcare resources, but also with a worse long-term prognosis [6-9]. In a retrospective analysis from a high-volume center, the rate of anastomotic leak was 5.1%. The 30-day mortality in patients with anastomotic leak was 35.7% compared to 4.2% for patients without this complication. Moreover, anastomotic leak accounted for 31.3% of the overall 30-day mortality [9].

In a study performed by Dimick at al. in hospitals in the USA, where the overall complication rate is 43%, the incidence of pulmonary failure, renal failure, aspiration, re-intubation, septicemia, and surgical complications was higher in patients undergoing esophagectomy at low-volume centers [7]. The same authors, in a larger series, reported that patients who underwent esophageal resection at low-volume hospitals (LVH), i.e., where less than seven esophagectomies are performed annually, had a higher risk of postoperative complications than those operated on at high-volume hospitals (HVH). The percentage of patients having at least one complication was 39% at HVH and 48% at LVH. Furthermore, the risk of postoperative mortality for patients with at least one complication was significantly higher (16.9%) than for those without complications (2.5%) [8]. Similar results were obtained by Wouters et al. in a study from The Netherlands, where morbidity is significantly higher in LVH, again defined as those annually performing less than seven esophagectomies per year [10].

A recent survey in Australian hospitals revealed an effect of hospital case volume on postoperative morbidity. The rates of post-resection complications were 19% for HVH (> 20 esophagectomies per year), 24% in LVH (≤ 10 esophagectomies per year), and 31% in mid-volume hospitals (between 11 and 20 esophagectomies per year) [11].

By contrast, Courrech Staal et al., analyzing the results obtained in a high-volume referral center with a low annual volume of esophagectomy (mean number < 10 per year), reported a morbidity rate of 53%, which was comparable to data published from high-volume centers [12].

9.2.2 Mortality

A trend toward a reduction in mortality rate after esophagectomy with increased hospital volume was demonstrated. In hospitals in the USA, Dimick et al. showed that the mortality rate was as high as 15.3% for LVH (performing less than seven esophagectomies annually) and 7.5% for HVH [13]. In The Netherlands, Wouters et al. reported a significantly lower mortality in HVH (mean volume of 56 resections a year) than in LVH (< 7 resections per year): 5% vs. 13% [10]. Similarly, in a Swedish study, hospital mortality was 10.4% in LVH (< 5 resections per year), 6.3% in hospitals of intermediate-volume (5-15 resections per year), and 3.5% in HVH (> 15 resections per year) centers [1].

There is still much debate on the cut-off number of esophagectomies necessary to define HVH or LVH. In a recent meta-analysis, the cut-off adopted was the following: very low-volume centers < 5 esophagectomies per year, low-volume centers 5–10 esophagectomies per year, medium- and high-volume centers 11–20 and > 20 procedures per year, respectively. According to these different classes, patients at hospitals where fewer than five esophagectomies were annually performed had a very high postoperative mortality (median 18%) compared to HVH (median 4.9%). The authors suggested a minimum number of 20 esophagectomies per year to reduce post-operative mortality [14].

Consistent with this data, in our institution we report a 3.3% mortality rate with a mean number of 40 esophagectomies performed per year.

9.2.3 Long-term Survival

There is still an ongoing debate about the relationship between surgical volume, however defined, and outcome. This is important because in many reports long-term prognosis seems to be influenced by hospital volume: Wouters et al. found that patients with stage I and II disease had a better 5-year survival in HVH [10]. In the above cited Australian series, 3-year overall survival in patients undergoing resection was 45.1% in LVH, 58.0% in mid-volume hospitals, and 64.4% in HVH [11]. Similar results were registered in Swedish hospitals, where overall 5-year survival was higher in HVH (> 15 resections per year) than in LVH (<5 resections per year): 22% vs. 17% [1]. Ultimately, the meta-analysis performed by Metzger at al. resulted in clear evidence that increasing the case volume leads to an improvement in long-term prognosis [14].

However not all authors agree with these conclusions. A recent analysis from the Netherlands failed to show better survival in patients treated in HVH (more than 20 resections per year) [15] and the same results were reported from a prospective population-based cohort of 3293 consecutive patients in Scotland [16]. In the latter study, however, the number of operations per year in LVH was < 13, which is a higher cut-off than in the other reported experience. Similarly, a Swedish nationwide population-based study was unable to find differences in long-term survival in patients undergoing esophageal cancer surgery at HVH (≥ 10 esophagectomies per year) and LVH (< 10 esophagectomies per year) after adjustment for clinically relevant covariates [17].

These apparently conflicting results show that volume itself does not guarantee a high quality of surgical care, and they draw attention to the importance of other relevant factors to improve the outcome of esophageal cancer patients

9.3 The Surgeon's Case Volume and Experience

Some studies have also suggested an association between the surgeon's case volume and postoperative morbidity-mortality after esophagectomy. Rouvelas et al. showed that the 30-day mortality in low-, medium-, and high-case-volume surgeon groups was 7.1, 2.1, and 2.6%, respectively [18]. Moreover, a recent retrospective study supported surgeon's experience as being potentially more significant than the absolute number of procedures performed at an institution per year. In a LVH (< 10 procedures per year), the patients of a single experienced surgeon had morbidity (48%) and 30-day mortality (3.6%) rates comparable to those reported from HVH [19].

A recent report from UK found that 30-day mortality after esophagectomy for cancer was significantly higher in patients treated by general surgeons than by cardiothoracic surgeons (9.0% vs. 6.1%), and that it was higher in LVH (mean case volume < 20 cases per year) than in HVH (mean case volume of 20 or more cases per year): 9.6% vs. 6.3%. Considering the combined effects of specialty and volume, postoperative mortality was significantly higher in low-volume than in high-volume general surgical units. Finally, mortality rates were similar in high-volume general surgical and high-volume cardiothoracic units. The authors argued that these findings regarding the two surgical specialties were related to differences in the training of the two types of surgeons: in particular, cardiothoracic training involves extensive experience in dealing with complications specific to operations of the chest, with a stronger emphasis on postoperative critical care than most general surgery programs [20].

In conflict with these results, a study population from Northern Ireland showed no significant surgeon-related difference in operative patient mortality, irrespective of the surgical case volume, nor were there differences between consultants and trainee surgeons (4.3% vs. 4.4%). No significant differences in long-term outcomes were found when taking into account the rate of major complications and the cancer stage amongst the patients. The authors attributed their findings to the fact that all of the patients were managed by a multidisciplinary team practiced in cancer management, such as available at HVH [21].

References

1. Wenner J, Zilling T, Bladstrom A, Alvegard TA (2005) The influence of surgical volume on hospital mortality and 5-year survival for carcinoma of the oesophagus and gastric cardia. Anticancer Res 25:419-424
2. Dimick JB, Cowan JA, Ailawadi G et al (2003) National variation in operative mortality rates for esophageal resection and the need for quality improvement. Arch Surg 138:1305-1309
3. Law S, Wong KH, Kwok KF et al (2004) Predictive factors for postoperative pulmonary complications and mortality after esophagectomy for cancer. Ann Surg 2004:791-800
4. Law S (2010) Esophagectomy without mortality: what can surgeon do? J Gastrointest Surg 14:S101-S107
5. Wouters MW, Karim-Kos HE, le Cessie S et al (2009) Centralization of esophageal cancer surgery: does it improve clinical outcomes? Ann Surg Oncol 16:1789-1798
6. Currech Staal EFW, Wouters MWJM, Boot H et al (2010) Quality-of-care indicators for oesophageal cancer surgery: a review. EJSO 36:1035-1043
7. Dimick JB, Pronovost PJ, Cowan JA Jr, Lipsett PA (2003) Surgical volume and quality of care for esophageal resection: do high-volume hospitals have fewer complications? Ann Thorac Surg 75:337-341
8. Dimick JB, Pronovost PJ, Cowan JA Jr (2003) Variation in postoperative complication rates after high-risk surgery in the United States. Surgery 134:534-540
9. Junemann-Ramirez M, Awan MY, Khan ZM, Rahamin JS (2005) Anastomotic leakage post-esophagogastrectomy for esophageal carcinoma: retrospective analysis of predictive factors, management and influence on long-term survival in high volume cantre. Eur J Cardiothorac Surg 27:3-7
10. Wouters MW, Wijnhoven BP, Karim-Kos HE et al (2008) High-volume versus low-volume for esophageal resections for cancer : the essential role of case mix adjustments based on clinical data. Ann Surg Oncol 15:80-87
11. Stavrou EP, Smith GS, Baker DF (2010) Surgical outcomes associated with oesophagectomy in New South Wales: an investigation of hospital volume. J Gastrointest Surg 14:951-957
12. Courrech Staal EF, van Coevorden F, Cats A et al (2009) Outcome of low-volume surgery for esophageal cancer in high-volume referral center. Ann Surg Oncol 16:3219-3226
13. Dimick JB, Wainess R, Upchurch G et al (2005) National trends in outcomes for esophageal resection. Ann Thorac Surg 79:212-218
14. Metzger R, Bollshweiler E, Vallböhmer D et al (2004) High volume centers for esophagectomy: what is the number needed to achieve low postoperative mortality? Dis Esophagus 17:310-314
15. Verhoef C, van de Weyer R, Schaapveld M et al (2007) Better survival in patients with esophageal cancer after surgical treatment in university hospitals: a plea for performance by surgical oncologist. Ann Surg Oncol 14:1678-1687
16. Thompson AM, Rapson T, Gilbert FG, Park KGM.(2007) Hospital volume does not influence long-term survival of patients undergoing surgery for oesophageal or gastric cancer. Br J Surg 94:578-584
17. Rouvelas I, Lindblad M, Zeng W et al (2007) Impact of hospital volume on long-term survival after esophageal cancer surgery. Arch Surg 142:113-117
18. Rouvelas I, Jia C, Viklund P et al (2007) Surgeon volume and postoperative mortality after oesophagectomy for cancer. Eur J Surg Oncol 33:162-168
19. Santin B, Kulwicki A, Price P (2008) Mortality rate associated with 56 consecutive esophagectomies performed at a "low-volume" hospital: is procedure volume as important as we are trying to make it? J Gastrointest Surg 12:1346-1350

20. Leigh Y, Goldacre M, McCulloch P (2009) Surgical speciality, surgical volume and mortality after oesophageal cancer surgery. Eur J Surg Oncol 35:825-825
21. Jeganathan R, Kinnear H, Campbell J et al (2009) A surgeon's case volume of oesophagectomy for cancer does not influence patient outcome in high volume hospital. Interact Cardiovasc Thorac Surg 9:66-69

Section II

Carcinoma of Hypopharynx and Cervical Esophagus

Surgical Treatment: Indications, Early and Long-term Results, and Disease Recurrence

10

Giovanni de Manzoni, Franco Barbieri, Andrea Zanoni, and Francesco Casella

Cancers of the hypopharynx and cervical esophagus used to be studied and treated together, due to the anatomical proximity of the two structures and the frequent infiltration of both. Nowadays, they are considered two different disease entities, with different symptoms, patterns of diffusion, and survival rates.

10.1 Hypopharynx

10.1.1 Introduction

Anatomically, the hypopharynx is the lower part of the pharynx and represents the link between the oropharynx and the esophagus. It lies posterior to the larynx and is divided into the pyriform sinuses, the posterior pharyngeal wall, and the postcricoid area.

Hypopharyngeal cancer (HC) represents 3–7% of all head and neck tumors [1, 2] and most of them are squamous cell carcinomas (SCCs). The prognosis for these patients is dismal, with a 5-year overall survival rate after radical treatment of 15–45%, especially because of late diagnosis [1, 2].

The symptoms of HC are nonspecific until the tumor is large enough to cause aspiration, hoarseness, or respiratory compromise. Between 70 and 80% of the patients have advanced disease at diagnosis, with 10–30% presenting with stage IV disease, due to distant metastases (usually the lung, bone, liver, and skin) [1, 2]. The cancer tends to spread transmurally, infiltrating the larynx and thyroid gland. It also tends to diffuse downwards to the cervical esophagus and, in very late stage disease, to the prevertebral fascia and mediastinal structures. Nodal involvement is present in more than 50% of the

G. de Manzoni (✉)
Dept. of Surgery, Upper G.I. Surgery Division, University of Verona, Verona, Italy

G. de Manzoni (Ed.), *Treatment of Esophageal and Hypopharyngeal Squamous Cell Carcinoma*,

patients and bilateral cervical and paratracheal node metastases are frequent [1, 2].

The main risk factors for the development of HC are smoking and alcohol assumption. Two interesting studies [3, 4] reported an increased risk of cancer both for smokers-non-drinkers and for drinkers-non-smokers. The risk of cancer increases with increasing number of smoked cigarettes and alcohol amount. The concept of "field cancerization," due to the multiple cancerogenic agents acting on the aero-digestive tract, is largely accepted. Accordingly, 10–20% of the patients with head and neck cancer will develop synchronous or metachronous esophageal cancer.

The treatment of HC aims at radical resection with the least mutilating procedure. Laryngeal preservation can be considered if oncological radicality is conserved. As described in the next chapter, the use of multimodal treatments is increasing and deserves further investigation.

10.1.2 Surgical Treatment

Traditionally, HC was treated by total laryngectomy with partial or circumferential hypopharyngectomy [1, 5, 6]. Today, the standard treatment consists of surgery and, in cases of advanced disease and all cases of pN+, adjuvant radiotherapy.

Patients treated with circumferential pharyngectomy must, due to the resulting substantial defects, undergo challenging reconstruction procedures. The type of reconstruction depends on the surgeon's expertise and preference. When the cancer invades the cervical esophagus, a gastric pull-up is the typical choice. In cancers limited to the neck area, there are different possibilities. A free jejunal graft (as described below in the section on cervical esophageal cancer) could be used for hypopharyngeal and for cervical esophageal defects. A pectoralis myocutaneous flap, either completely tubed or in a U-shape, can be used in hypopharyngeal reconstruction, without the need of microvascular anastomoses. Free fasciocutaneous flaps, such as radial forearm and anterolateral thigh free flaps, have been increasingly used for reconstruction, both in circumferential and partial resection, as they can be adapted as patches for partial defects or tubularized for circumferential resections. Even if the functional results seem to be better with free fasciocutaneous flaps than with free jejunal grafts for hypopharyngeal reconstruction, the leak rate of 33% is not negligible [1, 5, 6].

For selected cases, i.e., cT1 cancers of the upper part of the pyriform sinus, advanced but very lateralized tumors, or downstaged tumors in patients treated with neoadjuvant chemoradiation, a partial resection could be performed. This allows for functional preservation of the larynx, with significantly improved quality of life.

In cT1 cancers of the upper part of the pyriform sinus, a supraglottic hemilaryngo-pharyngectomy can be used. In very early stages, transoral (minimally invasive) laser surgery is an option.

In advanced but very lateralized tumors a hemilaryngo-pharyngectomy can be performed. However, for tumors of the upper part of the pyriform sinus or in case of fixation of the involved hemilarynx this procedure is contraindicated.

A small tumor (< 1 cm) located on the lateral wall of the pyriform sinus can be treated with partial pharyngectomy, with removal of the lateral side of the thyroid cartilage and of the ipsilateral large horn of the hyoid bone.

In summary, in HC, sacrifice of the larynx is relatively frequent, especially because late diagnosis prevents less destructive procedures. The increased role of multimodal treatments with downstaging of the neoplastic lesions might increase the number of patients eligible for laryngeal preservation.

10.1.3 Lymphatic Spread and Lymphadenectomy

At diagnosis, 75–80% of the patients present with nodal metastases [7]. The nodal stations involved in the lymphatic spread are levels II and III upwards (superior laterocervical nodes) and levels IV and VI downwards (inferior laterocervical nodes and recurrent nerve nodes). Level V (supraclavicular) nodes are affected only in more advanced stages, when nodal metastases are already present at other levels. Level I (submandibular nodes) is hardly involved by HC whereas involvement of the retropharyngeal nodes occurs in 20–60% of the cases. The risk of occult micrometastases in clinically negative patients (cN0) is quite high, with a mean reported prevalence of 44% [7].

Considering the high prevalence of nodal metastases even in cN0 patients and the significant impact on survival, a routine neck dissection is deemed mandatory to improve both local control and survival. In case of cN+ disease, radical dissection is needed, consisting of lymphadenectomy of levels I–V together with nodes of the central compartment (level VI). If the metastases infiltrate the internal jugular vein or the sternocleidomastoid muscle, the sacrifice of these structures is compulsory; otherwise, a radical modified type III dissection can be performed, sparing these structures.

In patients with cN0 disease, the lymphadenectomy should be selective instead of radical, to reduce morbidity, with dissection of the most frequently involved stations, i.e., levels II, III, IV, and VI.

Buckley and MacLennan [8] reported a 47% prevalence of contralateral nodal metastases in patients with cN0 disease. While their study considered selected patients, the high prevalence nonetheless supports bilateral neck dissection. Moreover, the procedure should be mandatory in any patient with clinical N+ disease, even in case of very lateralized tumors. Also, patients with cN0 disease in which there is central cancer should undergo bilateral neck dissection. In highly lateralized, early cancers, the absence of ipsilateral metastases at intraoperative cryostat might allow the avoidance of contralateral dissection.

10.1.4 Long-term Results and Disease Recurrence

In such cases, the prognosis is still dismal, even if HC has a better prognosis than cervical esophageal cancer. The reported overall survival is 18–48% [1, 9], but overall survival can reach 80% for patients with T1 cancers, even those treated with partial surgery. A multimodal approach may increase local control and survival, but definitive data are lacking.

The main causes of death after radical treatment are locoregional relapse and second tumor, especially in the aero-digestive tract. The mean interval between treatment and relapse is around 2 years, while between treatment and onset of the second primary tumor the interval is around 3 years [1, 9].

10.2 Cervical Esophagus

10.2.1 Introduction

Anatomically, the cervical esophagus extends from the hypopharynx to the thoracic inlet, at the level of the sternal notch. Although the length of the esophagus differs widely with gender and body size, normal measurements during endoscopy are from 15–20 cm, measured from the incisors, normally with a total length of less than 5 cm (Fig. 10.1) [10].

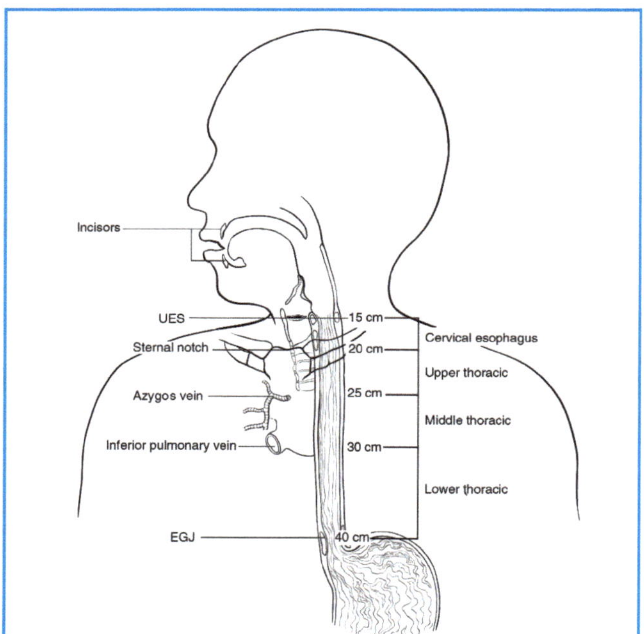

Fig 10.1 Normal anatomical subdivisions of the esophagus. Lengths measured from the incisors. (Reproduced from [10], with permission)

Cervical esophageal squamous cell carcinoma (CESCC) is rare, occurring in approximately 5–10% of patients with esophageal neoplasms. Survival is poor due to intrinsic disease aggressiveness, delayed diagnosis, and treatment difficulties. Moreover, given the rarity of this cancer, studies of significant power are difficult to carry out.

Historically, pharyngo-laryngo-esophagectomy (PLE) was considered the gold standard for these types of malignancies. However, the correct therapeutic strategy nowadays is a matter of debate. First, neither randomized trials nor meta-analyses have been reported in the recent literature, and all studies suffer from small sample size and different and not uniform types of treatment. Second, to expand the study population and because of the frequent involvement of the pharyngo-esophageal junction, cervical cancers are often considered together with hypopharyngeal neoplasms, even though treatment strategies and prognosis are quite different [11, 12], with hypopharyngeal cancers associated with significantly longer survival in most studies.

Despite some exceptions, surgery is still the mainstay of treatment, with R0 resection representing the aim of all therapies. Multimodal approaches with possible avoidance of surgical resection have also been proposed.

Controversies exist regarding definition of the adequate extent of esophagectomy, the criteria to preserve the larynx, the type of reconstruction, and the correct extent of lymphadenectomy. The use of multimodal treatments is also increasing and deserves investigation.

10.2.2 Type of Exeresis

The nature of the surgical tissue destruction significantly impacts morbidity and mortality, survival and recurrence, and the quality of residual life. Thus, all these issues influence therapeutic decision-making. Neither tailored treatments nor stage-adapted treatments are widely accepted in this relatively uncommon condition. The poor survival of these patients, even with radical surgery, and the highly mutilating procedures make the choice of treatment particularly challenging.

The hypopharynx and/or the upper thoracic esophagus are frequently involved, together with distant intramural lesions in the thoracic esophagus. This clinical picture makes resection of the entire esophagus mandatory. Organ-sparing has been suggested in patients with pure cervical esophageal cancer, but the risk of distant intramural metastases, which are hardly detectable endoscopically and surgically, makes this choice questionable, especially when upfront surgery without neoadjuvant chemoradiation is performed.

Furthermore, because of the local aggressiveness of cervical cancer, many if not most of the patients have locally advanced cancers at diagnosis, with cT4 representing 50% of the cases reported in the literature [12] and in our personal case load [14]. The most frequently infiltrated structures are the larynx, thyroid, trachea, and recurrent laryngeal nerves. All these structures are resectable, at the cost of more aggressive and mutilating surgery. A patient is considered to have inoperable disease when the spinal column or the great vessels of the neck are infiltrated, in case of distant metastases, or when poor performance status prevents radical surgery.

The problem of surgical mutilation and the devastating effects of aggressive surgery are particularely relevant since, as reported in the literature, the prognosis of patients treated accordingly is very poor. Previously, PLE was considered the gold standard, but the loss of voice and speech, due to laryngectomy, along with permanent tracheostomy are not often compensated by prolonged survival. Other therapeutic options have thus been proposed. The current options are PLE via a trans-hiatal or trans-thoracic approach and cervical esophagectomy with laryngectomy. Laryngeal preservation is possible in selected cases and reduces the degree of mutilation.

The surgical choices described in the recent literature are summarized in Table 10.1 [11, 12, 15-19]. As shown, more than one approach has been adopted, with cervical esophagectomy and laryngeal preservation increasingly performed. Of note, the number of patients studied in each therapeutic group has been quite small, especially considering only the pure cervical cases. This has two important implications: (1) It is difficult to draw conclusions with small sample sizes, especially when different surgical procedures were performed; (2) Treatment might have been chosen based on the cancer's location, i.e., hypopharyngeal or cervical, which adds further confusion.

Table 10.1 Type of surgical demolition in cervical esophageal squamous cell carcinoma

Author (year)	N.	Pure cervical	Total esophagectomy	Cervical esophagectomy
Triboulet et al. (2001) [10]	209 (1982-1999)	78	PLE: 132 L-P: 0	L: 77 L-P: 0
Wang et al. (2006) [11]	41 (1984-2002)	15	PLE:41 L-P: 0	L: 0 L-P: 0
Daiko et al. (2007) [14]	74 (1982-2002)	15	PLE: 19 L-P: 0	L: 55 L-P: 0
Ferahkose et al. (2007) [15]	52 (1996-2006)	33	PLE: 14 L-P: 24	L: 8 L-P: 6
Ott et al. (2009) [17]	109 (1986-2006)	109	PLE: 0 L-P: 0	L: 20 L-P: 89
Shirakawa et al. (2004) [18]	54 (1985-2003)	31	PLE: 0 L-P: 0	L: 47 L-P: 7
Kadota et al. (2009) [16]	32 (1984-2002)	17	PLE: 0 L-P: 0	L: 0 L-P: 32

PLE, Pharyngo-laryngo-esophagectomy; *L-P,* larynx preservation; *L,* laryngectomy.

Pharyngo-laryngectomy with total esophagectomy. PLE is a very destructive and mutilating operation, with permanent tracheostomy and definitive loss of voice. However, these patients, after a period of rehabilitation, can eat normally and the risk of aspiration is evidently absent. The procedure can be carried out without thorax opening, with the esophagus completely removed and the risk of involved margins annulled. Certainly, in case of massive involvement of the upper thoracic esophagus or in case of distant lesions in the thoracic esophagus, thorax opening is deemed essential (Chap. 13).

Without thoracotomy, a lymphadenectomy can be performed only in the cervical region and upper mediastinum; otherwise, an extended mediastinal lymphadenectomy necessitates a thoracotomy. As reported below, the problem of lymphadenectomy is relevant, with surgical resection a valid option only if it is radical, with clear margins and correct lymphadenectomy.

Cervical esophagectomy with laryngectomy. This procedure became feasible once the continuity of the digestive tract could be reconstructed without the need for a gastric tube as a conduit to replace the esophagus. The theoretical advantage of this procedure is the possibility to spare the residual esophagus and to avoid its blind dissection. Laryngectomy aims at achieving a radical resection at the proximal margin. This technique can only be used when the cancer is confined to above the sternal notch.

An interesting Japanese trial [13] compared the results of total vs. proximal esophagectomy in terms of survival and recurrence in two groups of patients. With the limit of being a retrospective study with small cohorts of patients (10 and 11, respectively), the extent of esophagectomy did not influence survival at multivariate analysis.

The major criticism of this procedure is the risk of resecting only a small portion of the upper esophagus, leaving in situ intramural distant metastases, which are not easily detectable either preoperatively or intraoperatively, especially during upfront surgery. Furthermore, the presence of laryngectomy does not make this procedure less mutilating than PLE in terms of residual quality of life.

Larynx-preserving esophagectomy. Cervical or total esophagectomy without laryngectomy has been proposed to reduce the impact on the quality of residual life. Opponents of laryngeal preservation claim that it leads to important risks in terms of early and long-term outcome. There is a theoretical risk of higher recurrence, due to a reduced proximal margin, with possible cancer involvement. Unfortunately, there are no comparative studies of laryngectomy and laryngeal preservation, and the significant rate of local recurrence in cervical esophageal cancer might be explained by a number of reasons, not only laryngeal preservation. The reported overall survival is similar to that achieved with laryngectomy; it may have been the case that, paradoxically, laryngectomy was performed in more advanced cases, resulting in worse outcome. In the above-mentioned Japanese trial [13], the addition of laryngectomy was an independent marker of worse outcome at multivariable analysis.

In terms of early outcomes, even if morbidity and mortality rates are reportedly similar to those achieved with laryngectomy, the types of complications are fairly different. Indeed, the necessity to preserve the laryngeal recurrent nerves makes the procedure more challenging, with the risk of monolateral or even bilateral vocal cord palsy. Bilateral vocal cord paralysis, with the necessity of definitive tracheostomy, represents the failure of larynx-preserving surgery. Monolateral paralysis increases the risk of aspiration pneumonia, which is considerable in these patients as they need swallowing rehabilitation. Moreover, transient tracheostomy is frequently performed to protect the airways from aspiration.

Based on the similar survival and recurrence rates, the superior quality of life, and the risks of complications, laryngeal preservation should be reasonably applied to all possible candidates. However, preservation might be indicated only in selected cases of upfront surgery, in which a clear proximal margin of 2 cm can be obtained [13, 20]. A recent indication may be the downstaging achieved with chemoradiation, which has importantly increased the number of candidates for laryngeal preservation. Meanwhile, there is considerable debate, as in rectal cancer, between those who advocate preservation, because of the increased quality of life, and those who oppose it, claiming that downstaging and downsizing do not exclude the risk of residual microfoci of cancer in the esophageal wall.

In summary, the most appropriate surgical demolitive procedure is still a matter of debate, but radical resection is the mainstay of any procedure. Total esophagectomy can guarantee the eradication of possible intramural metastases and should be the preferred approach, at least until comparative studies with sufficient sample sizes become available. Laryngeal preservation should be adopted whenever feasible, but the indications should be strict, to avoid non-radical operations. A safe margin of 2 cm during upfront surgery or at least clear margins after downstaging can theoretically permit both oncological radicality and better quality of life.

10.2.3 Type of Reconstruction

Historically, the most frequently used conduit after esophagectomy was the stomach, with the construction of a gastric tube along the greater curvature. In case of cancers of the cervical esophagus, other substitutes have been proposed. Among these, the technique that has gained the most resonance is the restoration of the continuity with a free jejunal graft transfer. This technique became widespread following the advent of microvascular anastomotic techniques.

While the surgical procedure to create a gastric tube is well known, recon-

Table 10.2 Type of surgical reconstruction in cervical esophageal squamous cell carcinoma

Author (year)	N.	Gastric pull-up	Free jejunal graft	Others (colon graft, flaps, etc.)
Triboulet et al. (2001) [11]	209 (1982-1999)	127	77	5
Wang et al. (2006) [12]	41 (1984-2002)	39	-	2
Daiko et al. (2007) [15]	74 (1982-2002)	19	50	5
Ferahkose et al. (2007) [16]	52 (1996-2006)	38	14	-
Ott et al. (2009) [18]	109 (1986-2006)	-	109	-
Shirakawa et al. (2004) [19]	54 (1985-2003)	-	54	-
Kadota et al. (2009) [17]	32 (1984-2002)	-	32	-

struction of the alimentary tract with a free jejunal graft merits discussion. A jejunal segment is divided together with its vascular pedicle and a jejunojejunostomy is performed. Then, the free jejunal graft is placed on the defect in an isoperistaltic position and the proximal and distal anastomoses are performed. Next, microvascular anastomoses are constructed between the jejunal vessels and superior thyroid artery or external carotid artery and internal or external jugular vein [16, 18].

Both methods are nowadays widely used. The results achieved with the study population of recent trials are displayed in Table 10.2 [11, 12, 15-19].

Both the gastric tube and the free jejunal graft have important advantages and disadvantages. In the gastric pull-up, a single anastomosis is needed and there are no problems of vascular supply. Moreover, the distal margin is safe, by definition. Nevertheless, this is a highly tissue-destructive procedure and it is associated with frequent cardiorespiratory morbidity. The advantages of the free jejunal graft are reduced invasiveness at the donor site, easy harvesting of the graft, good size approximation, the possibility to perform a limited esophageal resection with organ preservation, and the theoretically quicker functional recovery. Nonetheless, the need for two anastomoses between the residual esophagus and the graft and two microvascular anastomoses markedly increases the risk of leak and graft failure due to necrosis. There is also a higher risk of distal margin positivity.

It is difficult to compare the methods with respect to either the long-term results, as numerous factors are involved, or morbidity, as conflicting results are reported in the literature. In summary, each method has its proponents and opponents and the ideal type of reconstruction remains a matter of debate.

10.2.4 Morbidity and Mortality

The complications after these highly destructive procedures are considerable (Table 10.3) [11, 12, 15-19]. Total morbidity ranges from 30% to more than 70% and it is substantially equivalent to that described for thoracic esophageal cancer. The rates of anastomotic leak and graft necrosis resulting from gastric pull-up vs. free jejunal graft differ in the reported trials. In general, the anastomotic leak rate is 3–23% and 4–32% for gastric pull-up and free jejunal graft, respectively. The graft necrosis rate is 2–10% and 0–24% for gastric pull-up and free jejunal graft, respectively.

Graft necrosis is due to vascular inadequacy, often caused by venous thrombosis at the anastomotic level, especially if small recipient vessels are used. It is much more frequent in the case of free jejunal graft and accounts for most of the need for re-operation. Moreover, while conservative treatment is

Table 10.3 Morbidity and mortality in surgically treated cervical esophageal squamous cell carcinoma with different surgical procedures

Authors (year)	N.	Morbidity (% total)				Mortality
		Anastomotic leak		Graft necrosis		
		GP	FJG	GP	FJG	
Triboulet et al.	209	80 (38.3%)				
(2001) [11]	(1982-1999)	20 /127 (16%)	25/77 (32%)	2/127 (1.7%)	5/77 (6%)	10 (4.8%)
Wang et al.	41	19 (46.3%)				
(2006) [12]	(1984-2002)	9/39 (23%)	–	1/39 (3%)	–	4 (9.8%)
Daiko et al.	74	25 (34%)				
(2007) [15]	(1982-2002)	2/19 (10%)	2/50 (4%)	2/19 (10%)	3/50 (6%)	3 (4%)
Ferahkose et al.	52	27 (51.9%)				
(2007) [16]	(1996-2006)	1/38 (3%)	0/14 (0%)	2/38 (6%)	1/14 (7%)	3 (5.7%)
Ott et al.	109	81 (74.3%)				
(2009) [18]	(1986-2006)	–	29/109 (27%)	–	26/109 (24%)	3 (2.8%)
Shirakawa et al.	54	–				
(2004) [19]	(1985-2003)	–	–		5/54 (9%)	0 (0%)
Kadota et al.	32	16 (50%)				
(2009) [17]	(1984-2002)	–	4/32 (12%)	–	0/32 (0%)	0 (0%)

GP, gastric pull-up; *FJG*, free jejunal graft.

possible in most cases of anastomotic leak, surgical substitution of the graft is necessary when necrosis occurs. Ott and colleagues [18] reported that graft ischemia necessitated reoperation in 20% of the patients.

A Chinese trial using gastric pul-up [21] reported a 42% total morbidity rate, with a mortality of 1.9%. The most common complications were respiratory ones. Anastomotic leakage occurred in 9% of the patients, while no graft necrosis was described in the study population.

In summary, as in thoracic esophageal cancer, anastomotic leak is the main cause of surgical morbidity. Graft necrosis is the most severe surgical complication and the main cause of re-operation; it is much more frequent after reconstruction with free jejunal graft.

10.2.5 Multimodal Treatments

Multimodal treatments are considered an alternative to upfront surgery in CESCC and they are fully dealt with in the next chapter. In most of the aforementioned studies, some sub-groups of patients have been treated with neoadjuvant protocols (Table 10.4) [11, 12, 15, 17, 18]. However, the results of the various trials can be misinterpreted because of the heterogeneity of the study population and the small sample size. In thoracic esophageal cancer, multimodal treatments are increasingly adopted as the standard of care, but they are more difficult to evaluate in cervical cancer. The main advantage of neoadjuvant chemoradiation is the possibility to achieve a complete response or at least a downstaging and downsizing of the tumor. The reduced size of the cancer due to response to treatment has both a good impact on survival and makes laryngeal preservation, and thus the possibility to perform a less mutilating surgical procedure, more likely.

Table 10.4 Multimodal treatments in cervical esophageal squamous cell carcinoma

Author (year)	N.	Neoadjuvant treatment	Surgery alone	Adjuvant treatment
Triboulet et al. (2001) [11]	209 (1982-1999)	22 CRT 15 CT 5 RT	22	145 RT
Wang et al. (2006) [12]	41 (1984-2002)	6 RT	14	21 RT
Daiko et al. (2007) [15]	74 (1982-2002)	–	58	11 RT 5 CT
Ott et al. (2009) [18]	109 (1986-2006)	94 CRT	15	–
Kadota et al. (2009) [17]	32 (1984-2002)	4 previous RT	23	2 RT 3 CT

CRT, chemoradiation therapy; *RT*, radiation therapy.

10.2.6 Lymphatic Spread and Lymphadenectomy

The Japanese Classification of Esophageal Cancer [22] defines the regional nodes for the cervical esophagus as groups 100–104 for the neck and 105 and 106 for the upper thorax (Fig. 10.2). Paratracheal nodes and, in particular, recurrent nerve nodes are considered part of the primary drainage nodes [22-27].

As described for the thoracic esophagus (Chap. 13), lymphatic pathways in the submucosa run downwards and upwards, but a precise description of lymphatic spread in the cervical esophagus is lacking.

In a recent study [7], the rate of cervical metastases in patients with cervical esophageal cancer was 86%, while mediastinal metastases were found in 33% of the patients. Of note, even though the sample size was small, the rate of mediastinal node positivity increased to 56% in cancers infiltrating the upper thoracic esophagus. The rate of metastases in the upper mediastinum is between 40 and 70% according to a recent review [24]. A European study [27] described a 60% involvement rate of cervical or paratracheal nodes, with only paratracheal nodal involvement in 19% of the cases. A Japanese trial [28] proposed considering the nodal compartments based on the metastatic rate and overall survival after lymphadenectomy. Even with these subclassifications, which need evaluation with larger cohorts of patients, it seems clear that the recurrent-nerve nodes are among the primary drainage nodes.

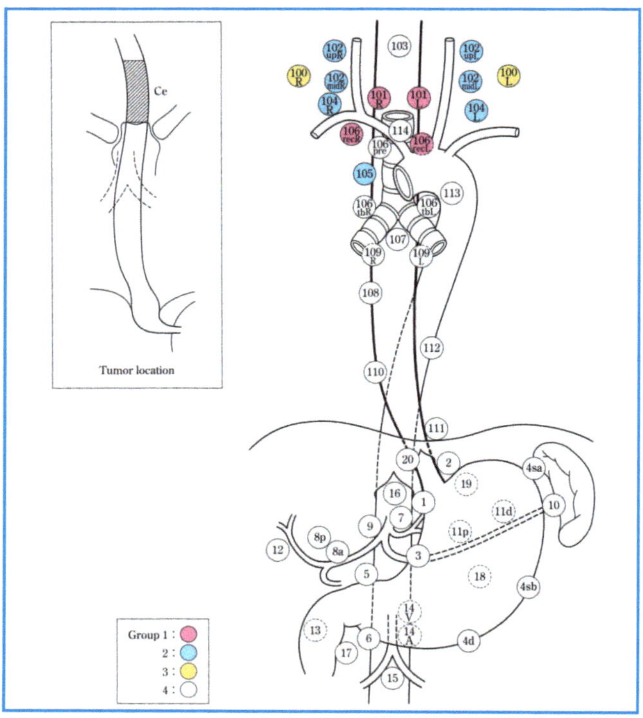

Fig 10.2 Drainage nodal stations for CESCC according to the Japanese Classification of Esophageal Cancer. (Reproduced from [22], with permission)

Table 10.5 Type of lymphadenectomy performed in cervical esophageal squamous cell carcinoma

Author (year)	N.	Neck dissection	Mediastinal dissection	pN+
Triboulet et al. (2001) [11]	209 (1982-1999)	n.r.	n.r.	n.r.
Wang et al. (2006) [12]	41 (1984-2002)	28 (68%)	n.r.	26 (93%)
Daiko et al. (2007) [15]	74 (1982-2002)	74 (100%)	n.r.	50 (67%)
Ferahkose et al. (2007) [16]	52 (1996-2006)	52 (100%)	n.r.	n.r.
Ott et al. (2009) [18]	109 (1986-2006)	67 (61%)	n.r.	21 (31%)
Kadota et al. (2009) [17]	32 (1984-2002)	29 (91%)	n.r.	n.r.

n.r., not reported or not performed.

N category, together with radical resection, is a major prognostic factor [15, 18, 27]; hence, lymphadenectomy is no doubt crucial in the treatment of CESCC as for SCC of the thoracic esophagus.

Neck dissection is normally performed, while upper mediastinal dissection is not routine. Upper mediastinal lymphadenectomy, as carried out by Hirano and coworkers [26], involves a cervical approach with possible sternal splitting. The authors claim that tracheal bifurcation is the lower limit of lymphadenectomy achievable without thoracotomy. The type of lymphadenectomy used in several recent trials is listed in Table 10.5 [11, 12, 15-18]. As mentioned above, only neck dissection was routinely performed.

In our institution, mediastinal lymphadenectomy is considered crucial to the treatment of CESCC; hence, we opt for thoracotomy with extensive mediastinal nodal dissection together with neck dissection. In our dataset, morbidity and mortality are low, thus making extended dissection feasible and safe.

When chemoradiation is performed, good knowledge of the lymphatic spread is needed to determine the fields of radiation. Paratracheal and recurrent-nerve nodes should be considered primary drainage stations, such that the fields of radiotherapy should include the upper mediastinum. This is especially true in definitive chemoradiation, with the aim to eradicate probable metastases.

In summary, N status is a main prognostic factor for CESCC. Lymphatic spread has not been described in detail in the literature, but upper mediastinal nodes are involved in a high percentage of cases. A correct lymphadenectomy could improve the poor prognosis of this rare and aggressive cancer and is therefore mandatory. Whether upper mediastinal dissection via the cervical route is sufficient is a matter of debate. We believe that probably a complete mediastinal dissection via a thoracotomy can eradicate skip and occult metastases in the mid-lower mediastinum, thus improving survival. Accordingly, we conclude that an upper mediastinal nodal dissection should be considered as the standard approach, together with neck lymphadenectomy. Lymphadenectomy of the mid-lower mediastinum should be considered in high-volume centers, as it may improve survival; it should also be performed in all the patients with cancer involving the upper thoracic esophagus.

10.2.7 Cervico-thoracic Junction Cancer

Cancer located at the cervico-thoracic junction creates relevant problems, both in terms of surgical strategy and oncological radicality [29]. A cancer that infiltrates the upper thoracic esophagus should be considered and treated as a thoracic cancer, with a surgical approach comprising thoracotomy and three-field lymphadenectomy. Infiltration of adjacent organs occurs more frequently and earlier than in upper thoracic cancer. Indeed, involvement of the cervical region makes total esophagectomy with hypopharyngogastric anastomosis mandatory. The proximity to the trachea posteriorly, the great vessels in the left neck, and the laryngeal recurrent nerves in the narrow thoracic inlet increase the chance of detecting T4 tumors, thus explaining the even worse prognosis of these cancers. The lymphatic diffusion is similar to that in cervical and thoracic carcinoma, with mediastinal nodes and in particular recurrent nerve nodes as primary drainage nodes. Both neck and mid-lower thoracic nodes are frequently involved, making three-field lymphadenectomy the mainstay in the treatment of these neoplasms. In cervico-thoracic junction cancer, the increased use of neoadjuvant or definitive chemoradiation has improved survival, as it is the case in cervical and thoracic cancer.

10.2.8 Long-term Results

The prognosis of patients with CESCC is poor, due to the cancer's aggressiveness, late diagnosis, and rarity, all of which have hampered the development of standardized treatment protocols. The ideal treatment, among upfront surgery, neoadjuvant chemoradiation + surgery, or definitive chemoradiation with possible salvage surgery, is still controversial.

The results of several trials published in the last years are summarized in Table 10.6 [11, 12, 15-19]. Five-year overall survival was 24–47% considering all of the study populations, which often included patients with hypopharyngeal cancer. Considering cervical carcinoma alone, survival ranged from 13% to 47%. However, all the reported studies suffer from the above-mentioned problems of heterogeneity.

The impact of radical resection (R0) and correct lymphadenectomy is intense. Indeed, locoregional relapse is a major cause of death, with 46% of the patients treated with radical intent dying due to recurrence, with locore-

Table 10.6 Overall survival after radical surgery for cervical esophageal squamous cell carcinoma

Author (year)	N.	Overall survival	Only cervical carcinomas
Triboulet et al. (2001) [11]	209 (1982-1999)	24% 5 years	14% 5 years
Wang et al. (2006) [12]	41 (1984-2002)	31.5% 5 years	13.3% 5 years
Daiko et al. (2007) [15]	74 (1982-2002)	33% 5 years	n.r.
Ferahkose et al. (2007) [16]	52 (1996-2006)	n.r.	n.r.
Ott et al. (2009) [18]	109 (1986-2006)	47% 5 years	47% 5 years
Shirakawa et al. (2004) [19]	54 (1985-2003)	47% 5 years	n.r.
Kadota et al. (2009) [17]	32 (1984-2002)	n.r.	45.9% 5 years

n.r., not reported.

Table 10.7 Recurrence after radical surgery for CESCC. Locoregional and systemic are considered as percentage of the total number of relapses

Author (year)	Recurrence (total)	Locoregional	Systemic or mixed
Triboulet et al. (2001) [11]	59%	80%	20%
Wang et al. (2006) [12]	47%	58%	42%
Daiko et al. (2007) [15]	59%	82%	18%
Ferahkose et al. (2007) [16]	n.r.	n.r.	n.r.
Ott et al. (2009) [18]	39%	65%	35%
Shirakawa et al. (2004) [19]	n.r.	n.r.	n.r.
Kadota et al. (2009) [17]	n.r.	n.r.	n.r.

n.r., not reported.

gional recurrence representing 60–80% of the relapses (Table 10.7) [11, 12, 15-19]. The late stage of the disease at diagnosis and non-radical intervention could be the main causes of the dismal results and the high rate of recurrence, especially locoregional relapses.

10.3 Conclusions and Flow-charts

The following flow-charts describing proposed treatment strategies can be drawn for cervical and cervico-thoracic cancers according to T stage.

For CESCC, we opt for upfront total esophagectomy with gastric pull-up, and cervical and upper mediastinal lymphadenectomy for T1 cancers. The lar-

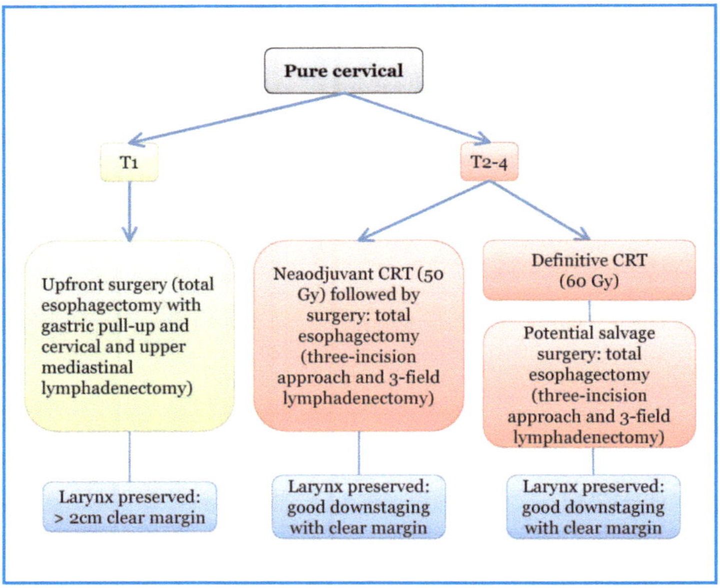

Fig. 10.3 Proposed flow-chart for the treatment of pure cervical cancers

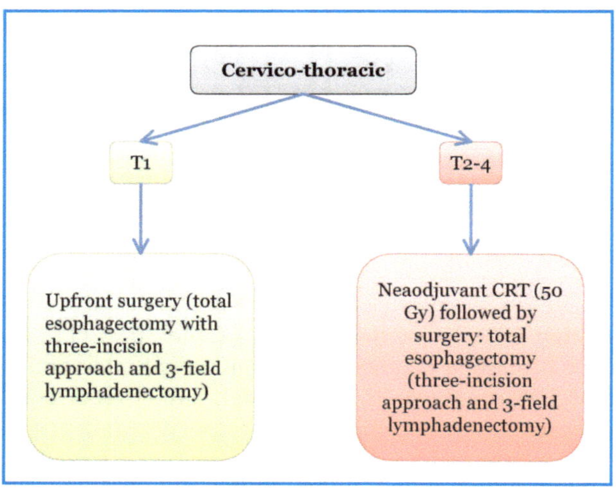

Fig. 10.4 Proposed flow-chart for the treatment of cervico-thoracic cancers

ynx is preserved if a safe 2-cm proximal margin can be obtained. In advanced cases, there are two choices: neoadjuvant chemoradiation therapy (50 Gy) followed by total esophagectomy, with a three-incision approach and three-field nodal dissection, or definitive chemoradiation therapy (60 Gy) with possible salvage surgery. The larynx might be preserved in case of excellent downstaging with a fairly safe, clear proximal margin. The normally used conduit to replace digestive tract continuity is a gastric tube (Fig. 10.3).

In patients with cervico-thoracic cancer, the strategy is the same as in thoracic cancer. The surgical procedure is a three-incision approach with three-field lymphadenectomy. In case of T1 cancers, upfront surgery is preferred, even if, due to clinical nodal involvement, neoadjuvant chemoradiation therapy is administered followed by surgery. Advanced cases may be treated with neoadjuvant CRT followed by surgery. As described in Chap. 14, we prefer neoadjuvant over definitive chemoradiation therapy (Fig. 10.4).

References

1. Takes RP, Strojan P, Silver CE et al (2010) Current trends in initial management of hypopharyngeal cancer: The declining use of open surgery. Head Neck. doi:10.1002/hed.21613
2. Wycliffe ND, Grover RS, Kim PD, Simental A, Jr. (2007) Hypopharyngeal cancer. Top Magn Reson Imaging 18:243-258
3. Blot WJ, McLaughlin JK, Winn DM et al (1988) Smoking and drinking in relation to oral and pharyngeal cancer. Cancer Res 48:3282-3287
4. Day GL, Blot WJ, Shore RE et al (1994) Second cancers following oral and pharyngeal cancers: role of tobacco and alcohol. J Natl Cancer Inst 86:131-137
5. de Bree R, Rinaldo A, Genden EM et al (2008) Modern reconstruction techniques for oral and pharyngeal defects after tumor resection. Eur Arch Otorhinolaryngol 265:1-9
6. Richmon JD, Brumund KT (2007) Reconstruction of the hypopharynx: current trends. Curr Opin Otolaryngol Head Neck Surg 15:208-212
7. Ferlito A, Shaha AR, Buckley JG, Rinaldo A (2001) Selective neck dissection for hypopharyngeal cancer in the clinically negative neck: should it be bilateral? Acta Otolaryngol 121:329-335
8. Buckley JG, MacLennan K (2000) Cervical node metastases in laryngeal and hypopharyngeal cancer: a prospective analysis of prevalence and distribution Head Neck 22:380-385
9. Carrasco Llatas M, Lopez Molla C, Balaguer Garcia R et al (2009) Hypopharyngeal cancer: analysis of the evolution and treatment results. Acta Otorrinolaringol Esp 60:3-8
10. Edge SB, Byrd DR, Compton CC, eds. (2010) AJCC Cancer Staging Manual, 7th ed., Springer, New York, NY
11. Triboulet JP, Mariette C, Chevalier D, Amrouni H (2001) Surgical management of carcinoma of the hypopharynx and cervical esophagus: analysis of 209 cases. Arch Surg 136:1164-1170
12. Wang HW, Chu PY, Kuo KT et al (2006) A reappraisal of surgical management for squamous cell carcinoma in the pharyngoesophageal junction. J Surg Oncol 93:468-476
13. Fujita H, Kakegawa T, Yamana H (1999) Total esophagectomy versus proximal esophagectomy for esophageal cancer at the cervicothoracic junction. World J Surg 23:486-491
14. Laterza E, Rodella L, Fersini A (2002) Chirurgia dei Carcinomi dell'Ipofaringe e dell'Esofago Cervicale. In: Battocchia A, Laterza E (eds) Le Malattie dell'Esofago: Diagnosi e Terapia. Piccin, Padova, pp 467-485
15. Daiko H, Hayashi R, Saikawa M et al (2007) Surgical management of carcinoma of the cervical esophagus. J Surg Oncol 96:166-172
16. Ferahkose Z, Bedirli A, Kerem M et al (2008) Comparison of free jejunal graft with gastric pull-up reconstruction after resection of hypopharyngeal and cervical esophageal carcinoma. Dis Esophagus 21:340-345
17. Kadota H, Sakuraba M, Kimata Y et al (2009) Larynx-preserving esophagectomy and jejunal transfer for cervical esophageal carcinoma. Laryngoscope 119:1274-1280

18. Ott K, Lordick F, Molls M et al (2009) Limited resection and free jejunal graft interposition for squamous cell carcinoma of the cervical oesophagus. Br J Surg 96:258-266
19. Shirakawa Y, Naomoto Y, Noma K et al (2004) Free jejunal graft for hypopharyngeal and esophageal reconstruction. Langenbecks Arch Surg 389:387-390
20. Peracchia A, Bonavina L, Botturi M et al (2001) Current status of surgery for carcinoma of the hypopharynx and cervical esophagus. Dis Esophagus 14:95-97
21. Shuangba H, Jingwu S, Yinfeng W et al (2011) Complication following gastric pull-up reconstruction for advanced hypopharyngeal or cervical esophageal carcinoma: a 20-year review in a Chinese institute. Am J Otolaryngol 32:275-278
22. Japanese-Esophageal-Society (2008) Japanese Classification of Esophageal Cancer. 10th edn. Kanehara & Co, Tokyo
23. Cense HA, van Eijck CH, Tilanus HW (2006) New insights in the lymphatic spread of oesophageal cancer and its implications for the extent of surgical resection. Best Pract Res Clin Gastroenterol 20:893-906
24. de Bree R, Leemans CR, Silver CE et al (2011) Paratracheal lymph node dissection in cancer of the larynx, hypopharynx, and cervical esophagus: The need for guidelines. Head Neck 33:912-916
25. Hermans R (2004) Imaging of hypopharyngeal and cervical oesophageal cancer. Cancer Imaging 4:7-9
26. Hirano S, Nagahara K, Moritani S et al (2007) Upper mediastinal node dissection for hypopharyngeal and cervical esophageal carcinomas. Ann Otol Rhinol Laryngol 116:290-296
27. Timon CV, Toner M, Conlon BJ (2003) Paratracheal lymph node involvement in advanced cancer of the larynx, hypopharynx, and cervical esophagus. Laryngoscope 113:1595-1599
28. Fujita H, Sueyoshi S, Tanaka T et al (2008) A new N category for cancer of the cervical esophagus based on lymph node compartments. Esophagus 5:19-26
29. Laterza E, Fersini A, Rodella L (2002) Chirurgia del Carcinoma dell'Esofago Cervico-Toracico. In: Battocchia A, Laterza E (eds) Le Malattie dell'Esofago: Diagnosi e Terapia, Piccin, Padova, pp 487-495

Multimodal Treatment: Early and Long-term Results and Recurrences

11

Antonio Grandinetti

11.1 Historical Background

In the past, the treatment of choice for hypopharyngeal and cervical squamous cell carcinoma (SCC) was radiotherapy alone, administered over large fields and using what have now become obsolete techniques. The early and late outcomes and quality of life of these patients were disappointing, since many often required additional palliative surgical treatment to control dysphagia or complications associated with radiotherapy (RT). A major advance occurred in 1960, with the adoption of pharyngolaryngoesophagectomy (PLE), with or without adjuvant RT, as the standard surgical approach for cervical esophageal carcinoma (CEC) [1]. However, despite significant improvements over the following decades, PLE has a high morbidity (49%) and mortality (9%), and the quality of life is compromised by "en bloc" laryngectomy [2].

A third and major improvement occurred in the 1980s, with the adoption of multimodality therapy, consisting of the administration of effective antineoplastic drugs together with RT. This new approach derived from preliminary results of larynx preservation protocols in advanced hypopharyngeal tumors, in which induction chemotherapy and definitive radiation therapy could be effective in preserving the larynx in a high percentage of patients, without compromising overall survival [3]. Nowadays, combined modality treatment with chemotherapy, radiotherapy, and surgery has been accepted as the best therapeutic option for most of these patients.

A. Grandinetti (✉)
Radiation Oncology Unit, Borgo Trento Hospital,
Verona, Italy

G. de Manzoni (Ed.), *Treatment of Esophageal and Hypopharyngeal Squamous Cell Carcinoma*,

11.2 Adjuvant Therapy

11.2.1 Postoperative Radiation Therapy

In R0 resected SCC of the esophagus, radiotherapy as the single adjuvant treatment has not shown any prognostic impact compared with surgery alone and is not routinely indicated, even if many papers report a reduction in local recurrence [4, 5]. Xiao et al. [6], in a large randomized trial, confirmed these findings but in a retrospective review also determined that the 5-year survival of patients with involved lymph nodes treated with postoperative RT was 34.1%, compared with a 17.6% survival rate of patients who received surgery alone.

Wang et al. [7] used PLE to treat 41 patients with SCC involving both the hypopharynx and the cervical esophagus. Adjuvant radiotherapy, with a mean dose of 47.5 Gy, was administered to 21 patients 3–4 weeks after surgery and was shown to improve outcome. Median survival was 37.2 months compared with 6.4 months in patients not receiving postoperative RT. The best results were reported in tumors < 5 cm and mainly located in the hypopharynx, probably because of the high rate of paratracheal node metastasis in CEC compared with hypoharyngeal tumors (71.4% vs. 8.3%). Since mediastinal node dissection is a technically very difficult operation, residual neoplastic cells in that area could lead to a high rate of locoregional recurrence. Accordingly, the authors concluded that in advanced CEC the "R" category might not reflect the exact status of residual disease. Thus, at present the only standard role of adjuvant RT is for patients with positive margins R1 and R2; however, on the basis of these data, the benefit of postoperative RT has yet to be clarified and remains an area of investigation.

11.2.2 Postoperative Chemotherapy

In the last decade, the role of adjuvant chemotherapy has not been investigated extensively, particularly with respect to new drugs, and specific data on SCC of the esophagus are therefore lacking. Three phase III trials compared adjuvant chemotherapy to surgery alone in patients with SCC, without distinction according to the cancer site, but none was able to show a benefit in terms of survival. Similarly, results from prospective randomized trials of the Japanese Esophageal Oncology Group failed to demonstrate an overall survival benefit, even though an improvement in 5-year disease-free survival was observed in N+ patients [8]. Adjuvant chemotherapy is poorly tolerated by patients already treated with chemotherapy as part of a combined neoadjuvant protocol, as reported in the RTOG 8501 study, in which only 54% of the patients completed the planned peri-operative schedule.

11.2.3 Postoperative Chemoradiotherapy

In patients undergoing surgery without receiving prior induction therapy, postoperative chemoradiotherapy (CRT) is of therapeutic interest, based on several retrospective studies suggesting a benefit for patients with SCC [9]. Bedard et al., in a retrospective review of 70 patients with node-positive esophageal carcinoma, compared adjuvant CRT with surgery alone. Patients treated with concurrent CRT received four cycles of chemotherapy (cisplatin, 5- FU with or without epirubicin) and a total of 50 Gy RT with standard fractionation and 3D planning. Median and 5-year overall survival were significantly better in the adjuvant CRT arm (47.5 months and 48%) than in the surgery-alone arm (14.1 months and 0%), with a high rate of locoregional recurrence in the latter subgroup (35% vs. 13%). Toxicities were acceptable in the CRT arm, with no treatment-related deaths [10].

A similar study, carried out at the Cleveland Clinic [11] on 31 patients with advanced disease, revealed that those who received adjuvant CRT had improved median survival (28 vs. 15 months) and four-year overall survival (44 vs. 0%) compared with patients treated with surgery alone ($p = 0.05$).

Another non-randomized study from Taiwan [12] compared adjuvant CRT (30 patients) and adjuvant RT (30 patients). Patients in the CRT arm had a mean survival of 31.7 months and a 3-year overall survival of 70% vs. 20.7 months and 33.7% for patients in the RT arm ($p = 0.003$). Locoregional and distant failure rates were also better in the combined therapy group: 40 vs. 60% and 27 vs. 57%, respectively, in favor of the CRT patients. The toxicity profile was acceptable.

A recent study [13] focused on the role of high-dose postoperative RT (66 Gy in 33 fractions) with concurrent low-dose cisplatin chemotherapy for patients with advanced CEC after cervical esophagectomy with or without laryngectomy (34 patients). Grade 3 toxicities during CRT were important but acceptable: leukopenia (36% of the patients), neutropenia (18%), and mucositis (9%). At a median follow-up of 39 months, 1- and 3-year overall survival rates were 91% and 71%, respectively. The authors concluded that concurrent CRT with low-dose cisplatin is well tolerated and has the potential to improve locoregional control and overall survival in patients with advanced CEC.

In conclusion, concurrent adjuvant CRT after R0 resection can be recommended in patients with CEC based on meaningful benefit in terms of locoregional control.

11.3 Neoadjuvant Therapy

11.3.1 Preoperative Radiation Therapy

Historical data from the literature comparing surgery with or without preoperative radiotherapy failed to show an improvement in the percentage of resection or overall survival. Among five randomized trials, only one reported a 3-year survival advantage for patients who received neoadjuvant RT. In addition, a more recent meta-analysis, from Arnott et al. [14], evaluating 1147 patients in five randomized clinical trials, showed no significant difference between patients treated with neoadjuvant RT followed by resection and those receiving surgery alone, although there was a trend in the former towards a reduction of risk of death, estimated to be 11% at 5 years. Therefore, preoperative RT alone currently has no role in the treatment of patients with resectable esophageal cancer.

11.3.2 Preoperative Chemotherapy

There have been three randomized trial on the use of neoadjuvant chemotherapy in patients with resectable esophageal SCC. In all of these series, however, in the majority of the patients the cancer was located in the thoracic esophagus. These cases are discussed in detail in Chap. 12. Briefly, however, in the US Intergroup trial, there was no difference in local control at 2 years (32% vs. 31%) or in overall survival (23% vs. 26%) [15] while in the largest randomized trial, that of the Medical Research Council, with a similar design, chemotherapy increased both the percentage of complete resections (54% vs. 60%, $p < 0.0001$), without postoperative side effects, and the 2-year overall survival (43% after chemotherapy + surgery compared to 34% after surgery alone) [16].

The third study was a Dutch phase III trial, reported by Kok in Abstract form [17]. The clinical and radiological response rates after two cycles of cisplatin plus etoposide were evaluated in 160 patients with operable SCC. Those with a major response were treated with two additional cycles of chemotherapy and then with surgery, while non-responders proceeded directly to surgery. Patients receiving the complete preoperative chemotherapy course had a better median survival than patients undergoing surgery alone: 18.5 vs. 11 months (p=0.002).

In summary, there are currently few data regarding the use of preoperative chemotherapy in patients with advanced hypopharyngeal and cervical esophageal cancers. Results from randomized and non-randomized trials are contradictory, with many authors concluding that chemotherapy alone cannot be routinely recommended for patients with resectable SCC.

11.3.3 Preoperative Chemoradiotherapy

Neoadjuvant CRT is discussed in detail in Chap. 12. Here it suffices to say that, among the many studies on preoperative CRT, it is not easy to distinguish the outcome of patients with hypopharyngeal and cervical esophageal cancers, since this subset is frequently incorporated under the denomination of "locally advanced esophageal cancer." Despite these limitations, there is no doubt that preoperative CRT is superior to RT or chemotherapy alone and can be delivered with acceptable toxicity. This approach may improve resectability and locoregional control, with a positive trend of increased overall survival in some reports.

In general, none of the most relevant randomized trials [18-23] showed a clear level A advantage for neoadjuvant CRT in SCC, although there was a trend in several studies supporting combined treatment. The meta-analysis of Gebski et al. [24], comprising more than 1200 patients recruited in ten randomized controlled trials, revealed that neoadjuvant concomitant CRT, compared to surgery alone, significantly improved 2-year overall survival (hazard ratio 0.81; 0.70-0.93, $p = 0.002$). In addition, this meta-analysis showed no benefit for patients who received sequential preoperative chemotherapy and radiotherapy.

11.4 Definitive Chemoradiotherapy

There are sufficient data from clinical studies supporting definitive CRT as the treatment of choice for patients with advanced hypopharyngeal and cervical esophageal cancers requiring an "en bloc" PLE, as the latter procedure is associated with a subsequent reduction in the quality of life. Thus, many patients would prefer the option of definitive CRT rather than surgery, with the hope of laryngeal preservation. Indeed, nowadays, most clinicians consider concurrent CRT alone as the standard treatment for these cancers, despite the lack of level A evidence from randomized trials.

The RTOG 85-01 trial, comparing CRT and RT alone, was the basis of support for non-operative treatment. Patients were randomized to either RT alone (64 Gy in 32 fractions over 6.4 weeks) or chemotherapy with cisplatin (75 mg/m^2 day 1) plus 5-FU (1000 mg/m^2/day continuous infusion/4 days) and 50 Gy concurrent RT with standard fractionation. Patients enrolled in the CRT arm also received two additional cycles of the same chemotherapy schedule after radiation. This trial showed that overall survival was significantly improved in the combined treatment arm (38% vs. 10% 2-year survival rate) with lower recurrence rates (16% vs. 24%). These significant prognostic differences were confirmed after the 5-year follow-up [25].

Recently, two European randomized trials compared definitive CRT with CRT followed by surgery in patients with locally advanced but potentially resectable SCC in all sites. The first, performed in Germany [21], randomized 172 patients to preoperative therapy consisting of induction chemotherapy followed by concurrent chemotherapy (cisplatin plus etoposide) and external-beam radiotherapy (40 Gy) followed by surgery, or to preoperative therapy alone with a higher radiation dose (at least 65 Gy). There was no survival benefit with the addition of surgery to combined CRT: median survival was 16 vs. 15 months and 3-year overall survival 31% vs. 24%. Progression-free survival at 2 years was improved with the addition of surgery (41% vs. 64%, $p = 0.003$) but at a price of higher treatment-related mortality (12% vs. 3.5%). The second study was the French FFCD 9102 trial [26], in which 444 patients underwent concurrent chemotherapy (cisplatin and 5 FU) and radiation therapy with two split courses of 15 Gy/3 Gy per fraction, 2 weeks apart, or with 46 Gy with standard fractionation. Those who responded to initial therapy (259 patients) were subsequently randomized either to surgery or to further combined CRT. The median survival rate was 19.3 vs. 17.7 months and overall survival was 40 vs. 34% without significant differences between the two groups ($p = 0.44$). Locoregional recurrence was higher in the CRT group (43% vs. 34%), while the 3-month mortality rates were significantly worse in patients operated on after CRT (9.3% vs. 0.8%). Thus, surgery can improve local control but at the cost of increased treatment-related mortality. On the basis of these data, Bedenne et al. concluded that patients with locally advanced SCC who respond to initial CRT do not have any survival advantage from subsequent surgery [26].

There are only a few single-institution studies specifically addressing the outcome of patients with advanced CEC who are treated with concurrent CRT. The best outcomes seem to be obtained with cisplatin plus 5-FU and concurrent radiation doses >50 Gy.

Wang et al. [27] reported a retrospective analysis of 22 patients with cervical and 13 with upper thoracic esophageal cancer treated at the M.D. Anderson Cancer Center with concurrent CRT. Radiotherapy was delivered with conventional or 3D technique to a median dose of 50.4 Gy: 11 patients received a dose under 50 Gy, seven 50 Gy, and 17 > 50 Gy. A complete response at the end of the CRT schedule was observed in 63% of the patients, with a 5-year survival of 18.6% and a disease-free survival of 22.4%. The response was better among patients receiving a dose ≥ 50 Gy than in those administered < 50 Gy (75% vs. 30%), with a better prognosis in terms of 5-year survival (29% vs. 0%).

Burmeister et al. [28] reported interesting results on 34 patients with CEC at early or intermediate stage (I-IIB) who were treated with definitive chemotherapy (cisplatin and 5 FU) and concurrent higher-dose RT (mean 61 Gy, range 50–65). A local complete response of 91% was determined based on follow-up endoscopy. At a median follow-up of 55 months, local control was 88% and actuarial 5-year survival 55%. The authors also reported several important side effects: grade 3 myelosuppression in 12% of the patients, aspiration pneumonia in 6%, need for tube feeling in 15%, and cardiac failure in 3%. A stricture developed in 44% of the patients and there were two complications-related deaths because of stricture (trachea-esophageal fistula and hemorrhage).

Soto Parra et al., in a study on more advanced CEC (54% stage III), reported the outcome of 37 patients treated with cisplatin/5-FU and concurrent radiation, with doses ranging from 50 to 60 Gy. There was a complete response in 24 patients (65%) and the 5-year survival was 32%, with one treatment-related death [29].

Bidoli et al. [30] treated 32 CEC patients with definitive concurrent CRT based on 5-FU and cisplatin plus 50 Gy RT with conventional fractionation. Larynx preservation was achieved in 15 of 32 patients and the 10-year disease-free and overall survival rates were 31% and 27%, respectively.

In another Italian study, Santoro et al. [31] treated 27 patients with four cycles of cisplatin/5-FU-based chemotherapy and split-course 50 Gy radiotherapy delivered as 30 Gy during the first cycle and 20 Gy during the third cycle of chemotherapy. This approach resulted in cure in one-fourth of the advanced lesions. Four patients with stage I disease were reported alive and disease-free after a follow-up of 43 months, without the need for salvage laryngectomy or esophagectomy.

A more recent work from Chiba University retrospectively evaluated the treatment approach for advanced CEC in 21 patients, with special emphasis on concurrent CRT with or without surgery. RT was delivered with a 3D technique at a median dose of 64 Gy (range 60–74) for definitive treatment and a lower median dose of 40 Gy if preoperative therapy was planned. Grade 3/4 toxicity was observed in 43% of the patients, with one death caused by radiation pneumonia. After a median follow-up of 19 months, the overall 2-year survival was 41%; in patients receiving definitive CRT, local control was worse (71% in T1-T3 tumors, 14% in T4 patients) than in patients who underwent subsequent surgery, in whom local control was obtained in five out of six. However, 2-year survival was not significantly different in the two groups: 50% CRT + surgery vs. 40% definitive CRT) [32].

The University of Hong Kong published the results of a retrospective study comparing PLE, with or without adjuvant radiotherapy, to up-front CRT [2]. Tong et al. studied 107 patients, of whom 62 underwent PLE as the primary therapy, 21 had up-front CRT, and the others only palliative treatment. In the PLE group, curative resection was achieved in 37 patients (59.7%), with an in-hospital mortality rate of 7.1%. In the CRT group, there was tumor downstaging in ten patients (46%) and six patients had a clinical complete response, while among the eleven patients with poor response, PLE was required in five for palliation of symptoms. The authors concluded that, even if direct comparison between the two modalities of treatment was difficult without a randomized controlled trial, definitive CRT could be a valid alternative to PLE. However, it has to be considered that, after definitive CRT, a significant proportion of patients require salvage surgery.

11.5 Radiation Therapy Technique

There are at least three studies focusing the optimal dose and fractionation of radiation therapy in the management of esophageal cancer. The first was performed by Minsky et al. [33], who reported the results of a phase III trial comparing high-dose vs. standard-dose radiation therapy. The 236 patients were randomly assigned to concurrent cisplatin/5-FU chemotherapy and radiation to a total dose of 50.4 Gy at 1.8 Gy per fraction (arm 1) or 64.8 Gy at 1.8 Gy per fraction (arm 2). There were no significant differences among the two groups in locoregional failure rates (56% vs. 52%), median survival (13 vs. 18 months), or 2-year overall survival (31% vs. 40%).

The second study, by Jacob et al. [34], addressed the choice of best fractionation in definitive concurrent CRT. Standard-course irradiation significantly improved local control (57% vs. 29%) and 2-year overall survival rates (37% vs. 23%) compared to split-course RT.

In the third study, Crehange [35] conducted a phase III trial of protracted CRT (26 Gy in 23 fractions) compared to split-course CRT (two 1-week courses of 15 Gy, 2 weeks apart). Although there was no statistically significant difference in overall survival, the 2-year relapse-free survival rate was 76.7% vs. 56.8% for protracted and split-course RT, respectively (p= 0002).

In conclusion, external-beam RT at a total dose of 50.4 Gy in 28 fractions (1.8 Gy/fraction) and 50 Gy in 25 fractions (2 Gy/fraction), in combination with concurrent cisplatin plus 5-FU chemotherapy, is considered the standard regimen for definitive treatment, with continuous-course RT is preferred over split-course radiation.

Particular attention must be paid to treatment simulation and planning, and to defining the exact extent of the tumor, which requires integrated information from a variety of radiological data. Modern treatment techniques involve computed tomography (CT)-based planning to detect radial extension of the primary lesion and nodal disease. The CT scan requires an individualized immobilization device, to be used during planning and treatment, thus ensuring uniform patient positioning day-to-day. Scans should be taken with the patient in the precise position of treatment, with his or her arms placed overhead. Oral and intravenuos contrast administration at the time of CT simulation enhances the visualization of gross tumor volume (GTV), allowing the delivery of an adequate dose to the target and limiting the dose to the spinal cord. Other useful diagnostic tests integrated in the planning procedure are esophagogram, endoscopy, and ultrasound. A sensitive improvement in planning precision comes from the recent utilization of positron emission tomography with 2-[fluorine-18] fluoro-2-deoxy-D-glucose (FDG-PET) and CT fusion simulation, which combine morphological and functional information. In a small prospective trial, Moureau et al. [36] reported the need for GTV adjustment in more than 50% of cases using this procedure.

The clinical target volume (CTV) usually includes the GTV, with a 1-cm radial margin and 4-cm proximal and distal margins, while the planning tumor volume (PTV) is defined as the CTV plus 1–2 cm to correct set-up errors and organ-movement shifting. If definitive RT is used in combined modality treatment at a dose > 50 Gy, reduction to a margin of 2 cm above and below the GTV should be considered in order to reduce toxicity.

In the planning of treatment for cervical primary tumors, patients are placed supine. Bilateral supraclavicular nodes and peri-esophageal nodes are usually included. The former are treated with a pair of anteroposterior fields to

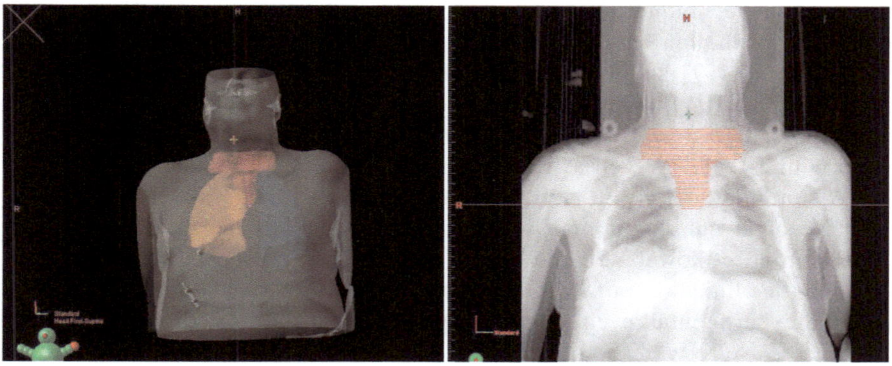

Fig. 11.1 Clinical target volume (CTV) in a patient with T2N1M0 squamous cervical esophageal cancer treated with definitive chemoradiotherapy

a total dose of 50 or 50.4 Gy, with electrons calculated 3 cm from the skin surface, while the latter are directly included in the GTV. Conversely, elective radiation to other clinically uninvolved lymph nodes is not usually performed (Fig. 11.1).

As far as field arrangement is concerned, various field designs are possible and their choice depends on the geometry of the primary tumor in relation to the spinal cord. Even if RT can be delivered in a number of ways, a three-field or four-field approach with an anterior and two posterior oblique off-cord fields (with or without the addition of another posterior field) has became the most common technique. Care should be taken to limit the radiation dose to dose-limiting critical normal structures near the GTV, such as the spinal cord, lungs, and heart. Thus, the V20 of the bilateral lung should be limited to 30%, as the probability of severe pneumonitis increases rapidly when this limit is exceeded. To avoid cardiac toxicity, the V40 of the heart should be limited to 50% or less and the total dose to the whole organ to 30 Gy [25, 33].

The dose to the spinal cord should be limited to 45 Gy and the dose to lung tissue minimized: the maximal possible dose to the spinal cord is delivered by the anterior or posterior fields and the remainder of the dose by oblique posterior off-cord fields. This beam arrangement is considered the standard technique for the treatment of CEC, since none of the beams enter laterally through the patient's arms and shoulders.

Intensity modulated radiation therapy (IMRT) has the possibility of improving dose conformality by shaping high-dose radiation around normal tissues while fully dosing the tumor and areas at risk. This is particularly useful in the treatment of hypopharyngeal and upper cervical esophageal carcinomas, in which the need to deliver doses of 60 Gy or greater are limited by the proximity of the cervical cord and the lungs. Studies comparing various IMRT plans with conventional 3-D radiotherapy for the treatment of upper esophageal tumors reported that an approach with four or five IMRT fields is the optimal technique to achieve both high conformality to the target and a reduction of the lung dose.

Wu et al. [37] studied the IMRT-plan target conformality in 15 patients treated with a simultaneous integrated IMRT boost. The authors found a better conformal high-dose distribution to the planning target volume with IMRT than with 3-D RT, as well as a lower mean dose to the lung and heart.

A similar study, by Fu et al. [38], specifically evaluated five patients with upper esophageal carcinomas, in which a simultaneous integrated boost with IMRT produced lower V20 and V30 in the lungs. At present, there are too few data on the clinical use of IMRT in CEC and this approach should still be considered experimental, even if promising.

11.6 Recurrent and Metastatic Disease

Approximately two-thirds of the patients treated with curative intent will require palliation due to symptoms from local recurrence, in particular a debilitating worsening dysphagia, pain, or tracheo-esophageal fistula. The main options include esophageal stent placement, intracavitary brachytherapy, radiotherapy, chemotherapy, and salvage surgery. Palliative strategies should be tailored according to each clinical situation, considering that in patients who have received prior definitive neoadjuvant or adjuvant CRT additional RT is limited and the response to drugs usually decreased. Conversely, when the site of recurrence is outside the previously irradiated area, with no local failure or distant metastasis, RT with or without chemotherapy might cure those single recurrences, as shown by Yorozu et al. [39]. They treated ten patients with single nodal recurrence after definitive CRT, with control of the irradiated relapse in eight of the ten patients. Two patients survived without disease for 5 years and three patients for 2 years.

At presentation, about half of the patients with hypopharyngeal and cervical esophageal carcinomas are not candidates for curative therapy, due to comorbidities, poor performance status, and the presence of bulky unresectable tumor with distant metastasis. The vast majority of them present with severe dysphagia, weight loss, and pain, so that palliation and quality of life become important clinical endpoints. These previously untreated patients can benefit from palliative interventions including the common therapies, used alone or in combination depending on the clinical picture.

The efficacy of external-beam radiation, either alone or in combination with chemotherapy, in medially fit patients with metastatic disease has been proven in several retrospective trials. This therapeutic option can offer relief of symptoms in more than 75% of these patients: palliation of dysphagia is achieved in 50–90% of patients with radiation alone and most of them (60%) remain dysphagia-free until death. Compared to other palliative strategies, RT has the disadvantage of a longer duration and a longer time to onset of symptom palliation. Another drawback is a transient exacerbation of dysphagia, due to peritumoral edema after radiation-induced esophagitis, that usually resolves shortly after treatment completion. This side effect is mainly observed when accelerated fractionation or hypofractionation schemes are used.

Coia et al. [40], in a retrospective analysis of 120 patients treated with concurrent CRT, reported a symptomatic relief of dysphagia in 43 and 83% of the patients within 2 and 6 weeks after treatment start, respectively.

Hayter et al. [41] treated 22 patients with severe dysphagia with palliative radiation (30 Gy/10 fraction) and a single concomitant chemotherapy course (5-FU plus mitomycin-C). The regimen was well tolerated and nearly 70% of the patients had a complete response, with a median time to normalization of symptoms of 5 weeks.

A more recent phase I/II trial [42] from Princess Margaret Hospital evaluated the toxicity and efficacy of accelerated fractionation radiotherapy (40 Gy/20 fractions twice a day over 2 weeks) for the palliation of dysphagia. This study demonstrated a dysphagia response rate of 69%, with a median duration of 5.5 months and an acceptable toxicity.

The Cochrane Review [43] identified four randomized trials reporting the outcomes of palliation in the treatment of dysphagia. This review compared combined chemotherapy and RT with RT alone, reporting no significant difference in dysphagia relief between the two treatment arms.

A fistulous tract between the esophagus and trachea or bronchus is not uncommon in advanced esophageal cancer, either as a result of radiation-induced necrosis of the tumor infiltrating the airway or because of natural disease progression. Tracheo-esophageal fistula is an unfavorable prognostic feature, even though some patient may survive for a prolonged period. Although trachea-esophageal fistula has historically been considered a contraindication to begin or continue RT, based on the fear that it will compromise healing and worsen clinical condition, there are data supporting the efficacy of radiation with merely palliative intent. Burt et al. [44] observed that if the fistula is untreated survival is only 4% at 6 months and 1% at 1 year, while patients who undergo palliative RT have a better survival rate: 15% at 6 months and 5% at 1 year. A report of the Mayo Clinic showed a median survival of 4.8 months without fistula worsening [45], and Malik et al. [46] observed fistula closure in two patients treated with CRT, concluding that the presence of a fistula should not necessarily exclude a patient from receiving palliative concurrent CRT.

In summary, external-beam radiation therapy is effective and routinely employed for palliation. The most common schedules are 50.4 Gy with standard fractionation, 30 Gy/10 fractions, 20 Gy/5 fractions, or an 8 Gy single fraction.

Brachytherapy (BT) is a useful tool for palliative treatment of advanced and recurrent esophageal cancer. In selected cases, it can be used in addition to external-beam RT or as an alternative in previously irradiated patients. BT can also be safely given after laser therapy (with a 4- to 6-week gap) and may improve the dysphagia-free interval. The major limit of BT is the effective treatment distance, since the primary isotope is iridium 192, which is usually prescribed to treat at a distance of 1 cm from the source. Therefore, any part of the tumor at a distance > 1 cm from the source will receive a suboptimal radiation dose. This limit has also been confirmed by pathological analysis of treated specimens.

Appropriate regimens recommended by the American Brachytherapy Society [47] include a dose of 15–20 Gy, with a high-dose rate in two to four applications, while in unfit patients with poor short-term prognosis a single high-dose rate of 15 Gy can achieve palliation of dysphagia in 70% of patients, with a low rate of complications.

In a randomized trial (209 patients), Homs [48] et al. compared single-dose BT (12 Gy) with metal stent placement for the palliation of dysphagia. While dysphagia improved more rapidly after stent placement, long-term relief was better after BT. In addition, BT had significantly fewer complications than stent placement (21 vs. 33%, respectively).

11.7 Conclusions

Hypopharyngeal cancer and CEC are usually very aggressive, such that patients with advanced disease have a limited survival regardless of therapy. The clinical setting is complicated by the fact that results reported in the literature are unclear for at least four reasons: (1) Cancers of the cervical esophagus and those of the hypopharynx (pyriform fossae, posterior wall, and retrocricoid region) and even laryngeal recurrences are often pooled under the same denomination. (2) In advanced stages, it is difficult to detect the exact site of origin of the lesion and therefore to properly evaluate the most appropriate therapy. (3) Second primaries and co-morbidities strongly impair the outcome of patients, making it more difficult to clearly demonstrate the benefit of treatments. (4) There is a lack of phase III randomized trials addressing the choice between surgery and definitive CRT therapy.

Therefore, our understanding about the ideal treatment of hypopharyngeal and cervical esophageal cancers is far from satisfactory, and the decision-making process remains complex, since the available data comparing multimodal therapy with surgery alone (or surgery plus adjuvant radiotherapy) are conflicting. Nonetheless, several non-randomized studies from single institutions have been reported in recent years and there are several indications regarding the optimal therapeutic approach. Surgery, which was historically regarded as the gold standard of treatment, still plays a curative as well as a palliative role. Due to the complexity of the resection technique, it requires a team with great skill and experience and should be performed only in specialized institutions.

Some authors suggest that an aggressive surgical approach with PLE followed by adjuvant RT is a feasible option for SCC simultaneously involving the hypopharynx and the cervical esophagus, when the major tumor localization is in the hypopharynx [2, 8, 24, 29]. Conversely, poor surgical outcomes are observed for tumors > 5 cm in size or those mainly located below the pharyngo-esophageal junction. In these cases, surgery might not be an effective treatment and is not recommended. However, salvage surgery after failure of primary CRT is feasible and achieves good palliation of symptoms in the majority of patients. Finally, surgery alone is also preferred in patients more likely to have increased toxicity and reduced quality of life after multimodal therapy [49-51].

Definitive CRT is at present a valid alternative to surgery and in many countries it is considered the standard treatment for CEC with hypopharyngeal involvement, even in the absence of level A statistical evidence [52-54]. Direct comparison between the two modalities is objectively difficult since a randomized trial is unlikely to be feasible. However, similar survival rates are achieved in patients who respond to combined modality treatment and those who undergo R0 resections after PLE [55, 56]. Another important point in favor of definitive CRT is the possibility of larynx preservation and, consequently, improved quality of life. Therefore CRT as primary treatment is the most widely used therapeutic strategy in most oncological centers.

In the era of targeted therapy, newer chemotherapeutic drugs and biological agents, such as epidermal growth factor receptor blockers, vascular endothelial growth factor, and antisense oligonucleotides, need to be incorporated into multimodality strategies. At the same time, modern radiotherapy may contribute to achieve better response rates, with the use of more aggressive schedules (hypo- or hyperfractionation) associated with sophisticated techniques (IMRT, IG-IMRT), in order to deliver higher doses to the target volume without increasing the side effects to the adjacent organs.

At present, in the absence of conclusive phase III trials, the choice between definitive CRT and PLE should be based on clear information and on the patient's preference. Thus, a multicenter randomized study comparing surgery with definitive CRT and surgery with CRT followed by surgery is required.

References

1. Ong GB, Lee TC (1960) Pharyngogastric anastomosis after oesophagopharyngectomy for carcinoma of the hypopharynxand cervical oesophagus. Br J Surg 48:193-200
2. Tong DKH, Law S, Wan Kwong DL et al (2011) Current management of cervical esophageal cancer. World J Surg 35:600-607
3. Department of Veterans Affairs Laryngeal Cancer Study Group (1991) Induction chemotherapy plus radiation compared with surgery plus radiation in patients with advanced laryngeal cancer. N Eng J Med 324:1685-1690
4. Bernier J, Domenge C, Ozsahin M et al (2004) Postoperative irradiation with or without concomitant chemotherapy for locally advanced head and neck cancer. N Engl J Med 350:1945-1952
5. Zieren HU, Müller JM, Jacobi CA et al (1995) Adjuvant postoperative radiation therapy after curative resection of squamous esophageal cell carcinoma: a prospective randomized study. World J Surg 19:444-449
6. Xiao ZF, Yang ZY, Miao YJ et al (2005) Influence of number of metastatic lymph nodes on

survival of curative resected thoracic esophageal cancer patients and value of radiotherapy: report of 549 cases. Int J Radiat Oncol Biol Phys 62:82-90
7. Wang HW, Chu PY, Kuo KT et al (2006) A reappraisal of surgical management for squamous cell carcinoma in the pharyngoesophageal junction. J Surg Oncol 93:468-476
8. Ando N, Iizuka T, Ide H et al (2003) Surgery plus chemotherapy compared with surgery alone for squamous cell carcinoma of the esophagus: a Japan Clinical Oncology Group Study. J Clin Oncol 21:4592-4596
9. MacDonald JS, Smalley SR et al (2001) Chemoradiotherapy after surgery compared with surgery alone for adenocarcinoma of the stomach or gastroesophageal junction. N Eng J Med 345:725-730
10. Bedard EL, Inculet RI, Malthaner RA et al (2001) The role of surgery and postoperative chemoradiation therapy in patients with lymph node positive esophageal carcinoma. Cancer 91:2423-2430
11. RiceTW, Adelstain DJ, Chidel MA et al (2003) Benefit of postoperative adjuvant chemoradiotherapy in locoregionally advanced esophageal carcinoma. J Thorac Cardiovasc Surg 126:1590-1596
12. Liu HC, Hung SK, Huang CJ et al (2005) Esophagectomy for locally advanced esophageal cancer, followed by chemoradiotherapy and adjuvant chemotherapy. World J Gastoenterol 11:5367-5372
13. Dalko H, Hayashi R, Sakuraba M et al (2011) A pilot study of postoperative radiotherapy with concurrent chemotherapy for high-risk squamous cell carcinoma of the cervical esophagus. Japanese J Clin Oncol 41:508-513
14. Arnott SJ, Duncan W, Gignoux M et al (2000) Preoperative radiotherapy for esophageal carcinoma. Cochrane database Syst Rev (4):CD001799
15. Kelsen DP, Winter Ka, Gunderson LL et al (2007) Long-term results of RTOG trial 8911 (USA Intergroup 113): a random assignment trial comparison of chemotherapy followed by surgery compared with surgery alone for esophageal cancer. J Clin Oncol 25:3719-3725
16. Bancewicz JCP, Clark PI, Smith DB, et al (2002) Surgical resection with or without preoperative chemotherapy in oesophageal cancer: a randomized controlled trial. The Lancet 359:1727-1733
17. Kok TC, Siersema PD, Lanschot JV et al (1997) Neoadjuvant chemotherapy in operable esophageal squamous cell cancer: final report of a phase III multicenter randomized controlled trial. Proc Am Soc Clin Oncol 16:277
18. Bosset J, Grignoux M, Triboulet J et al (1997) Chemoradiotherapy followed by surgery compared with surgery alone in squamous cell cancer of the esophagus. N Engl J Med 337:161-167
19. Urschel JD, Vasan H (2003) A meta-analysis of randomized controlled trials that compared neoadjuvant chemoradiation and surgery to surgery alone for resectable esophageal cancer. Am J Surg 185:538-543
20. Urba S, Orringer M, Turrisi A et al (2001) Randomized trial of preoperative chemoradiation versus surgery alone in patients with locoregional esophageal carcinoma. J Clin Oncol 19:305-313
21. Stahl M, Sttuschke M, Lehman N et al (2005) Chemoradiation with and without surgery in patients with locally advanced squamous cell carcinoma of the esophagus. J Clin Oncol 23:2310-2317
22. Burmeister BH, Smithers BM, Gebski V et al (2005) Surgery alone versus chemoradiotherapy followed by surgery for resectable cancer of the oesophagus: a randomized controlled phase III trial. Lancet Oncol 6:659-668
23. Tepper J, Krasna MJ, Niedzwiecki D et al (2008) Phase III trial of trimodality therapy with cisplatin, fluorouracil, radiotherapy, and surgery compared with surgery alone for esophageal cancer: CALGB 9781. J Clin Oncol 26:1086-1092
24. Gebski V, Burmeister B, Smithers BM et al (2007) Survival benefits from neoadjuvant chemoradiotherapy or chemotherapy in oesophageal carcinoma:a meta-analysis. Lancet Oncol 8:226-234
25. Cooper JS, Guo MD, Herskovic A et al (1999) Chemoradiotherapy of locally advanced

esophageal cancer: long term follow-up of a prospective randomized trial (RTOG 85-01). JAMA 281:1623-1627
26. Bedenne L, Michel P, Bouche O et al (2007) Chemoradiation followed by surgery compared with chemoradiation alone in squamous cancer of the esophagus: FFCD9102. J Clin Oncol 25:1160-1168
27. Wang S, Liao Z, Chen Y et al (2006) Esophageal cancer located at the neck and upper thorax treated with concurrent chemoradiation: a single-institution experience. J Thorac Oncol 1:252-259
28. Burmeister BH, Dickie G, Smithers BM et al (2000) Thirty-four patients with carcinoma of the cervical esophagus treated with chemoradiation therapy. Arch Otolaryngol Head and Neck Surg 126:205-208
29. Soto Parra H, Valente M, Bidoli P et al (1997) Definitive chemoradiotherapy in cervical esophageal carcinoma. Proc Am Soc Clin Oncol 16:A929
30. Bidoli P, Bajetta E, Stani SC et al (2002) Ten-year survival with chemotherapy and radiotherapy in patients with squamous cell carcinoma of the esophagus. Cancer 94:352-361
31. Santoro A, Bidoli P, Salvini PM et al (1993) Larynx preservation with combined chemotherapy plus radiotherapy in upper squamous cell carcinoma of the esophagus. Proc Am Soc Clin Oncol 12 (Abstract 899)
32. Uno T, Isobe K, Kawakami H et al (2007) Concurrent chemoradiation for patients with squamous cell carcinoma of the cervical esophagus. Dis Esophagus 20:12-18
33. Minsky BD, Pajak TF, Ginsberg RJ et al (2002) INT0123(Radiation Therapy Oncology Group 94–05) Phase III trial of combined-modality therapy for esophageal cancer: high-dose versus standard-dose radiation therapy. J Clin Oncol 20:1167-1174
34. Jacob J, Seitz JF, Langlois C et al (1999) Definitive concurrent chemoradiation therapy in squamous cell carcinoma of the esophagus: preliminare results of a French randomized trial comparing standard versus split-course irradiation (FN-CLCC-FFCD9305) Proc Am Soc Clin Oncol 18:1035a
35. Crehange G, Maingon P, Peignaux K et al (2007) Phase III trial of protracted compared with split-course chemoradiation for esophageal carcinoma: Federation Francophone de Cancerologie Digestive 9102. J Clin Oncol 25:4895-4901
36. Moureau-Zabotto L, Touboul E, Lerouge D et al (2005) Impact of CT and 18F-deoxyglucose positron emission tomography image fusion for conformal radiotherapy in esophageal carcinoma. Int J Radiat Oncol Biol Phys 63:340-345
37. Wu Q, Mohan R, Morris M et al (2003) Simultaneous integrated boost intensity-modulated radiotherapy for locally advanced head-and-neck squamous cell carcinoma. Int J Radiat Oncol Biol Phys 56:573-585
38. Fu WH, Wang LH, Zhou ZM et al (2004) Comparison of conformal and intensity-modulated techniques for simultaneous integrated boost radiotherapy of upper esophageal carcinoma. World J Gastroenterol 10:1098-1102
39. Yorozu A (2005) Radiotherapy for nodal recurrence after chemoradiotherapy for esoophageal carcinoma. Esophagus 2:21-23
40. Coia LR, Soffen EM, Schultheiss TE et al (1993) Swallowing function in patients with esophageal cancer treated with concurrent radiation and chemotherapy. Cancer 71:281-286
41. Hayter CR, Huff-Winters C, Paszat L et al (2000) A prospective trial of short-course radiotherapy plus chemotherapy for palliation of dysphagia from advanced esophageal cancer. Radiother Oncol 56:329-333
42. Kassan Z, Wong RK, Ringash J et al (2008) A phase I/II study to evaluate the toxicity and efficacy of accelerated fractionation radiotherapy for the palliation of dysphagia from carcinoma of the oesophagus. Clin Oncol 20:53-60
43. Wong R, Malthaner R (2006) Combined chemotherapy and radiotherapy (without surgery) compared with radiotherapy alone in localized carcinoma of the esophagus. Cochrane Database Syst Rev (1):CD002092
44. Burt M, Diehl W, Martini N et al (1991) Malignant esophagorespiratory fistula: management options and survival. Ann Thorac Surg 52:1222-1228

45. Gschossmann JM, Bonner JA, Foote RL et al (1993) Malignant tracheoesophageal fistola in patients with esophageal cancer. Cancer 72:1513-1521
46. Malik SM, Krasnow SH, Wadleigh RG (1994) Closure of tracheoesophageal fistulas with primary chemotherapy in patients with esophageal cancer. Cancer 73:1321-1323
47. Gaspar LE, Nag S, Herskovic A et al (1997) American Brachytherapy Society consensus guidelines or brachitherapy of esophageal cancer. Int J Radiat Oncol Biol Phys 38:127-132
48. Homs MY, Steyerberg EW, Eijkenboom WMH et al (2004) Single-dose brachytherapy versus metal stent placement for the palliation of dysphagia from oesophageal cancer: multicenter randomized trial. Lancet 364:1497-1504
49. Graham AJ, Shrive FM, Ghali WA et al (2007) Defining the optimal treatment of locally advanced esophageal cancer: a systematic review and decision. analysis.Ann Thorac Surg 83:1257-1264
50. Fujita H, Sueyoshi S, Tanaka T et al (2005) Esophagectomy: is it necessary after chemoradiotherapy for a locally advanced T4 esophageal cancer? Prospected nonrandomized trial comparing chemoradiotherapy with surgery versus without surgery. World J Surg 29:25-31
51. Tachimori Y, Kanamori N, Uemura N et al (2009) Salvage esophagectomy after high-dose chemoradio-therapy for esophageal squamous cell carcinoma. J Thorac Cardiovasc Surg 137:49-54
52. Pignon JP, Bourhis J, Domenge C et al (2000) Chemotherapy added to locoregional treatment for head and neck squamous-cell carcinoma: three meta-analyses of updated individual data. MACH-NC Collaborative Group. Meta-Analysis of Chemotherapy on Head and Neck Cancer. Lancet 355: 949-955
53. Takagawa R, Kunisaki C, Makino H et al (2008) Efficacy of chemoradiotherapy with low-dose cisplatin and continuous infusion of 5-fluorouracil for unresectable squamous cell carcinoma of the esophagus. Dis Esophagus 22:482-489
54. Akutsu Y, Matsubara H, Shuto K et al (2009) Clinical and pathologic evaluation of the effectiveness of neoadjuvant chemoradiation therapy in advanced esophageal cancer patients. World J Surg 33:1002-1009
55. Pasini F, de Manzoni G, Grandinetti A et al (2009) Effect of neoadjuvant combined modality therapy with weekly docetaxel and cisplatin, 5-fluorouracil continuos infusion and concurrent radiotherapy on pathological responce rate in esophageal cancers: a phase II study. J Clin Oncol 27:213s(4548)
56. Agarwala AK, Hanna N, McCollum A et al (2009) Preoperative cetuximab and radiation (XRT) for patients (pts) with surgically resectable esophageal and gastroesophageal junction (GEJ) carcinomas: a pilot study from the Hoosier Oncology Group and the University of Texas Southwestern. J Clin Oncol 27:216s(4557)

Section III

Carcinoma of Thoracic Esophagus

Neoadjuvant Treatment 12

Felice Pasini, Anna Paola Fraccon, and Giovanni de Manzoni

12.1 Preoperative Chemoradiotherapy

To date, the benefits and risks of neoadjuvant chemoradiotherapy (CRT) in esophageal cancer have been investigated in randomized phase III clinical trials, phase II trials, and retrospective studies [1-3]. Randomized clinical trials [4-15] compared neoadjuvant CRT with surgery alone and, although most of them demonstrated higher survival rates in the combination arm, overall survival (OS) and disease-free survival (DFS) were statistically improved in only four [4-7] and two trials [8-9], respectively (Table 12.1).

Walsh et al [4] randomized 113 patients with adenocarcinoma (AC) to two courses of neoadjuvant chemotherapy with cisplatin and fluorouracil (PF) for 5 days with concurrent radiotherapy (RT) or to surgery. The median OS was 16 vs. 11 months (p= 0.01) with a 3-year OS of 32% vs. 6% (p = 0.01), favoring the combination arm. The criticisms of this single-institution trial were the poor outcome of the surgical arm, far inferior to historical controls, and the unreported pre-treatment tumor stage.

The CALGB 9781 trial [5] was prematurely closed with only 56 (25% squamous cell carcinoma, SCC) of an expected 500 patients enrolled. The poor accrual was reportedly due to the unwillingness of many patients but also physicians to enroll in the surgery alone arm. Patients were randomly assigned to either two preoperative cycles of PF for 4 days with concurrent RT or to surgery. The pathological complete response (pCR) rate in the combination arm was 34%. A 5-year OS of 39% vs. 16% and a median survival of 4.48 vs. 1.79 years (p= 0.002) were reported in the combination and surgery arm, respectively.

F. Pasini (✉)
Dept. of Medical Oncology, "Santa Maria della Misericordia" Hospital, Rovigo, Italy

G. de Manzoni (Ed.), *Treatment of Esophageal and Hypopharyngeal Squamous Cell Carcinoma*,

Table 12.1 Characteristics of the principal studies

Author (year)	Histology	Schedule of radiotherapy	Schedule of chemotherapy	Concurrent or sequential	Number of patients CRT/S	pCR (%)	MS (months) CRT/S	3[a]-5-year OS (%) CRT	S	p
Nygaard et al. (1992) [10]	SCC	35 Gy, 1.75 Gy/d 5 d/wk for 4 wks	Cisplatin: 20 mg/m^2 d1-5, 15-19 Bleomycin: 10 mg/m^2 d1-5, 15-19	sequential	47/41	n.r.	8/7	17*	9*	n.s.
Apinop (1994) [11]	SCC	40 Gy, 2 Gy/d 5 d/wk for 4 wks	Cisplatin: 100 mg/m^2 d1, 29 FU: 1000 mg/m^2 d1, 29-32	concurrent	35/34	20	10/7	24	10	n.s.
Le Prise et al. (1994) [12]	SCC	20 Gy, 2 Gy/d d8-19	Cisplatin: 100 mg/m^2 d1, 21 FU: 600 mg/m^2 d2-5, 22-25	sequential	41/45	10	10/11	19*	14*	n.s.
Walsh et al. (1996) [4]	AC	40 Gy, 2.67 Gy/d d1-5, 8-12, 15-19	Cisplatin: 75 mg/m^2 d7 FU: 15 mg/kg d1-5 wks 1 and 6	concurrent	58/55	22	16/11	32*	6*	< 0.05
Bosset et al. (1997) [8]	SCC	37 Gy, 3.7 Gy/d 5 d/wk for 2 wks	Cisplatin: 80 mg/m^2 d0-2	sequential	143/139	20	19/19	7	9	n.s.
Urba et al. (2001) [13]	AC/SCC	45 Gy, 1.5 Gy bid d1-5, 8-12, 15-19	Cisplatin: 20 mg/m^2 d1-5, 17-21 FU: 300 mg/m^2 d1-21 Vinblastin: 1 mg/m^2 d1-4,17-20	concurrent	50/50	28	17/18	30*	16*	n.s.
Lee et al. (2004) [14]	SCC	45.6 Gy, 1.2 Gy bid d1-28	Cisplatin: 60 mg/m^2 d1, 21 FU: 1000 mg/m^2 d2-5	concurrent	51/50	n.r.	28/27	49*	41*	n.s.
Burmeister et al. (2005) [9]	AC/SCC	35 Gy, 2.33 Gy/d 5 d/wk for 3 wks	Cisplatin: 80 mg/m^2 d1 FU: 800 mg/m^2 d2-5	concurrent	128/128	15	22/19	17	13	n.s.
Natsugoe et al. (2006) [15]	SCC	40 Gy, 2 Gy/d 5 d/wk for 4 wks	Cisplatin: 7 mg/m^2 FU: 350 mg/m^2 5d/wk for 4-6 wks	concurrent	22/23	n.r.	not reached/27	57	41	n.s.

(*cont.* ↓)

Table 12.1 (*continued*)

Tepper et al. (2008) [5]	AC/SCC	50.4 Gy, 1.8 Gy/d 5 d/wk for 5.5 wks	Cisplatin: 100 mg/m^2 d1, 29 FU: 1000 mg/m^2 d1-4, 29-32	concurrent	30/26	34	54/21	39	16	< 0.01
Cao et al. (2009) [6]	SCC	40 Gy, 2 Gy/d d1-5, 8-12, 15-19, 22-26	Mitomycin:10 mg/m^2 d1, 8 Cisplatin 20 mg/m^2/d d1-5, 8-12 c.i. FU: 500 mg/m^2/d d1-5, 8-12 c.i.	concurrent	118/118	23	n.r.	73	53	<0.05
Van der Gaast et al. (2010) [7]	AC/SCC	41.4 Gy, 1.8 Gy/d 5 d/wk for 4.5 wks	Carboplatin: AUC2 d1, 8, 15, 22, 29 Paclitaxel: 50 mg/m^2 d1, 8, 15, 22, 29	concurrent	188/175	33	49/26	59	48	0.011

AC, Adenocarcinoma; *CRT*, chemoradiotherapy; *FU*, fluorouracil; *MS*, median survival; *n.r.*, non reported; *n.s.*, non significant; *OS*, overall survival; *pCR*, pathologic complete remission; *S*, surgery.

In the study of Cao et al. [6], 473 patients with SCC were randomly divided into four groups: preoperative chemotherapy, preoperative RT, preoperative CRT, and surgery alone. The radical resection rate in the preoperative CRT arm was 98%, significantly higher than the 73% of the surgery group. The pCR rate in the combination arm was 23%. The 3-year OS rate of the CRT group was significantly better than that of the control group (73% vs. 53%, respectively, $p < 0.05$).

The CROSS trial [7] was conducted in 363 patients (74% AC): preoperative weekly carboplatin (AUC 2) and paclitaxel (50 mg/m^2) with concurrent RT (41.4 Gy) resulted in statistically better OS than achieved with surgery alone. Median survival was 49 vs. 26 months and the 3-year survival rate 59% vs. 48% in the combination and surgery arm, respectively. The pCR rate was 32%. The regimen was well tolerated, with 95% of patients completing all five cycles; postoperative complications and mortality were similar in the two arms.

In two randomized clinical trials, the benefit was limited to DFS [8, 9]. In the EORTC study [8], comprising 100% SCC, the DFS gain of the combination arm was related to a longer local disease-free period (RR 0.60, 95% CI 0.4-0.9; $p= 0.003$). The study was critically flawed by an unusual schedule of sequential CRT: the high single-dose fraction delivered (3.7 Gy) likely caused excess postoperative mortality, obscuring any OS benefit. The better DFS of the Australian study [9] was restricted to the SCC subset (HR 0.47, 95% CI 0.25–0.86, $p = 0.014$); however, since SCC patients represented only 35% of the study population, the trial was underpowered to determine the real magnitude of benefit in this subgroup. Another possible criticism was the schedule, which consisted of a single cycle of PF and doses of RT of only 35 Gy. All of the other randomized clinical trials enrolled about 100 patients or less and were therefore not adequately statistically powered (Table 12.1).

In the attempt to overcome the inconsistencies of the results, a few meta-analyses have been performed over the last decade [16-19]. However, these are biased by the low number and quality of the randomized clinical trials that were analyzed: i.e., lack of individual data, inadequate sample size, treatment heterogeneity in terms of chemotherapy and RT schedules, old staging methods, variation in clinical practice over the years, different surgical procedures, and different histological types enrolled (AC, SCC, or both).

The most recent meta-analysis [19] evaluated 11 randomized clinical trials published from 1980 to 2008, comprising 1308 patients. OS was statistically higher after neoadjuvant CRT; the effect was maintained over time and the OR for survival at 3 years was 1.78 (95% CI 1.20-2.6, $p < 0.004$). Moreover, the combination arm showed: (a) a lower incidence of local recurrence (OR: 0.64, 95% CI: 0.41-0.99, $p = 0.04$), but a similar distant recurrence rate; (b) a higher R0 resection rate (OR: 2.16, 95% CI: 1.58-2.97, $p < 0.001$), despite a lower resection rate (OR: 0.36, 95% CI: 0.24-0.54, $p < 0.001$); (c) a higher postoperative mortality (OR: 1.68, 95% CI: 1.03-2.73, $p = 0.04$), although this difference disappeared when two studies were excluded [8, 10]; (d) not statistically different postoperative complications, both fatal and non-fatal. Subgroup analysis showed that the survival benefit was limited to patients receiving concurrent and not sequential CRT (OR 2.12, 95% CI 1.20-3.76 $p = 0.01$ at 3 years), as previously reported [16, 18]; however, the survival gain was lost in Asian patients. The pCR rate in the 11 randomized clinical trials ranged between 10% and 34%. The survival benefit for the combination arm demonstrated in this meta-analysis is likely to be further reinforced in future analyses that also consider the new data of the CROSS trial.

Additional information has been provided by a recent systematic review reporting the data of 38 papers (23 retrospective, 12 prospective, 3 randomized clinical trials) published from 2000 onwards and including 3640 patients [3]. Nearly all reported the use of cisplatin-based regimens, mostly in combination with fluorouracil (28 studies), but the doses, timing, and fractionation of the RT varied widely. Doses ranged from 30 to 60 Gy, with a total dose of at least 45 Gy in 22 studies and some studies using more than one schedule. Conventional fractionation was reported in 28 studies, hyperfractionation in three, hypofractionation in four, a split-course in three, and an accelerated schedule in two. In five studies, the type of fractionation was not reported.

Data regarding CRT-related toxicity G3/4 were reported only in 10 studies: neutropenia occurred in 1–60%, neutropenic fever in 1–6%, nausea/vomiting in 0–16%, and esophagitis in 0–43%. Nutritional support (enteral or parenteral) was required in 6–35% of the patients. Preoperative and postoperative CRT-related mortality rates were 2.3 and 5.2%, respectively. The incidence of postoperative complications (mainly anastomotic leakage, pulmonary and cardiac problems, surgical re-interventions, dehydration, and thrombosis) was 1–44%, perhaps related to the timing of surgery. Although mostly scheduled 4–7 weeks after completion of CRT, the proper timing of surgery has yet to be definitively determined. Postoperative complication rates were not statistically different between the combination and the surgery arm.

About 83% of the patients underwent esophagectomy following CRT; the remaining were progressing (6%), unfit for surgery (5%), refused surgery (4%), or died during or shortly after CRT (1.5%). The mean R0 resection rate was 88%. Five-year survival rates varied from 16 to 59% in all patients and from 34 to 62% in those achieving pCR. Neoadjuvant CRT had a worsening effect on most aspects of health-related quality of life, even though this was a temporary effect and there was a recovery or even an improvement one year after surgery. The pCR rate, probably the most important prognostic factor, was in the range of 13–49%, with a mean of 26% in evaluable operated patients, apparently not different from the 24% reported by a previous review [1].

Recently our institution reported a phase II study [20] that used an intensive protocol of neoadjuvant combined modality therapy with weekly docetaxel and cisplatin, fluorouracil continuous infusion, and concurrent RT. Median survival was 55 months in the whole group, with a 5-year survival rate of 73% in the subset of complete responders. The pCR rate was 47%: the median follow-up was about 5 years, demonstrating that these pCRs were durable. G3/4 toxicities were non-hematological (mainly asthenia and esophagitis) and neutropenia in 32% and 13% of the patients, respectively.

12.2 Chemotherapy

The Intergroup trial 113, carried out in the USA, randomized 440 eligible patients with clinical stage I–III (54% AC and 46% SCC) to three cycles of PF followed by surgery and an additional two cycles of postoperative chemotherapy vs. surgery alone [21]. No significant differences for preoperative chemotherapy vs. surgery in terms of R0 resection rate (59% vs. 63%, respectively), median survival (1.3 years in both arms), or 3-year survival (23% vs. 26%, respectively) were reported. The long-term update confirmed the absence of a significant difference in OS [22]. The pCR was only 2.5% in the preoperative group, while postoperative mortality was 6% in both arms. Only 38% of the patients actually received both cycles of the planned postoperative chemotherapy. Subgroup analysis found an improvement in the 5-year survival rate of R0 patients (32% vs. 5%) and the 19% of patients responding to chemotherapy.

The British Medical Research Council (MRC) [23] randomized 802 patients (66% AC) to two cycles of PF plus surgery vs. surgery alone. A 9% absolute survival improvement (43% vs. 34%, $p = 0.004$) was detected at 2 years in the neoadjuvant group, along with a higher R0 resection rate (60% vs. 54%, $p < 0.0001$). Median survival was also significantly improved (16.8% vs. 13.3 months), irrespective of histology.

The conflicting survival results reported between these two large trials using similar chemotherapy schedules may be explained by multiple factors. The larger sample size of the MRC trial may have allowed the detection of a statistically small, yet clinically significant survival advantage. The histologies were different: in the MRC trial about two-thirds of the patients had AC as opposed to 54% in the Intergroup trial. The follow-up in the MRC trial was substantially shorter than that reported in the Intergroup trial, and the initial differences in survival may not persist over time. Moreover, the less toxic schedule of chemotherapy of the MRC trial likely improved patient compliance.

12.3 Conclusions

The optimal treatment strategy for resectable esophageal cancer is still a controversial topic. Neoadjuvant CRT has been accepted by many, although not all, as the standard of care, because it increases the rates of R0 resection and local tumor control; but, above all, it is the only way to achieve a pCR, which highly correlates with improved OS. On the whole, however, the absolute OS gain is about 13% at 2 years [18]. This small benefit must be balanced against the toxicity of the treatment.

Although neoadjuvant and peri-operative chemotherapy have also been found to be effective approaches, there is reasonable evidence that such treatments are inferior to neoadjuvant CRT. Only clinically well designed and statistically powered randomized clinical trials will help to solve the problem.

References

1. Geh JI, Crellin AM, Glynne-Jones R (2001) Preoperative (neoadjuvant) chemoradiotherapy in oesophageal cancer. Br J Surg 88:338-356
2. Jin L, Xiu-Feng C, Bin Z et al (2009) Effect of neoadjuvant chemoradiotherapy on prognosis and surgery for esophageal carcinoma. World J Gastroenterol 15:4962-4968
3. Courrech Staal EFW, Aleman BMP, Boot H et al (2010) Systematic review of the benefits and risks of neoadjuvant chemoradiation for oesophageal cancer. Br J Surg 97:1482-1496
4. Walsh TN, Noonan N, Hollywood D et al (1996) A comparison of multimodal therapy and surgery for esophageal adenocarcinoma. N Engl J Med 335:462-467
5. Tepper J, Krasna MJ, Niedzwiecki D et al (2008) Phase III trial of trimodality therapy with cisplatin, fluorouracil, radiotherapy, and surgery compared with surgery alone for esophageal cancer: CALGB 9781. J Clin Oncol 26:1086-1092
6. Cao XF, He XT, Ji L et al (2009) Effects of neoadjuvant radiochemotherapy on pathological staging and prognosis for locally advanced esophageal squamous cell carcinoma. Dis Esophagus 22:477-481
7. Van der Gaast A, Van Hagen P, Hulshof M et al (2010) Effect of preoperative concurrent chemoradiotherapy on survival of patients with resectable esophageal or esophagogastric junction cancer: Results from a multicenter randomized phase III study. J Clin Oncol 28:15s, (abstr 4004)
8. Bosset JF, Gignoux M, Triboulet JP et al (1997) Chemoradiotherapy followed by surgery compared with surgery alone in squamous-cell cancer of the esophagus. N Engl J Med 337:161-167
9. Burmeister BH, Smithers BM, Gebski V et al (2005) Surgery alone versus chemoradiotherapy followed by surgery for resectable cancer of the oesophagus: a randomised controlled phase III trial. Lancet Oncol 6:659-668
10. Nygaard K, Hagen S, Hansen HS et al (1992) Pre-operative radiotherapy prolongs survival in operable esophageal carcinoma: a randomized, multicenter study of pre-operative radiotherapy and chemotherapy. The second Scandinavian trial in esophageal cancer. World J Surg 16:1104-1109
11. Apinop C, Puttisak P, Preecha N(1994) A prospective study of combined therapy in esophageal cancer. Hepatogastroenterology 41:391-393
12. Le Prise E, Etienne PL, Meunier B et al (1994) A randomised study of chemotherapy, radiation therapy, and surgery versus surgery for localized squamous cell carcinoma of the esophagus. Cancer 73:1779-1784
13. Urba SG, Orringer MB, Turrisi A et al (2001) Randomized trial of preoperative chemoradiation versus surgery alone in patients with locoregional esophageal carcinoma. J Clin Oncol 19:305-313
14. Lee J, Park S, Kim S et al (2004) A single institutional phase III trial of preoperative chemotherapy with hyperfractionation radiotherapy plus surgery versus alone for resectable esophageal squamous cell carcinoma. Ann Oncol 15:947-954
15. Natsugoe S, Okumura H, Matsumoto M et al (2006) Randomized controlled study on preoperative chemoradiotherapy followed by surgery versus surgery alone for esophageal squamous cell cancer in a single institution. Dis Esophagus 19:468-472
16. Urschel JD, Vasan H (2003) A meta-analysis of randomized controlled trials that compared neoadjuvant chemoradiation and surgery to surgery alone for resectable esophageal cancer. Am J Surg 185:538-543
17. Fiorica F, Di Bona D, Schepis F et al (2004) Preoperative chemoradiotherapy for oesophageal cancer: a systematic review and meta-analysis. Gut 53:925-930
18. Gebski V, Burmeister B, Smithers BM et al (2007) Survival benefits from neoadjuvant chemoradiotherapy or chemotherapy in oesophageal carcinoma: a meta-analysis. Lancet Oncol 8:226-234
19. Jin HL, Zhu H, Ling TS et al (2009) Neoadjuvant chemoradiotherapy for resectable esophageal

carcinoma: A meta-analysis. World J Gastroenterol 15:5983-5991

20. Pasini F, de Manzoni G, Stievano L et al (2009) Effect of neoadjuvant combined modality therapy with weekly docetaxel (D) and cisplatin (P), 5-fluorouracil (5-FU) continuous infusion (c.i.), and concurrent radiotherapy (RT) on pathological response rate in esophageal cancers (EC): A phase II study. J Clin Oncol 27:15s, (abstr 4548)
21. Kelsen DP, Ginsberg R, Pajak TF et al (1998) Chemotherapy followed by surgery compared with surgery alone for localized esophageal cancer. N Engl J Med 339:1979-1984
22. Kelsen DP, Winter KA, Gunderson LL et al (2007) Long-term results of RTOG trial 8911 (USA Intergroup 113): a random assignment trial comparison of chemotherapy followed by surgery compared with surgery alone for esophageal cancer. J Clin Oncol 25:3719-3725
23. Medical Research Council Oesophageal Cancer Working Group (2002) Surgical resection with or without preoperative chemotherapy in oesophageal cancer: a randomised controlled trial. Lancet 359:1727-1733

Controversial Issues in Esophageal Cancer: Surgical Approach and Lymphadenectomy

13

Giovanni de Manzoni, Andrea Zanoni, and Simone Giacopuzzi

13.1 Introduction

Surgery is still the mainstay in the curative treatment of resectable esophageal cancer. Nevertheless, controversies and debate exist about the optimal management in terms of surgical approach, extent of resection, location of the anastomosis, and optimal nodal dissection. Moreover, the correct role of multimodal treatments, whose use is constantly increasing, has still to be defined, as well as their impact on surgical approach and lymphadenectomy.

The ability to cure esophageal cancer depends primarily on whether a radical removal of the tumor, achieving a R0 resection, is possible. The aim of this chapter is to define the surgical options and the role of lymphadenectomy in the management of esophageal cancer.

13.2 Proximal and Distal Resection Margins

R0 resection is the mainstay in the management of resectable esophageal cancer. Indeed, inadequate resection may result in histologically involved margins (R1-2) and hence in locoregional recurrence [1]. The incidence of recurrence is closely related to the margin of clearance during the surgical procedure, which is established by taking into account the extent of intramural spread of the primary tumor [1, 2]. The tendency of esophageal cancer to spread intramurally is well recognized [1].

Intramural metastases are defined as metastatic lesions clearly separated from the primary tumor, which originate from intramural vascular spread and

G. de Manzoni (✉)
Dept. of Surgery, Upper G.I. Surgery Division, University of Verona,
Verona, Italy

G. de Manzoni (Ed.), *Treatment of Esophageal and Hypopharyngeal Squamous Cell Carcinoma*,

lymphatic or blood vessel invasion [1, 3]. The frequency of intramural metastases is between 9% and 42% and increases with increasing depth of tumor invasion. In one study [2], intramural metastases were found only in T2 or more advanced cancers, while in another trial [3] intramural metastases, although increasing in number with increasing depth of invasion, were found also in 10% of T1 cancers. The number of cases with intramural metastases on the proximal and distal sides is almost the same [2-4]. In addition, nodal involvement is more frequently reported in patients with intramural metastases [2].

Subepithelial accessory lesions consist of cancer nests beneath the non-cancerous epithelium and include direct extension by invasion and intramural metastases [3, 5]. Subepithelial direct extension normally does not exceed 2–2.5 cm, while intramural metastases can be found beyond 5 cm from the main lesion [3]. The presence of subepithelial lesions is quite impressive, occurring in almost 50% of T1sm3-T2 cancers, and half of them are located at least 5 mm beyond from the main lesion [5].

Esophageal specimens tend to shrink after their removal, and especially after formalin fixation. This phenomenon can lead to underestimates of the actual in situ length of the specimen, making it difficult to precisely define subepithelial spread and resection margins. Some authors [2, 3] report that shrinkage from the in situ (before removal) length is about 10%, but an almost normal esophageal length can be estimated if the specimen is measured fresh, stretched and pinned onto a cork board. In another trial [4], measurements were performed in fresh, contracted specimens; shrinkage was more pronounced, with lengths representing 45% of the in situ lengths.

In fresh specimens, the most distant metastases were found at 9.5–10.5 cm from the main lesion [2, 3]. Subepithelial accessory lesions are the most important cause of positive resection margins, as these lesions are difficult to detect even during intraoperative observation of the resected esophagus [3]. As anastomotic recurrence is strongly related to the presence of subepithelial lesions, safe margins, both proximally and distally from primary tumor, are of utmost importance. If the risk of involved margins were only related to direct subepithelial invasion, as in rectal cancer, a safe margin of 2.5 cm would be enough; but because of intramural distant metastases, much wider margins are required. To completely annul the theoretical risk of positive resection margins, removal of the entire esophagus would be necessary. To avoid total esophagectomy, various authors have proposed resection margins wide enough to cope with the risk of positive margins [3] or anastomotic recurrence [2, 4].

In one trial, the risk of anastomotic recurrence was as high as 20% if the resection margin in situ was < 5 cm, decreasing to 8% with a margin of 8–10 cm [2]. In another trial, anastomotic recurrence never occurred when the margin was ≥ 8 cm [4]. A 10-cm in situ margin was thus proposed.

The risk of a positive margin was found to be $< 5\%$ according to a trial [3] adopting a margin from the main lesion of 1 cm in T1-2 cancers and 3 cm in more advanced cases. These measurements were done in resected specimens, so that an in situ margin of 5 cm was inferred as sufficiently safe. The proximal margin is more difficult to determine but also prognostically more relevant than the distal margin; however, a safe distal margin is also of importance. The above-mentioned studies, as well as a trial focused on distal margins [6], support a safe distal margin of 5 cm.

Obviously, cancer site is also important in defining the location of resection and anastomosis. In the surgical treatment of upper thoracic cancers a cervical anastomosis is necessary, while in mid-lower cancers an intrathoracic anastomosis is sufficiently safe [1]. In the latter, a high supra-azygotic anastomosis allows an increased free resection margin as well as reduced gastroesophageal reflux symptoms.

Even if the ideal resection margin in thoracic squamous cell carcinoma (SCC) has not been clearly established, in our institution we aim at achieving a 10-cm proximal in situ margin above and a 5-cm in situ distal margin underneath the main lesion.

13.3 Circumferential Resection Margin

The concept of circumferential resection margin (CRM) is used in rectal cancer surgery. This entity is defined as the radial margin of resection after removal of the rectum and surrounding mesorectum. It has been shown that a CRM < 1 mm corresponds to a positive or involved CRM, that is to say, R+ resection and thus a high local recurrence rate and dismal survival [7]. While it is unclear whether the same concept can be applied to esophageal cancer, two different classifications have been proposed [8]. The first, by the Royal College of Pathologists (RCP), considered only two classes, i.e. CRM positive (CRM+), if the CRM is involved or cancer is detected within 1 mm of the margin, and CRM negative (CRM-) otherwise. The second classification, proposed by the College of American Pathologists (CAP), divided patients into three categories: CRM involved, cancer within 1 mm of the CRM, and cancer far from the CRM by > 1 mm. Clearly, a CRM that is directly involved implies R+ resection. Furthermore, it is important to study the CRM only for pT3 cancers [7, 9, 10], because finding a circumferential positive margin in pT1 and pT2 cancers indicates inadequate surgery, leaving in situ part of the esophageal wall involved with cancer, meaning R2 resection. For pT4a cancers, it is also difficult to define the prognostic significance of CRM positivity, which is probable occurrence in all cases.

In the late 1990s, the application of CRM was proposed for esophageal cancer, even though the difficulties in evaluating CRM made the number of trials quite small. Some features of the studies in the recent literature are shown in Table 13.1 [7-15]. Sample size was quite good, ranging between 100 patients and over 300, depth of tumor invasion was pT3 in 60–100% of the study populations, and histology was prevalently adenocarcinoma in all but one study. This is not surprising, considering that most trials were performed in Europe, particularly in the UK, where adenocarcinoma occures more fre-

Table 13.1 Circumferential resection margin (CRM) positivity and its correlation with local recurrence and survival

Author [Reference]	N.	T3	Histology	Induction therapy	CRM+ (pT3)	Local recurrence	CRT independent prognostic factor
Dexter et al. [14]	135	70%	73% AdenoCa	0%	63%	n.r.	Yes
Khan et al. [15]	329	81%	61% AdenoCa	0%	20%	n.r.	No (only RCP used)
Griffith et al. [12]	249	62%	71% AdenoCa	13% CT	51%	n.r.	Yes
Sujedran et al. [10]	242	60%	76% AdenoCa	59% CT	39%	42% vs. 59% ($p = 0.032$)	Yes
Scheepers et al. [9]	110	78%	75% AdenoCa	28% CT	48%	n.r.	Yes
Saha et al. [11]	105	67%	100% AdenoCa	100% CT	53%	n.r.	Yes
Deeter et al. [8]	135	100%	87% AdenoCa	44% CT or CRT	54%	n.r.	Yes CAP, no RCP
Chao et al. [7]	151	100%	100% SCC	100% CRT	51%	21% vs. 39% (p=0.021)	Yes
Pultrum et al. [13]	98	59%	76% AdenoCa	0%	74%	Independent[a]	Yes (RCP)

n.r., not reported; *CAP*, College of American Pathologists; *RCP*, Royal College of Pathologists; *CT*, chemotherapy; *CRT*, chemoradiotherapy.
[a]CRM + independent factor for increased local recurrence.

quently. The only trial recruiting only SCC cases was a recent Chinese one [7], which was also the only one to evaluate the relationship between CRM and neoadjuvant chemoradiotherapy. As displayed in the table, a percentage of the patients were treated with neoadjuvant chemotherapy, but only two trials investigated the role of chemotherapy in modifying CRM positivity rate [10, 11]. CRM positivity evaluated with the RCP system for pT3 patients ranged between 20% and 63%, with a median value of 51%. According to the CAP system, a lower rate of CRM positivity was intuitively found in some studies [7, 8]. The relationship between CRM positivity and local recurrence rate was statistically significant in favor of CRM-negative patients in the only two studies that investigated the subject [7, 10].

CRM, along with nodal status, was demonstrated by multivariable analysis to be an independent prognostic factor in all but two studies, a finding that deserves further and more in-depth inspection. The largest published study, by Khan et al., was the only one that failed to find a significant relationship between CRM and survival. However, in this study, the author reported the lowest rate results of CRM positivity in the current literature. Moreover, only the RCP system was used in the evaluation of CRM.

It has been suggested that en-bloc esophagectomy reduces the percentage of CRM involvement, since the resulting tissue envelope surrounding the esophagus is much thicker than without the application of this technique [12]. That en-bloc esophagectomy can reduce CRM positivity is also supported by the Chinese study [7], as opposed to the proposed use of CRM even after a trans-hiatal approach [9]. However, even though the reduced rate of CRM-involved cases may be explained by use of the en-bloc technique, this does not elucidate the non-significant connection with survival. A highly informative study by Deeter and colleagues [8] used both CAP and RCP criteria to examine a cohort of patients. An involved CRM was found in 12% of the patients based on the CAP criteria and 61% of the patients based on the RCP criteria. This difference translated into statistically different survival using CAP compared with RCP. The authors concluded that the group of patients with uninvolved but close CRM should probably be considered as distinct from the group of patients with involved CRM, and that the CAP criteria better account for the CRM.

The study by the Chinese group [7] investigated the role of CRM in SCC of the esophagus after neoadjuvant chemoradiotherapy using both CAP (group 1: CRM > 1 mm; group 2: uninvolved but < 1 mm CRM; group 3: involved CRM) and RCP criteria. The CRM-positive rate was 51% with RCP and 17% with CAP criteria. According to the latter, the locoregional recurrence rate was significantly higher in groups 2 and 3, with a higher rate of systemic relapses in group 3. This tendency translated into statistically significant differences in 5-year survival, which resulted in rates of 40, 23, and 6%, respectively, for groups 1, 2, and 3 ($p < 0.05$).

Even though the circumferential margin can be analyzed after every type of esophageal resection, like trans-hiatal esophagectomy [9], the more extensive the resection, i.e., en-bloc technique, the better the results in terms of reduced CRM involvement.

The role of neoadjuvant therapy in CRM determination has not been clarified yet, because of the discordant results reported after chemotherapy. In fact, in two studies [9, 12] there was no difference in CRM+ rate between patients treated with surgery alone and those receiving neoadjuvant therapy, while in another trial [10] CRM positivity was significantly more frequent after surgery alone.

The possible difference in behavior between SCC and adenocarcinoma also has not been investigated completely.

The local control and low locoregional recurrence rate achieved by chemoradiotherapy (CRT), because of the local effect of radiation, could reduce the impact of en-bloc resection and the importance of CRM. However, this also has not been confirmed so far.

CRM seems to be a prognostic indicator for pT3 patients. Furthermore, the CAP criteria (CRM > 1 mm; uninvolved but < 1 mm CRM; involved CRM) seem to more correctly reflect the true significance of CRM involvement, in which probably an intermediate assessment class needs to be used.

It is probable, but not certain, that CRM involvement retains its significance even after neoadjuvant chemotherapy, but its role after chemoradiotherapy is under study. In summary, even though CRM is not routinely used by most institutions, it seems to be promising and deserves further investigation.

13.4 Lymphadenectomy

The extent of lymphadenectomy depends on one's perspective regarding esophageal cancer. If SCC is considered to be a systemic disease from its very beginning, then a more radical resection with extended lymphadenectomy would be unnecessary if not harmful. The view that locally advanced cancers are still curable justifies a radical resection along with lymphadenectomy with cure intent. It is obvious that the more nodes harvested, the more complete and precise the staging. An extended lymphadenectomy, with its inherently higher morbidity-mortality risk, would be justified only if it conferred a survival advantage.

Two important aspects favor lymphadenectomy as a therapeutic tool: first, the survival of patients with involved nodes (N+) is much poorer than that of patients with negative nodes, but the number of involved nodes and/or the ratio of involved to total resected nodes correlate with different survival rates [16-21]. This suggests that nodal dissection has a therapeutic role in patients with limited nodal involvement. The second aspect is the fact that also the absolute number of resected nodes, whether involved or not, correlates with survival [22-27].

13.4.1 Number of Involved Nodes and Lymph Node Ratio

Nodal involvement is a strong predictor of survival. As reported in Chap. 2, the new TNM staging system (7th edn.), in contrast to all previous versions in which nodal involvement was considered simply as positive (N1) or negative (N0), now takes into consideration the number of involved nodes, defining four categories for regional nodes: N0, N1 (1–2 nodes involved), N2 (3–6), N3 (≥ 7). Actually, there is an important difference in the definition of regional nodes between the AJCC-TNM and UICC-TNM classifications. The former considers regional nodes as those from the celiac trunk to the supraclavicular area, while the latter explicitly excludes the supraclavicular nodes. In a study by Tachimori and colleagues [28], it was claimed that it is absolutely correct to consider the number of involved nodes, which is the strongest prognostic factor for esophageal cancer. The authors affirmed that the site of metastasis is not so important, not even if positive nodes are located in the supraclavicular area. They concluded their report by saying that the supraclavicular nodes should be considered as regional nodes for esophageal cancer, in which case they are N and not M.

Table 13.2 Number of positive nodes and lymph node ratio cut-offs: correlation with reduction in overall survival and increased death risk

Author [Reference]	N.	Neoadjuvant	Fields of dissection	Cut off of N+ number	Cut off of lymph node ratio	5-year overall survival reduction	Increased hazard ratio
Shimada et al. [16]	133	0%	3 field	≥3	n.r.	Yes	Yes
Peyre et al. [17]	1053	0%	n.r.	≥8	n.r.	n.r.	Yes[a]
Liu et al. [18]	1325	0%	n.r.	≥4	≤25%	Yes	n.r.
Mariette et al. [19]	536	51% CRT	2 field	≥5	>20%	Yes	Yes
Kelty et al. [20]	218	30% CT	2 field	≥4	>20%	Yes	n.r.
Hsu et al. [21]	1069	0%	n.r.	≥4	≥20%	Yes	Yes
Smit et al. [29]	220	0%	2 field	>4	>20%	Yes	Yes

n.r., not reported.
[a]Risk of systemic disease.

A number of studies have investigated the precise role of the number of nodal metastases and/or the ratio between involved and total resected nodes [16-21]. The main characteristics and results of these recent trials are shown in Table 13.2 [16-21, 29]. The number of patients varied from 133 to 1325. The fields of nodal dissection were not uniform in the vast majority of the studies, only Shimada et al. [16], in their study of a smaller sample size, performed a radical 3-field lymphadenectomy in all the patients. Mariette et al. [19] and Kelty et al. [20] considered patients with and without induction treatments but only Mariette considered chemoradiation. Predictably, all studies described a significantly worse prognosis and/or a higher risk of death with an increasing number of involved nodes or higher ratio. The cut-off was defined as between 3 and 8 positive nodes and a ratio > 20% in almost all trials.

Recently, Peyre et al. [17] described their results in terms of risk of systemic disease, claiming that with the involvement of 8 or more nodes the probability of systemic disease reaches almost 100%, i.e., radical surgery is not indicated. This tendency is in line with two recent trials focusing only on esophageal adenocarcinoma [30, 31], in which there was no benefit from surgery when > 8 lymph nodes were involved.

The number of involved nodes and the lymph node ratio retains its role also after CRT, according to Mariette and colleagues [19], even if the number of dissected nodes in their trial was significantly lower after radiation therapy. By subdividing patients in adequately staged (≥ 15 nodes harvested) and inadequately staged (< 15 nodes analyzed), the authors found that, in patients with adequately staged disease, the number of involved nodes correlated with survival, whereas in inadequately staged disease the ratio was more relevant.

In the new TNM, the number of involved nodes is considered a strong prognostic factor, provided that an adequate number of lymph nodes are resected. Thus, there is a role for lymph node ratio in N+ patients, especially in cases in which a correct lymphadenectomy has not been performed.

13.4.2 Total Number of Resected Nodes

The total number of resected nodes is a good marker of lymphadenectomy success. The more nodes harvested, the more precise the staging. This can be related to survival in terms of stage migration. With a sufficient number of resected nodes, indeed, the inclusion of patients with correctly staged disease allows for almost perfect survival analyses. However, if the only advantage of extended lymphadenectomy is to obtain better staging, it would not be justified. Various trials have investigated whether increasing the number of resected nodes was related to better long-term outcome. The results of several recent trials are shown in Table 13.3 [22-24, 26, 27, 32, 33]. Most of these studies had very large study populations for both SCC and adenocarcinoma, ranging from 264 to 4882, with five out of seven trials comprising more the 1,000 patients. A 5-year overall survival advantage and/or a reduced hazard of death was found in all these studies. The cut-off of harvested nodes ranged from ≥ 6 to ≥ 30. In some of the reports, sub-stratifications were proposed. Rizk et al. [22] proposed to resect at least 10, 20, and 30 nodes, respectively, for T1, T2, and T3. Altorki et al. [23] instead claimed that for N+ patients 16 nodes are enough for staging and to obtain a survival benefit, while for N0 patients some advantage is gained when > 40 nodes are resected. Groth et al. [27] affirmed that even if 12 nodes are sufficient, the maximum survival advantage is obtained with 30 harvested nodes.

Table 13.3 Cut off number of harvested lymph nodes to obtain a survival advantage or a reduced hazard of death

Author [Reference]	N.	Cut off number of harvested lymph nodes	5-year OS advantage	Hazard of death reduced
Rizk et al. [22]	4627	≥30	Yes	n.r.
Altorki et al. [23]	264	≥25	n.r.	Yes
Peyre et al. [24]	2303	≥23	Yes	Yes
Hu et al. [26]	1098	≥6	Yes	n.r.
Groth et al. [27]	4882	≥12	n.r.	Yes
Twine et al. [32]	237	≥10	Yes	Yes
Schwartz et al. [33]	2597	≥30	Yes	Yes

OS, overall survival; *n.r.*, not reported

The multicenter study of Peyre et al. [24] consisted of nine centers distributed all over the world. The researchers found that the number of resected nodes is a strong and independent predictor of outcome, along with the number of involved nodes and the depth of invasion in both SCC and adenocarcinoma. Being a multicenter study, the surgical technique used at the various participating centers differed. The researchers discovered that en-bloc resection was the best technique to reach the threshold of 23 nodes (achieved in 66% of the patients compared with 14–24% of those treated using other techniques). Moreover, even after adequate lymphadenectomy, survival was significantly better after en-bloc than after other types of resection. An interesting remark by the authors was that both tumor depth and the number of involved nodes are predetermined, while the ability of the surgeon to improve survival was limited to ensuring an adequate lymphadenectomy.

Another important point was made by Groth et al. [27], who affirmed the importance of a correct lymphadenectomy even after chemoradiation. In fact, radiotherapy probably reduces the total number of resected nodes or at least downsizes them, making harvesting more difficult for the pathologist. In contrast with this view, a recent German trial [34] reported an equal number of resected nodes comparing one group of patients undergoing surgery alone and another receiving preoperative chemoradiation, but the harvested nodes, especially the metastatic ones, were significantly smaller in the latter group, making pathological examination harder.

One possible explanation for the survival advantage gained with extended nodal dissection is the possibility to eliminate occult metastases and micrometastases. Occult metastases are those undetected with preoperative work-up, especially after induction treatments. Micrometastases are defined as metastases detectable only with immunostaining but considered negative with imaging and by routine histological examination. The presence of micrometastases in supposed node-negative patients could explain the improved survival after extended lymphadenectomy in these patients [35].

An interesting study by Qubain and coworkers [36] found that micrometastases were present in 19% of cervical histologically negative nodes. There was a correlation between the presence of other metastases, in particular, mediastinal recurrent nerve metastases and cervical metastases and micrometastases. Thus, extended lymphadenectomy also in the cervical region may reduce the risk of micrometastases. Cervical nodal metastases could be predicted by exploring the mediastinal recurrent nerve area, thereby probably avoiding useless cervical lymphadenectomy.

13.4.3 Type of Lymphadenectomy

Considerable debate remains regarding the optimal type of lymph node dissection [28]. An appreciation of the anatomical lymphatic drainage system of the esophagus is essential to understanding the pathways of neoplastic diffusion

[28, 37] and thus to achieving an adequate field of dissection [28]. The lymphatic channels between the lamina propria and submucosa have been fully described. Recent anatomical studies, in particular by Kuge et al. [38], described the presence of very evident, long, longitudinal lymphatic pathways in the esophageal submucosa. Lymphatic routes to the periesophageal lymph nodes originate instead from the intermuscular area of the muscularis propria. The submucosal route explains the presence of skip metastases, while the intermuscular path is related to peri-esophageal metastases. Nodal diffusion thus depends on both the cancer site and intramural diffusion, i.e., T status [28].

Nodal Spread by Cancer Site

The pattern of nodal diffusion differs when patients are categorized on the basis of lesion location, even if the lymphatic metastasis rates are quite similar, over 55% for upper and mid-lower cancers [39, 40].

A number of recent studies [28, 39, 40] described the lymphatic flow depending on the site of the lesion. These studies were carried out in China and Japan, where three-field dissection (cervical, thoracic, and abdominal) is widely performed. In these trials, diffusion to cervical nodes was broadly present at all cancer sites; in one study [39] it reached 17% from lower thoracic cancer, which is the site of lower risk of upwards metastases (Table 13.4) [16, 39, 41, 42]. The percentage of patients with lower thoracic SCC and metastases in the upper mediastinum and supraclavicular area reached 27 and 6%, respectively, in advanced cancers (pT2-4) according to a recent Japanese trial [28]. For upper thoracic cancers, metastases in the upper mediastinum and supraclavicular area are a frequent occurrence.

In superficial cancers, even with tumors located in the mid- and lower esophagus, upper mediastinal and perigastric nodes are more often involved than nodes of the mid and lower mediastinum. For more advanced cancers, the frequency of metastases in the mid and lower mediastinum dramatically increases. However, Tachimori and co-workers found that node metastases in the mid and lower mediastinum are still less frequent than in the upper mediastinum and perigastric area, even for advanced cancers [28]. This pattern of nodal diffusion upwards and downwards from the primary tumor raises the problem of the extent of nodal dissection.

Table 13.4 Cervical nodal involvement by site of cancer in the thoracic esophagus

Author [Reference]	Upper (%)	Middle (%)	Lower (%)
Shimada et al. [16]	48	28	13
Nakagawa et al. [41]	56	16	12
Lerut et al. [42]	44	26	16
Chen et al. [39]	49	35	17

Table 13.5 Nodal involvement according to T stage

	Lerut et al. [42]	Mariette et al. [44]	Altorki et al. [46]	Ancona et al. [45]	Tachibana et al. [43]	Tachimori et al. [28]	Our data
T1 m	0%	17%	33%	0%	8%	47%	14%
T1 sm (sm1)				8%	7%		
T1 sm (sm2)	35%		50%	29%	19%		
T1 sm (sm3)				54%	47%		
T2	71%	53%	75%	/	/		41%
T3	78%	/	83%	/	/	82%	65%
T4	50%	/	50%	/	/		65%

Nodal Spread by T Status

While nodal spread depends on the tumor site, the incidence of nodal metastases correlates with depth of tumor invasion (pT). In this view, superficial cancers, defined as cancers confined to the mucosa or submucosa, can have distant metastases, due to the longitudinal path. In submucosal cancer, skip metastases may be more frequent than locoregional ones; thus, isolated distant lymph node metastases are not necessarily a sign of advanced disease [28]. If, instead, the tumor penetrates the muscle layer, the rate of peri-esophageal metastases increases and is thus a sign of more advanced cancer.

The frequency of nodal metastases is quite high in T1sm cancers, ranging from 21% to 54% in different trials [28, 40]. Of course, the incidence of nodal metastases in more advanced cancers is much higher (T2-4), ranging from 41 to 82% (Table 13.5) [28, 42-46].

Skip Metastases

Metastatic involvement of distant lymph nodes without infiltration in regional nodes is called skip metastasis [47]. As mentioned above, the presence of skip metastases depends on the lymphatic flow in the esophageal submucosa. In the study by Tachimori et al. [28], there was no difference in survival according to the areas of involved nodes, leading the authors to conclude that isolated distant lymph node involvement from superficial cancers is not necessarily a sign of advanced disease [28].

A recent German study [47] examined nodal involvement and skip metastases in a cohort of patients with either SCC or adenocarcinoma who underwent two-field lymphadenectomy, with partial recurrent-nerve-chain nodal dissection for upper thoracic cancers. The authors staged the harvested nodes according to the Japanese Society for Esophageal Disease staging system. Skip metastases were defined as the involvement of N2-N4 nodes, without infiltration of N1 nodes (see chap. 2, Fig. 2.1).

The authors found that 20% of N+ patients had skip metastases. The incidence of skip metastases in early cancers was higher than in more advanced stages: 39% in pT1 to 14% in pT3. Moreover, patients with skip metastases had significantly fewer infiltrated lymph nodes than N+ patients without skip metastases. Survival was found to be positively influenced by the presence of skip metastases. In fact, patients with skip metastases had a 53% 5-year overall survival compared with 15% for patients with continuous metastases (p = 0.0001). Moreover, compared with pN0 patients, patients with skip metastases with only one lymph node involved had a similar prognosis. Of note, while the authors applied the Japanese system, they did not perform extensive lymphadenectomy, thus a higher number of skip metastases may have been missed, especially in the cervical region.

In conclusion, skip metastases do not indicate advanced disease and these patients have a good prognosis. This mandates the use of adequate lymphadenectomy also in early cancers, to potentially cure the disease.

13.4.4 Extended Lymphadenectomy

At the 1995 Consensus Conference of the International Society for Diseases of the Esophagus (ISDE), the terms and types of lymphadenectomy were defined (Fig. 13.1) [48]. The area of lymphadenectomy was divided into three fields: abdomen (field I), thorax (field II), and neck (field III). For the thorax, nodal dissection was subdivided into three ranks: "standard" lymphadenectomy included mid and lower mediastinal dissection; "extended," also the upper mediastinum on the right side; and "complete" or "total," bilateral upper mediastinal dissection. Three-field consisted of a combination of field I, "complete" field II, and field III lymphadenectomy [48, 49].

The concept of en-bloc resection was also introduced, dealing with extended lymphadenectomy.

In the current literature, extended lymphadenectomy in SCC refers substantially to two types of nodal dissection: two-field "extended" or "complete," with or without en-bloc resection, and three-field dissection. Two-field "complete" lymphadenectomy consists of the thorough removal of bilateral upper mediastinal nodes along with abdominal nodes (D1+ abdominal dissection). It can be achieved with or without en-bloc resection.

En-bloc resection was first proposed by Logan and later re-introduced by Skinner [50, 51], especially for adenocarcinoma of the esophagogastric junction. This type of resection aims at maximizing local tumor control by removing the esophagus together with an envelope of surrounding tissue. In particular, the tumor-bearing esophagus is resected with both pleural surfaces laterally, the pericardium anteriorly, and all tissues between the esophagus and aorta or vertebral bodies, i.e., the thoracic duct, azygos vein, and segments of the intercostal arteries and veins. In minor modifications, the intercostal vessels and the trunk of the azygos vein or the thoracic duct can be spared. If necessary, a cuff of diaphragm is dissected with the esophagus. Ten centimeters of free proximal and distal margins must be preserved. Even if two-field lym-

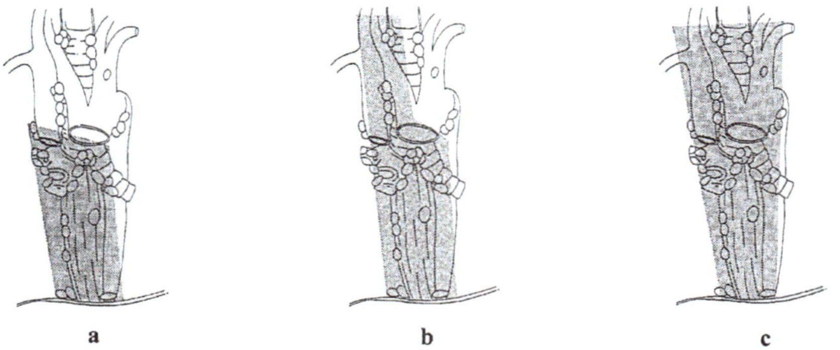

Fig. 13.1 Extent of lymphadenectomy according to the ISDE classification proposed at the consensus conference in Milan (1995) [48]. Areas of standard (a), extended (b) and total (c) mediastinal lymphadenectomy

phadenectomy and en-bloc resection are not synonymous, normally, in en-bloc esophagectomy, a middle and lower mediastinal node dissection along with an abdominal dissection is carried out.

En-bloc esophagectomy is indicated for mid-lower cancers, while in the upper esophagus this is almost impossible due to the presence of the surrounding unresectable vital organs.

It is difficult to compare en-bloc resection with complete nodal dissection in the mediastinal area, as comparative studies are lacking. Furthermore, the upper mediastinal nodes normally cannot be dissected en-bloc with the esophagus but have to be resected separately. A possible role of en-bloc esophagectomy is in the determination of circumferential margins.

Whether en-bloc has any use after induction CRT remains a matter of debate. However, CRT offers good local control, which may reduce the utility of this demanding technique. Thus, two-field complete lymphadenectomy without en-bloc, especially after CRT, is an alternative, but whether complete two-field dissection with en-bloc is superior to two-field dissection without en-bloc remains to be determined.

The other concept of extended lymphadenectomy is the three-field lymphadenectomy, developed by Japanese surgeons in the 1980s in response to the high incidence of cervical metastases for SCC of the esophagus. Technically, it consists of lymphadenectomy of the abdomen, thorax, and neck [46, 50]. Actually, the "third field" consists not only of the cervical nodes but also a continuous, anatomically inseparable chain of nodes from the superior mediastinum (recurrent nerve nodes) to the lower neck. These nodes can be referred to as the cervicothoracic nodes [46]. Three-field dissection can be performed along with or without en-bloc resection [46, 50].

Three-field dissection is justified only if it has a prognostic impact. In fact, while in dedicated centers the complication rate of this major surgical operation has been significantly reduced over the years, morbidity-mortality is still a concern [52]. Pulmonary complications, vocal cord palsy, caused by recurrent nerve injury, and anastomotic leaks account for most of the morbidity and mortality in surgically treated patients, especially those undergoing three-field dissection. Recurrent nerve paralysis is described in 12–60% [42, 41, 49, 53, 54-57] of the patients, with permanent paralysis in 3–31% [42, 49] and bilateral palsy in 5% [53].

The higher risk of complications associated with three-field dissection explains why this approach is so controversial. In fact, theoretically, the more extended the lymphadenectomy, the better the results achieved, as noted above. But this highly destructive surgery should be performed only if a real advantage in survival is obtained.

A number of studies have compared the results of three-field and two-field dissection, but most were non-randomized retrospective studies. Moreover, it is probably incorrect to consider all SCC together, since the cancer site is related to different lymphatic patterns.

An interesting retrospective Japanese trial [49] investigated the results of four approaches with the aim of defining the "optimal lymphadenectomy." Only 8% of the patients had a SCC of the upper esophagus and most were treated with three-field dissection. The researchers did not find differences in mortality, but recurrent nerve palsy was frequent after two-field complete and three-field dissection, reaching almost 30% for permanent paralysis. It is noteworthy that the rate of permanent paralysis was 15% also in the standard and extended groups. This is a very high percentage and is not consistent with other, more recent reports in the current literature [42, 53, 55, 56]. Also, anastomotic leakage, tracheal ischemia, and phrenic nerve paralysis were observed only after three-field dissection.

The distribution of recurrence and survival did not differ among the four groups. The only patients that showed a survival advantage with two-field complete or three-field lymphadenectomy were those with upper and middle SCC with nodal metastases (pN+).

The only randomized trial comparing two-field and three-field dissection was performed in the late 1990s in Japan, by Nishihira and colleagues [57]. Their small sample size study consisted of 30 and 32 patients in the two arms. Two-field dissection was defined as "extended" mediastinal dissection, according to ISDE definition. The presence of metastases in the superior mediastinum was noteworthy in both groups, while cervical metastases were almost absent. The authors suggested that selection bias explained this finding.

Regarding short-term outcome, a higher rate of recurrent nerve paralysis, with significantly more frequent need of tracheostomy, was seen in the three-field dissection group, with an equal rate of pulmonary complications in the two-field and three-field dissection groups. Leakage was instead more frequent in the two-field group. As for long-term outcome, a non-significant difference in survival was seen between the two arms and the difference in recurrence rate was not statistically significant. Of note, the study population included mainly patients with mid-lower cancers, with only one case of upper SCC.

Law and Wang [58] proposed a "complete" thoracic dissection with a two-field lymphadenectomy as a good and sufficient approach to SCC. In fact, they claimed that the most important field of dissection is the cervicothoracic node group and not cervical dissection, provided that a complete lymphadenectomy of the superior mediastinum is performed. The cervicothoracic nodes around the recurrent nerve can be dissected out from the thorax.

In summary, among the proponents of extended lymphadenectomy, there are two main points of view: proponents of the three-field dissection, because of the pattern of lymphatic diffusion, which includes the supraclavicular as regional nodes, and the proponents of "extended/complete" two-filed lymphadenectomy. The problem can also be approached by subdividing patients according to cancer site and depth of invasion: upper versus mid-lower cancers and T1sm versus more advanced cancers.

According to studies on lymphatic spread, superficial cancers have an involvement of the cervical nodes that is equal to that of advanced disease [42]. For the proponents of three-field dissection, this is further confirmation of its usefulness. Skeptics [59], however, claim that the present literature does not demonstrate enough advantage for the use of three-field dissection in superficial cancers. The question is still unanswered.

Somewhat less debate is generated regarding upper SCC. In the 1995 ISDE Consensus Conference, the panelists agreed on "complete" mediastinal dissection for supracarinal cancers. The most frequently used approach for upper SCC is three-field lymphadenectomy [16, 41, 60]. In a recent non-randomized study [60] comparing three-field with complete two-field dissection for upper SCC, the latter approach was an independent risk factor of reduced survival, prompting the use of the former. On the contrary, complete two-field dissection was proposed if the cervical nodes are clinically negative at preoperative staging [55]. This second view is contradicted by the frequent involvement of cervical nodes in the neck by upper SCC and because of the high rate of occult metastases and micrometastases.

The main debate arises with respect to mid-lower cancers. It may well be that cancers close to the carina should be treated like upper cancers, based on the lymphatic pattern. More problematic is the treatment of other mid-lower tumors. Few studies have compared three-field with total two-field lymphadenectomy for lower SCC only. One was a Japanese non-randomized trial [56] in which three-field lymphadenectomy could not be shown to provide a survival benefit considering the two approaches, except in patients with nodal metastases in the upper-middle mediastinum, in whom there was a statistically significant survival advantage in favor of the three-field approach. The researchers explained this observation by the better lymphadenectomy achieved using the three-field approach in the cervicothoracic region, although it should also be noted that the authors are strenuous proponents of three-field lymphadenectomy.

The major criticism of extended lymphadenectomy is its high rate of complications. Since mid-lower cancers are those in which three-field lym-

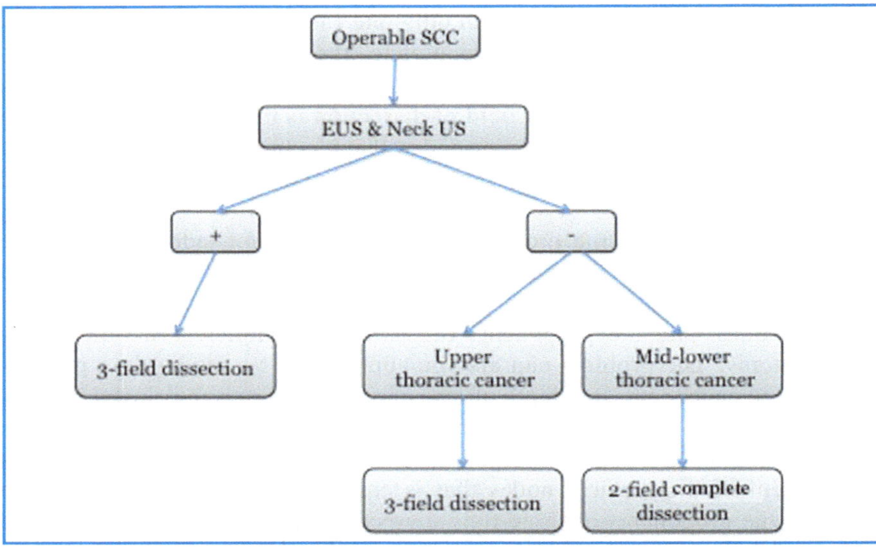

Fig. 13.2 Flow-chart of lymphadenectomy type according to cancer site and ultrasound (US) positivity in operable squamous cell carcinoma (SCC) of the thoracic esophagus. *EUS*, Endoscopic ultrasound

phadenectomy could be avoided, it would be useful to be able to predict the patients who would benefit from extended dissection, thus undergoing selective three-field lymphadenectomy.

Neck ultrasound (US) appears to be an accurate and reliable method of evaluating neck node metastases [61, 62]. US examination coupled with fine-needle aspiration shows a high accuracy (89–97%) [54, 61-63] in detecting nodal metastases. As a relation was found between recurrent nerve node metastases and cervical metastases [64-67], clinical detection of upper mediastinal involvement could be useful along with US to decide whether a three-field lymphadenectomy is appropriate. In a recent meta-analysis [68], endoscopic ultrasound (EUS) demonstrated a high sensitivity and specificity for mediastinal lymph node staging, particularly when associated with FNA. The combined approach improved sensitivity from 85% to 97% and specificity from 85 to 95% compared with EUS alone.

In summary, the debate on lymphadenectomy continues, the preferred type of nodal dissection has yet to be defined, and a number of questions remain unanswered. However, principles of treatment can be assumed and conclusions drawn: First, the number of resected nodes correlates with survival, perhaps because it also results in the elimination of occult metastases and micrometastases; thus, an extended lymphadenectomy is of utmost importance in the therapy of esophageal cancer. Second, the number of harvested lymph nodes retains its significance even after CRT, such that node dissection and node search during pathological examination after radiotherapy must be carried out, even if technically more demanding. The main criticism for the use of extended dissections is the higher risk of complication, without evidence in the current literature of a clearly detectable survival advantage.

Figure 13.2 is a flow chart diagramming the conclusions discussed herein and their implications. After excluding inoperable patients (metastatic or T4b), EUS and neck US should be carried out on those eligible for surgery. In patients with upper SCC or neck US and/or EUS positivity, a three-field lymphadenectomy should be performed. Mid-lower cancers with negativity of the US examination can be treated with two-field complete dissection. In our opinion, this approach could provide the best results in terms of oncological radicality, avoiding unnecessary neck dissections.

13.5 Surgical Approach

Two different surgical approaches are used in the treatment of esophageal cancer: trans-hiatal esophagectomy (THE) and trans-thoracic esophagectomy (TTE). The aim of TTE is to achieve radical surgery both on T and N, performing a radical lymphadenectomy of the thorax. This approach substantially consists of either the Ivor-Lewis procedure, with an intrathoracic anastomosis, or the McKeown procedure, with a cervical anastomosis after a thoracic and abdominal approach. THE consists of a gastric pull-up with an abdominal and a cervical access, avoiding thorax opening; thus, theoretically, it should have a lower morbidity-mortality rate. The philosophical starting point is that thoracic lymphadenectomy should have a minor effect on survival. Actually a higher morbidity-mortality rate for TTE has been reported in a few trials [69, 70], but in most others the complication rate for the two approaches was essentially the same [30, 31, 71-73].

Even if debate is still ongoing regarding the surgical route, a significantly larger number of nodes can be harvested with TTE [74, 75]. As stated throughout this chapter, correct lymphadenectomy is one of the cornerstones of treatment of esophageal cancer.

In the current literature, improved overall survival for SCC treated with TTE has been reported for cases with a limited number of involved nodes or micrometastases [72, 75, 76]. An important recent randomized trial compared TTE and THE in adenocarcinoma only patients [31]. No statistically detectable differences were found in terms of morbidity-mortality and overall survival, but there was an ongoing trend towards better overall 5-year survival with TTE. A statistically significant advantage in survival was instead seen in patients with a small number of involved nodes ($\leq$ 8 nodes) treated with a TTE approach. This is in line with another trial on adenocarcinoma [30], in which patients with $\leq$ 8 nodes involved who were treated via a trans-thoracic route had a significantly longer survival. In summary, TTE, when performed in dedicated centers, offers better oncological results, allowing a complete lymphadenectomy, with tolerable morbidity and mortality. The trans-thoracic route should therefore be used in every case of treatable esophageal cancer to obtain the best oncological radicality, especially after preoperative chemoradiotherapy. THE, however, can be quite safely used in critically ill patients to offer a survival advantage over palliation.

References

1. Law S (2009) Surgery techniques: anastomotic technique and selection of location In: Blair A. Jobe CRT, Jr, John G. Hunter (ed) Esophageal cancer principles and practice. Demos Medical, New York, pp 525-534
2. Lam KY, Ma LT, Wong J (1996) Measurement of extent of spread of oesophageal squamous carcinoma by serial sectioning. J Clin Pathol 49:124-129
3. Tsutsui S, Kuwano H, Watanabe M et al (1995) Resection margin for squamous cell carcinoma of the esophagus. Ann Surg 222:193-202
4. Law S, Arcilla C, Chu KM, Wong J (1998) The significance of histologically infiltrated resection margin after esophagectomy for esophageal cancer. Am J Surg 176:286-290
5. Kuwano H, Masuda N, Kato H, Sugimachi K (2002) The subepithelial extension of esophageal carcinoma for determining the resection margin during esophagectomy: a serial histopathologic investigation. Surgery 131:14-21
6. Casson AG, Darnton SJ, Subramanian S, Hiller L (2000) What is the optimal distal resection margin for esophageal carcinoma? Ann Thorac Surg 69:205-209
7. Chao YK, Yeh CJ, Chang HK et al (2011) Impact of circumferential resection margin distance on locoregional recurrence and survival after chemoradiotherapy in esophageal squamous cell carcinoma. Ann Surg Oncol 18:529-534
8. Deeter M, Dorer R, Kuppusamy MK et al (2009) Assessment of criteria and clinical significance of circumferential resection margins in esophageal cancer. Arch Surg 144:618-624
9. Scheepers JJ, van der Peet DL, Veenhof AA, Cuesta MA (2009) Influence of circumferential resection margin on prognosis in distal esophageal and gastroesophageal cancer approached through the transhiatal route. Dis Esophagus 22:42-48
10. Sujendran V, Wheeler J, Baron R et al (2008) Effect of neoadjuvant chemotherapy on circumferential margin positivity and its impact on prognosis in patients with resectable oesophageal cancer. Br J Surg 95:191-194
11. Saha AK, Sutton C, Rotimi O et al (2009) Neoadjuvant chemotherapy and surgery for esophageal adenocarcinoma: prognostic value of circumferential resection margin and stratification of N1 category. Ann Surg Oncol 16:1364-1370
12. Griffiths EA, Brummell Z, Gorthi G et al (2006) The prognostic value of circumferential resection margin involvement in oesophageal malignancy. Eur J Surg Oncol 32:413-419
13. Pultrum BB, Honing J, Smit JK et al (2010) A critical appraisal of circumferential resection margins in esophageal carcinoma. Ann Surg Oncol 17:812-820
14. Dexter SP, Sue-Ling H, McMahon MJ et al (2001) Circumferential resection margin involvement: an independent predictor of survival following surgery for oesophageal cancer. Gut 48:667-670
15. Khan OA, Fitzgerald JJ, Soomro I et al (2003) Prognostic significance of circumferential resection margin involvement following oesophagectomy for cancer. Br J Cancer 88:1549-1552
16. Shimada H, Okazumi S, Matsubara H et al (2006) Impact of the number and extent of positive lymph nodes in 200 patients with thoracic esophageal squamous cell carcinoma after three-field lymph node dissection. World J Surg 30:1441-1449
17. Peyre CG, Hagen JA, DeMeester SR et al (2008) Predicting systemic disease in patients with esophageal cancer after esophagectomy: a multinational study on the significance of the number of involved lymph nodes. Ann Surg 248:979-985

18. Liu YP, Ma L, Wang SJ et al (2010) Prognostic value of lymph node metastases and lymph node ratio in esophageal squamous cell carcinoma. Eur J Surg Oncol 36:155-159
19. Mariette C, Piessen G, Briez N, Triboulet JP (2008) The number of metastatic lymph nodes and the ratio between metastatic and examined lymph nodes are independent prognostic factors in esophageal cancer regardless of neoadjuvant chemoradiation or lymphadenectomy extent. Ann Surg 247:365-371
20. Kelty CJ, Kennedy CW, Falk GL (2010) Ratio of metastatic lymph nodes to total number of nodes resected is prognostic for survival in esophageal carcinoma. J Thorac Oncol 5 :1467-1471
21. Hsu WH, Hsu PK, Hsieh CC et al (2009) The metastatic lymph node number and ratio are independent prognostic factors in esophageal cancer. J Gastrointest Surg 13:1913-1920
22. Rizk NP, Ishwaran H, Rice TW et al (2010) Optimum lymphadenectomy for esophageal cancer. Ann Surg 251:46-50
23. Altorki NK, Zhou XK, Stiles B et al M (2008) Total number of resected lymph nodes predicts survival in esophageal cancer. Ann Surg 248:221-226
24. Peyre CG, Hagen JA, DeMeester SR et al (2008) The number of lymph nodes removed predicts survival in esophageal cancer: an international study on the impact of extent of surgical resection. Ann Surg 248:549-556
25. Herrera LJ (2010) Extent of lymphadenectomy in esophageal cancer: how many lymph nodes is enough? Ann Surg Oncol 17:676-678
26. Hu Y, Hu C, Zhang H et al (2010) How does the number of resected lymph nodes influence TNM staging and prognosis for esophageal carcinoma? Ann Surg Oncol 17:784-790
27. Groth SS, Virnig BA, Whitson BA et al (2010) Determination of the minimum number of lymph nodes to examine to maximize survival in patients with esophageal carcinoma: data from the Surveillance Epidemiology and End Results database. J Thorac Cardiovasc Surg 139:612-620
28. Tachimori Y, Nagai Y, Kanamori N et al (2011) Pattern of lymph node metastases of esophageal squamous cell carcinoma based on the anatomical lymphatic drainage system. Dis Esophagus 24:33-38
29. Smit JK, Pultrum BB, van Dullemen HM et al (2010) Prognostic factors and patterns of recurrence in esophageal cancer assert arguments for extended two-field transthoracic esophagectomy. Am J Surg 200:446-453
30. Johansson J, DeMeester TR, Hagen JA (2004) En bloc vs transhiatal esophagectomy for stage T3 N1 adenocarcinoma of the distal esophagus. Arch Surg 139:627-631
31. Omloo JM, Lagarde SM, Hulscher JB (2007) Extended transthoracic resection compared with limited transhiatal resection for adenocarcinoma of the mid/distal esophagus: five-year survival of a randomized clinical trial. Ann Surg 246:992-1000
32. Twine CP, Lewis WG, Morgan MA (2009) The assessment of prognosis of surgically resected oesophageal cancer is dependent on the number of lymph nodes examined pathologically. Histopathology 55:46-52
33. Schwarz RE, Smith DD (2007) Clinical impact of lymphadenectomy extent in resectable esophageal cancer. J Gastrointest Surg 11:1384-1393
34. Bollschweiler E, Besch S, Drebber U (2010) Influence of neoadjuvant chemoradiation on the number and size of analyzed lymph nodes in esophageal cancer. Ann Surg Oncol 17:3187-3194
35. Jamieson GG, Lamb PJ, Thompson SK (2009) The role of lymphadenectomy in esophageal cancer. Ann Surg 250:206-209
36. Qubain SW, Natsugoe S, Matsumoto M (2001) Micrometastases in the cervical lymph nodes in esophageal squamous cell carcinoma. Dis Esophagus 14:143-148
37. Tachibana M, Kinugasa S, Hirahara N, Yoshimura H (2008) Lymph node classification of esophageal squamous cell carcinoma and adenocarcinoma. Eur J Cardiothorac Surg 34:427-431
38. Kuge K, Murakami G, Mizobuchi S et al (2003) Submucosal territory of the direct lymphatic drainage system to the thoracic duct in the human esophagus. J Thorac Cardiovasc Surg 125:1343-1349

39. Chen J, Liu S, Pan J et al (2009) The pattern and prevalence of lymphatic spread in thoracic oesophageal squamous cell carcinoma. Eur J Cardiothorac Surg 36:480-486
40. Motoyama S, Maruyama K, Sato Y et al (2009) Status of involved lymph nodes and direction of metastatic lymphatic flow between submucosal and t2-4 thoracic squamous cell esophageal cancers. World J Surg 33:512-517
41. Nakagawa S, Nishimaki T, Kosugi S et al (2003) Cervical lymphadenectomy is beneficial for patients with carcinoma of the upper and mid-thoracic esophagus. Dis Esophagus 16:4-8
42. Lerut T, Nafteux P, Moons J et al (2004) Three-field lymphadenectomy for carcinoma of the esophagus and gastroesophageal junction in 174 R0 resections: impact on staging, disease-free survival, and outcome: a plea for adaptation of TNM classification in upper-half esophageal carcinoma. Ann Surg 240:962-972
43. Tachibana M, Hirahara N, Kinugasa S, Yoshimura H (2008) Clinicopathologic features of superficial esophageal cancer: results of consecutive 100 patients. Ann Surg Oncol 15:104-116
44. Mariette C, Piessen G, Balon JM et al (2004) Surgery alone in the curative treatment of localised oesophageal carcinoma. Eur J Surg Oncol 30:869-876
45. Ancona E, Rampado S, Cassaro M et al (2008) Prediction of lymph node status in superficial esophageal carcinoma. Ann Surg Oncol 15:3278-3288
46. Altorki N, Kent M, Ferrara C, Port J (2002) Three-field lymph node dissection for squamous cell and adenocarcinoma of the esophagus. Ann Surg 236:177-183
47. Prenzel KL, Bollschweiler E, Schroder W et al (2010) Prognostic relevance of skip metastases in esophageal cancer. Ann Thorac Surg 90:1662-1667
48. Fumagalli U, Akiyama H, DeMeester T (1996) Resective Surgery for Cancer of the Thoracic Esophagus: Results of a Consensus Conference held at the VIth World Congress of the International Society for Diseases of the Esophagus. Diseases of the Esophagus 9:30-38
49. Fujita H, Sueyoshi S, Tanaka T et al (2003) Optimal lymphadenectomy for squamous cell carcinoma in the thoracic esophagus: comparing the short- and long-term outcome among the four types of lymphadenectomy. World J Surg 27:571-579
50. Altorki N (2005) En-bloc esophagectomy-the three-field dissection. In: Landreneau RJ, Martin RF (eds) Esophageal surgery, vol 85. Elsevier-Surgical Clinics of North America, pp 611-619
51. Tachibana M, Kinugasa S, Yoshimura H et al (2004) En-bloc esophagectomy for esophageal cancer. Am J Surg 188:254-260
52. Fang W, Kato H, Tachimori Y et al (2003) Analysis of pulmonary complications after three-field lymph node dissection for esophageal cancer. Ann Thorac Surg 76:903-908
53. Tachibana M, Kinugasa S, Yoshimura H (2005) Clinical outcomes of extended esophagectomy with three-field lymph node dissection for esophageal squamous cell carcinoma. Am J Surg 189:98-109
54. Fang WT, Chen WH, Chen Y, Jiang Y (2007) Selective three-field lymphadenectomy for thoracic esophageal squamous carcinoma. Dis Esophagus 20:206-211
55. Shim YM, Kim HK, Kim K (2010) Comparison of survival and recurrence pattern between two-field and three-field lymph node dissections for upper thoracic esophageal squamous cell carcinoma. J Thorac Oncol 5:707-712
56. Igaki H, Tachimori Y, Kato H (2004) Improved survival for patients with upper and/or middle mediastinal lymph node metastasis of squamous cell carcinoma of the lower thoracic esophagus treated with 3-field dissection. Ann Surg 239:483-490
57. Nishihira T, Hirayama K, Mori S (1998) A prospective randomized trial of extended cervical and superior mediastinal lymphadenectomy for carcinoma of the thoracic esophagus. Am J Surg 175:47-51
58. Law S, Wong J (2001) Two-field dissection is enough for esophageal cancer. Dis Esophagus 14:98-103
59. Nozoe T, Kakeji Y, Baba H, Maehara Y (2005) Two-field lymph-node dissection may be enough to treat patients with submucosal squamous cell carcinoma of the thoracic esophagus. Dis Esophagus 18:226-229

60. Shimada H, Okazumi S, Shiratori T et al (2009) Mode of lymphadenectomy and surgical outcome of upper thoracic esophageal squamous cell carcinoma. J Gastrointest Surg 13:619-625
61. Griffith JF, Chan AC, Ahuja AT et al (2000) Neck ultrasound in staging squamous oesophageal carcinoma - a high yield technique. Clin Radiol 55:696-701
62. van Vliet EP, van der Lugt A, Kuipers EJ (2007) Ultrasound, computed tomography, or the combination for the detection of supraclavicular lymph nodes in patients with esophageal or gastric cardia cancer: a comparative study. J Surg Oncol 96:200-206
63. Natsugoe S, Matsumoto M, Okumura H (2010) Clinical course and outcome after esophagectomy with three-field lymphadenectomy in esophageal cancer. Langenbecks Arch Surg 395:341-346
64. Tachibana M, Kinugasa S, Yoshimura H et al (2003) Extended esophagectomy with 3-field lymph node dissection for esophageal cancer. Arch Surg 138:1383-1389
65. Tabira Y, Yasunaga M, Tanaka M et al (2000) Recurrent nerve nodal involvement is associated with cervical nodal metastasis in thoracic esophageal carcinoma. J Am Coll Surg 191:232-237
66. Shiozaki H, Yano M, Tsujinaka T et al (2001) Lymph node metastasis along the recurrent nerve chain is an indication for cervical lymph node dissection in thoracic esophageal cancer. Dis Esophagus 14:191-196
67. Sato F, Shimada Y, Li Z et al (2002) Paratracheal lymph node metastasis is associated with cervical lymph node metastasis in patients with thoracic esophageal squamous cell carcinoma. Ann Surg Oncol 9:65-70
68. Puli SR, Reddy JB, Bechtold ML et al (2008) Staging accuracy of esophageal cancer by endoscopic ultrasound: a meta-analysis and systematic review. World J Gastroenterol 14:1479-1490
69. Chang AC, Ji H, Birkmeyer NJ et al (2008) Outcomes after transhiatal and transthoracic esophagectomy for cancer. Ann Thorac Surg 85:424-429
70. Barreto JC, Posner MC (2010) Transhiatal versus transthoracic esophagectomy for esophageal cancer. World J Gastroenterol 16:3804-3810
71. Connors RC, Reuben BC, Neumayer LA, Bull DA (2007) Comparing outcomes after transthoracic and transhiatal esophagectomy: a 5-year prospective cohort of 17,395 patients. J Am Coll Surg 205:735-740
72. Junginger T, Gockel I, Heckhoff S (2006) A comparison of transhiatal and transthoracic resections on the prognosis in patients with squamous cell carcinoma of the esophagus. Eur J Surg Oncol 32:749-755
73. Rentz J, Bull D, Harpole D (2003) Transthoracic versus transhiatal esophagectomy: a prospective study of 945 patients. J Thorac Cardiovasc Surg 125:1114-1120
74. Wolff CS, Castillo SF, Larson DR (2008) Ivor Lewis approach is superior to transhiatal approach in retrieval of lymph nodes at esophagectomy. Dis Esophagus 21:328-333
75. Yekebas EF, Schurr PG, Kaifi JT et al (2006) Effectiveness of radical en-bloc-esophagectomy compared to transhiatal esophagectomy in squamous cell cancer of the esophagus is influenced by nodal micrometastases. J Surg Oncol 93:541-549
76. Grotenhuis BA, van Heijl M, Zehetner J (2010) Surgical management of submucosal esophageal cancer: extended or regional lymphadenectomy? Ann Surg 252:823-830

Treatment of Resectable Esophageal Cancer: Indications and Long-term Results

14

Giovanni de Manzoni, Andrea Zanoni, and Jacopo Weindelmayer

14.1 Introduction

The therapeutic strategy in squamous cell carcinoma of the esophagus depends on the possibility to obtain a R0 resection, which is deemed essential in the cure of this disease. An understanding of the routes of neoplastic diffusion is thus the first step in planning treatment strategy. This chapter addresses both the indications for surgical resection and the long-term results with respect to survival and patterns of recurrence.

The surgical strategy depends on the extent of neoplastic diffusion, evaluated in terms of intramural diffusion (T) and nodal status (N) [1, 2]. Nodal spread is a main prognostic determinant, considering both the site and the number of involved nodes, and is also strictly correlated with intramural diffusion of the cancer [1]. Lymphatic diffusion is discussed in detail in Chap. 13. Briefly, there are two routes of lymphatic drainage: (a) longitudinal submucosal, involved in the presence of skip metastases even in early cancers, and (b) intermuscular, through the muscularis propria. Different patterns of nodal diffusion can be seen according to the site of the cancer and the depth of tumor invasion through the esophageal wall.

14.2 Indications

Treatment strategy depends on three main points, all related to the neoplasm: site of primary tumor, depth of tumor invasion, and nodal involvement. Also of utmost importance is the performance status of the patient: a poor clinical

G. de Manzoni (✉)
Dept. of Surgery, Upper G.I. Surgery Division, University of Verona,
Verona, Italy

G. de Manzoni (Ed.), *Treatment of Esophageal and Hypopharyngeal Squamous Cell Carcinoma*,

condition might prevent the use of multimodal treatments or limit the surgical approach.

If clinical conditions allow the use of the best treatment possibility, a practical flow-chart for this disease can be drawn. By subdividing the patients on the basis of T stage, it is possible to dichotomize the tumors as either superficial or early cancers, if the neoplasm is confined to the mucosa and submucosa, independent of nodal involvement, or advanced cancers, from T2 to T4.

14.2.1 Superficial Cancer

T1m-T1sm

A superficial cancer of the esophagus is defined as a cancer with invasion within the submucosa [3-5]. The depth of invasion of superficial cancers can be classified into six categories based on the pathological examination of specimens obtained with surgery or endoscopic resection (endoscopic mucosal resection, EMR; endoscopic submucosal dissection, ESD). Mucosal cancers can be intraepithelial (m1), invade the lamina propria (m2), or infiltrate the muscularis mucosae (m3). Submucosal cancers are instead classified into those invading the upper third of the submucosa up to 200 µm (sm1), those invading the middle third (sm2), and those invading the deeper third (sm3) (Fig. 14.1) [3-5].

The rate of superficial squamous cell carcinoma (SCC) in Japan is between 15% and 30% [4-6]. In Western countries, the incidence is much lower than in Japan because of the lack of screening programs for upper-gastrointestinal malignancies [4].

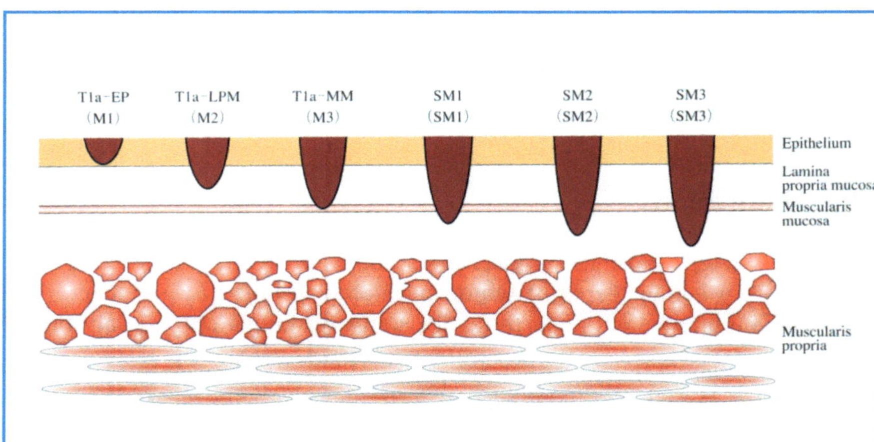

Fig. 14.1 Depth of tumor invasion in superficial squamous cell carcinoma (SCC) of the esophagus. (Reproduced from [5], with permission)

T1m1-m2 tumors do not reach the lymphatic vessels; thus excluding lymphatic metastases or systemic diffusion. T1m3 tumors reach the lymphatic pathways, with a non-negligible rate of node metastases of 16% in some reports [7], with a mean value of 10% [3-9].

Some studies report that in T1sm1 the probability of N+ is similar to that for T1m3 but in other trials nodal involvement was a significant 53% [7, 8].

T1sm2-3 tumors have a high incidence of nodal involvement, with a metastasis rate of up to 75% [3, 4, 7-9].

Endoscopic resection can be performed only if the lymphatic metastasis risk is absent or at least very low, because of the impossibility to carry out any type of lymphadenectomy. The indications for the treatment of superficial SCC thus consist of endoscopic resection for m1-m2, while for sm a surgical resection with lymphadenectomy is mandatory. The deeper mucosal cancers (m3) are controversially discussed. The more conservative approach to m3 is to avoid lymphadenectomy [3], but usually a more aggressive approach is preferred, because of the non-ignorable incidence of nodal metastases.

ESD can achieve a high R0 rate (78–95% [3]) with respect to T stage if applied with the correct indications, and is associated with a low perforation rate (0–6.4%) [3]. After ESD, if m1-m2 is confirmed histologically, a strict follow-up is feasible; if, instead, the cancer is m3 or sm, an esophagectomy with nodal dissection is necessary [3, 4].

Neoadjuvant treatments are a therapeutic option even for cT1sm, particularly if nodal involvement is clinically evident preoperatively. In our institution, we prefer to treat patients with neoadjuvant chemoradiation followed by surgery, even for cT1sm tumors or in any case of preoperatively detected nodal metastases.

In summary, endoscopic resection is the preferred option for m1-m2 cancers, while surgical resection with lymphadenectomy remains the standard treatment for m3 and sm cancers. Neoadjuvant treatment for early cancers is still a matter of debate, but it has been used with some success by dedicated centers.

14.2.2 Advanced Cancer

T2-T3

Locally advanced cancers (T2-3Nx) can be treated either with surgery alone or with multimodal treatments, consisting of neoadjuvant or definitive chemotherapy, radiotherapy, or both. An upfront surgical resection with radical intent is sometimes hardly applicable, resulting, in some trials, in lower survival than after neoadjuvant treatment. Mariette et al. [10] reported that in dedicated centers good survival can be achieved with surgery alone for T2-3N0 patients, reaching a 5-year overall survival of 49%. Survival decreases rapidly in patients with N+ disease: 27% for T1-2 and 17% for T3-4. The poor survival rates have prompted the use of multimodal treatments to improve the long-term results. The use of neoadjuvant therapies, particularly chemo- and radiotherapy (CRT) combined, has led to the creation of a new histological class: pathological complete responders (pCR), i.e., patients with no residual cancer both at the site of the primary tumor and at nodal status after lymphadenectomy. Neoadjuvant therapies are fully described in Chap. 12. Briefly, according to the current literature and our personal experience, pCR patients show an improved survival and a lower recurrence rate than either partial responders or non-responders.

In our institution, patients with T2-3 cancers are administered neoadjuvant treatment consisting of CRT (50 Gy of RT along with 5-fluorouracil, cisplatin, and docetaxel [11]). Surgery, with radical intent and extended lymphadenectomy, is performed 6-8 weeks after completion of CRT.

T4

The surgical approach to T4 carcinomas depends on the possibility to obtain a R0 resection. T4b cancers (unresectable tumors invading vital adjacent structures, such as the aorta, vertebral body, and trachea) can hardly be surgically resected and are instead frequently treated with definitive palliative chemotherapy or CRT.

A T4a cancer (resectable tumor invading the pleura, pericardium, or diaphragm) can be treated either with surgical resection or multimodal treatments. As upfront surgery is in most cases highly demanding, the use of chemotherapy or CRT might be advantageous, by downsizing the tumor, making resection less invasive with a higher chance to obtain R0, and by sterilizing nodal metastases, which are very common in T4 cancers.

The role of neoadjuvant therapy in patients with clinical evidence of adjacent organ invasion (cT4) has been investigated. As described in a paper from our institution [12], a number of cT4b tumors involving the aorta and trachea were treated with induction CRT and surgery. R0 resection was possible in 39% of the patients, with pathologic downstaging and pCR in 35% and 14% of the cases, respectively. The 5-year overall survival of the whole study population was only 5.9%. However, the best results were obtained in patients with aortic invasion, in whom 3-year survival was 31%. Dismal results were found for all other types of infiltration. A significantly detectable survival benefit was noted in R0 patients and responders to therapy compared with R+ and non-responders, respectively. In summary, patients with cT4b treated with CRT followed by surgery can obtain some benefit, even if the prognosis remains poor.

14.2.3 Definitive CRT

Definitive CRT has been proposed by some authors as a substitute for neoadjuvant treatment for locally advanced SCC. Two recent phase III randomized studies [13, 14] compared neoadjuvant CRT and surgery with definitive CRT.

In both studies, patients had cT3-4Nx SCC of the thoracic esophagus. In the German study, patients in the neoadjuvant arm were treated with 40 Gy, and those in the definitive CRT arm with 60 Gy, compared with 45 Gy and 66 Gy, respectively, for patients in the French trial. Of note, in both studies a suboptimal dose of RT was delivered in the neoadjuvant arms. The two studies achieved comparable results in terms of survival; indeed, an equivalent survival was obtained for both arms. The 2-year overall survival was 40% and 35%, respectively, for neoadjuvant and definitive CRT in the German study, and 34% and 40%, respectively, for the French one.

Treatment-related mortality was significantly higher in both studies for the neoadjuvant + surgery group, which nevertheless had a longer period of freedom from local progression. Stahl et al., however, showed that non-responders to chemoradiation who were treated with surgery with radical intent had an improved survival, compared with non-surgical cases. The conclusion drawn by the authors of these trials was that equivalent survival with less toxicity makes definitive CRT a feasible treatment strategy for responders to CRT, while surgery is still the only reasonable option for non-responders. Salvage surgery after such a high dose of RT remains an open question. Randomized studies comparing a definitive CRT with a neoadjuvant arm consisting of 50 Gy of RT could be useful to better define the role of this kind of treatment.

14.2.4 Salvage Surgery

Salvage surgery [15-20] has been proposed for persistent or recurrent local disease in esophageal cancer after definitive CRT. It is mainly offered to patients with SCC, but studies are limited and with a low volume of patients.

As mentioned previously, in definitive CRT a higher RT dose is delivered, reaching 65 Gy in many trials. Recently, in the USA, RT protocols consisted of a lower dose of 50.4 Gy as the maximum, while in Japan the standard is still 65 Gy.

After definitive CRT, as after neoadjuvant therapy, patients may have a complete response, partial response, or persistent disease. Difficulties in distinguishing the three groups based on imaging, endoscopy, and PET-CT findings explain the very high rate of persistent or recurrent local disease. The reported value of early treatment failure is 40–60% within the first year. After local disease appearance, surgery is the only viable therapeutic possibility, as the maximum dose of RT has already been reached.

As determined from the current literature, there are many more potential candidates for salvage surgery than patients treated with this approach. According to the best trials, 30% of the patients with local recurrence are eligible for salvage surgery; instead, these patients are often treated with palliative care regardless of the possibility of curative treatment. This is probably due to lack of defined follow-up protocols and selection criteria and it often leads to tumor progression to an inoperable state in case of ineffective follow-up.

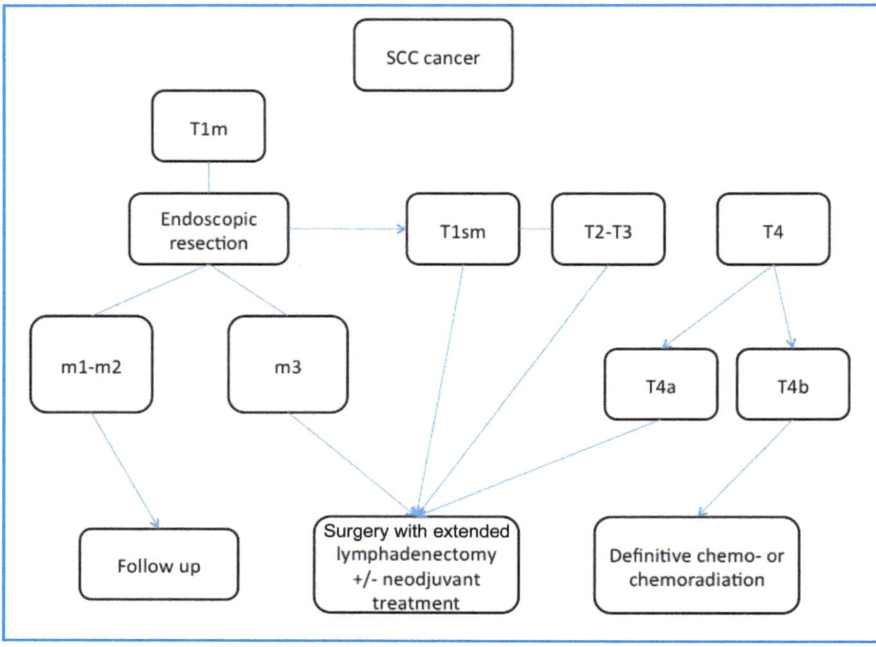

Fig. 14.2 Proposed flow-chart according to T stage

The most important limit of salvage surgery is the technical difficulty due to inflammation in the early period after CRT and to fibrosis later on. Both conditions make surgery more difficult and dangerous, accounting for the higher morbidity and mortality (8–20%) than following neoadjuvant therapy preceding immediate surgery.

R0 resection is the main prognostic factor associated with long-term survival. The 5-year overall survival for R0 patients is between 25 and 35%.

Although the high frequency of complications is a concern, salvage surgery is probably the only treatment that offers any chance of long-term survival in locally recurrent SCC after definitive CRT.

14.2.5 Conclusions

In summary, it is possible to draw a simple flow-chart of the approach to SCC of the esophagus (Fig. 14.2). For T1m1-m2 cancers, endoscopic resection or limited surgical resection is indicated. T1m3 and T1sm cancers should be treated using radical surgery with lymphadenectomy. Neoadjuvant CRT can be evaluated, especially in case of clinical nodal involvement. Locally advanced T2-3 cancers are treated either with surgery alone or, probably more appropriately, with neoadjuvant therapy followed by surgery. Extended lymphadenectomy is anyway mandatory.

To improve surgical resectability, neoadjuvant therapy followed by surgery is indicated for T4a and selected cases of T4b (aorta limited invasion) tumors, while palliative chemo- or chemoradiation is the treatment of choice for all other T4b tumors.

The role of definitive chemoradiotherapy with potential salvage surgery for SCC is still undefined. The difficulties related to salvage surgical resection and lymphadenectomy after high dose of RT (60–65 Gy), the inability to define clinical complete response to treatment, and the high rate of recurrences within the first year make this approach less well accepted than surgery alone or neoadjuvant CRT followed by surgery.

14.3 Long-term Results

14.3.1 Surgery Alone

Esophageal SCC has a poor prognosis, although some steps have been taken in improving survival. Survival with surgery alone is 10–35% at 5 years [7, 9] and recurrence reaches 50% within 12 months [21-23]. Survival data, dividing patients in groups according to T, N and stage, are reported in Tables 14.1, [24-26] and 14.2 [27-29].

Nodal status is a main prognostic feature; in fact, in all trials, N+ patients have a dismal 5-year survival, reaching 37% in the best case, compared to an overall survival of 46–75% in node-negative patients.

Survival decreases with increasing depth of tumor invasion. Patients with pT1is and T1m cancers treated with surgical resection have a 5-year survival of around 100%, while survival between 50% and 80% is reported for those with all pT1 tumors. Survival decreases for pT2 to 37–62% and to 19–31% for pT3. Where reported, pT4 patients did not show a 5-year survival over 10%.

Table 14.1 5-year overall survival according to T, N and pTNM stage with surgery alone

<table>
<tr><th></th><th>Mariette et al. [24]</th><th>Hsu et al. [25]</th><th>Lerut et al. [26]</th></tr>
<tr><td>T1</td><td>74%</td><td>49%</td><td></td></tr>
<tr><td>T2</td><td>37%</td><td>39%</td><td></td></tr>
<tr><td>T3</td><td>50%</td><td>23%</td><td></td></tr>
<tr><td>T4</td><td></td><td>10%</td><td></td></tr>
<tr><td>N0</td><td>68%</td><td>46%</td><td></td></tr>
<tr><td>N+</td><td>27%</td><td>21%</td><td></td></tr>
<tr><td>Stage I</td><td>84%</td><td></td><td>100%</td></tr>
<tr><td>Stage IIA</td><td>49%</td><td></td><td rowspan="2">59%</td></tr>
<tr><td>Stage IIB</td><td>27%</td><td></td></tr>
<tr><td>Stage III</td><td></td><td></td><td>37%</td></tr>
</table>

Table 14.2 5-year overall survival according to T, N and pTNM stage (neoadjuvant therapy in a percentage from 20% to 50% of the cases)

	Mariette et al. [27]	Law et al. [28]	Thompson et al. [29]	Altorki et al. [30]
T0	74%		63%	
T1	69%		53%	
T2	49%		42%	
T3	19%		25%	
N0	61%		53%	
N+	22%		18%	
Stage 0	76%	59%	63%	
Stage I	79%	38%	64%	88%
Stage IIA	46%	34%	43%	84%
Stage IIB	41%		42%	30%
Stage III	13%	9%	12%	54%

14.3.2 Multimodal Treatments

In meta-analyses, chemoradiation proved to be the best treatment choice, especially when concurrent chemoradiation was used [31-34]. This led many centers to adopt neoadjuvant concurrent chemoradiotherapy as the standard of care [35, 36]. In our institution, the protocol consists of 5-fluorouracil (5-FU) administered by protracted intravenous infusion (PVI) with weekly administration of i.v. cisplatin and docetaxel [11]. The first cycle consists of chemotherapy alone and is followed by a second cycle of concurrent chemoradiotherapy (50 Gy in total). The surgical procedure is performed between the 6th and the 8th weeks after completion of the treatment.

Re-staging after induction treatment is difficult, because of the pathological modifications in the esophageal wall and lymph nodes. Moreover, TNM staging after therapy has important limitations (Chap. 2).

To our knowledge, only two trials evaluated the importance of downstaging N status after neoadjuvant therapy [37, 38] for esophageal cancer, one of which was based on adenocarcinoma only. Both studies compared retrospectively a group of patients with downstaged N0 cancers after induction treatment with a group of surgery-only patients. Both trials found a statistically detectable survival advantage in favor of "real" N0 patients, i.e., those with both clinical and pathological N0, compared with the downstaged patients. Also, downstaged N0 patients had a better outcome than N+ patients. The results of these studies indicate an improvement in survival for patients with downstaged compared with N+ disease, even if the tumors in the former group cannot be considered as "real" N0.

A significant response to treatment, especially pCR, consisting of complete regression of the neoplasm with the absence of residual cancer, both at the primary site and the nodal level, is related to better outcome [31]. The pCR rate is between 11% and 43% where reported [38-40], with a mean R0 resection rate of 76% [39-41]. The lower pCR rate was obtained in trials using a lower radiation dose (20 Gy of RT), which is now considered suboptimal. In our experience, R0 resection was achieved in 95% of the patients who were operated on and underwent tumor resection. Our pCR rate was 47% in patients with resected disease and 40% of all patients treated who received induction CRT.

Between 1987 and 2000 [42], patients treated with induction CRT followed by surgery at our institution underwent the Al-Sarraf protocol (with cisplatin and 5-FU), initially with 40 Gy of RT. The 5-year overall survival of patients with R0 resected disease was 37%, which increased to 43% in those administered a 50-Gy dose of RT. Patients with a pCR had a 5-year overall survival rate of 75%. For pT4 patients, a survival advantage, even of low power, was seen in responders to therapy and R0 resection [42].

The current protocol of concurrent CRT with 5-FU, cisplatin, and docetaxel has been implemented since 2000, achieving a 44% 5-year overall survival for SCC and a more impressive 58% in disease-related survival. Considering pCR, the 5-year overall survival has remained 75%, with 87% disease-related survival. Dismal results are seen in non-responders to treatment, while an intermediate survival rate is suggested in partial responders to treatment (Fig. 14.3).

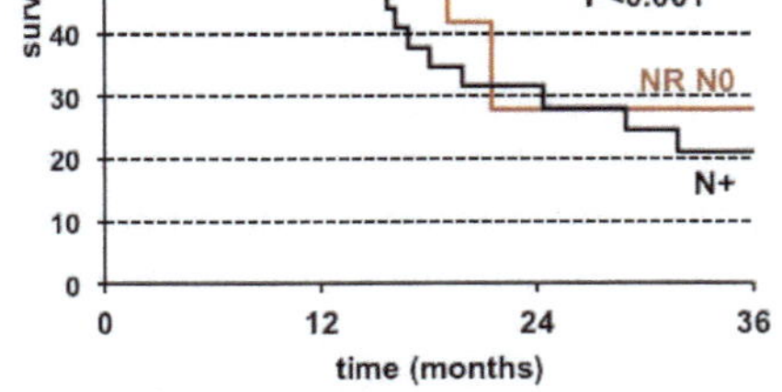

New classification

	0	12	24	36
ypT0	44	38	29	22
MRD	16	12	7	6
NR	9	4	2	1
N+	39	21	9	6

Fig. 14.3 Three-year disease-related survival curves for patients staged with SPR (size-based pathological response) classification of response ($p < 0.001$) [43]. *ypT0*, Pathological tumor category 0 after chemoradiotherapy (complete response); *N0*, no nodal involvement; *MRD*, minimal residual disease; *NR*, non response; *N+*, nodal involvement

Table 14.3 5-year survival after chemoradiotherapy and surgery according to response. Only one study considered the nodal status

	Mariette et al. [27]	Verlato et al. *[43]	Meredith et al. [44]
pCR	75%	85%	52%
pPR	55%	58%	36%
pNR	24%	28%	22%
pN+		21%	

*survival expressed as 3-year disease related survival.

Survival according to response to induction treatment, however, is still a matter of debate. Table 14.3 [27, 43, 44] presents the distinction made in terms of response: complete, partial, or no response. Only a study, published by our group [43], reported survival according to nodal status, which we believe to be a main prognostic parameter. Survival in this trial was defined as 3-year disease-related survival.

Non-responders demonstrated a dismal prognosis, not surpassing a 30% survival rate in any study. The table shows that there is indeed a class consisting of partial responders; these patients have an intermediate prognosis to that of complete responders and non-responders.

As neoadjuvant treatments are increasingly adopted in numerous centers, it becomes crucial to analyze the definition of response to treatment.

14.4 Recurrence

In the current literature, the recurrence rate of any site after surgery alone is between 34 and 79%, most commonly around 50% [21-23]. The recurrence rate after neoadjuvant CRT is similar to that achieved with surgery alone in past studies, but recent trials have shown a reduced recurrence rate at any site, with an American trial reporting 31.5% [44].

14.4.1 Timing and Diagnosis

Recurrence can become evident either in the presence of clinical symptoms or during follow-up in asymptomatic patients. Recurrence is diagnosed with imaging and endoscopy (gastroscopy and bronchoscopy). The most frequently used imaging tools are CT, typically in investigations of the neck, chest, and abdomen, and ultrasonography of the cervical region. If recurrence is suspected, PET-CT is a viable tool to better identify relapse but is still a second-line option in the follow-up of patients operated on for SCC. The correct timing of follow-up examinations has not been defined but most recurrences become evident within the first 2 years after surgery. Some authors propose very frequent controls for the first few years, for instance every 3 months for the first 2 years [21]. Others recommend annual checks [23, 46]. We recommend controls every 6 months for the first 5 years, followed by annual controls for the subsequent 5 years. The rationale of follow-up is to allow for the early detection of recurrence, since therapy for disease relapse is possible in selected cases with localized disease.

14.4.2 Type of Recurrence

Recurrence can be locoregional, systemic, or mixed. Locoregional relapse comprises recurrence at the anastomotic site into the esophageal wall, at the esophageal bed, or at locoregional nodes. Lymph node involvement is by far the most common cause of locoregional recurrence.

Systemic relapse refers to the involvement of non-regional nodes and to hematological spread of the cancer, with the liver and lungs as the mainly involved sites, followed by bone and brain. A very recent trial [47] investigated the pattern of disease recurrence in nearly 300 patients with non-metastatic esophageal SCC who underwent transthoracic esophagectomy without previous neoadjuvant CRT. The authors found that, among the distant recurrences, 47% consisted of lung relapse, 31% liver, 24% bone, 7% brain, and other rare metachronous metastases for the remaining cases. A similar incidence of hematogenous recurrence is reported in the recent literature.

Mixed relapse consists of the concomitant detection of locoregional and systemic disease, regardless of which appeared first.

14.4.3 Recurrence after Surgery Alone

The pattern of recurrence in patients treated with surgery alone is equally distributed between locoregional and systemic or mixed relapse, with 50/50 reported in numerous studies [21-23]. There have also been a number of studies, published over the last 10 years, in which the rate and the pattern of recurrence were described (Table 14.4) [21, 23, 46, 48-53]. Japanese and French trials refer mainly to SCC, while studies from other Western countries pertain mainly to adenocarcinoma. In most centers today, adjuvant therapies are administered in a large number of cases. The employment of chemotherapy, radiotherapy, or both has confounded the interpretation of data on recurrence. In the above-cited trials, lymphadenectomy, consisting of either two-field or three-field dissection, was always performed. As shown in Table 14.4, the median recurrence rate for these trials was 49% (range: 25–59%) and the median time-to-recurrence 11–12 months.

The recurrence pattern reported in the above-mentioned studies is shown in Table 14.5 [21, 23, 46, 48-53]. Among the patients with recurrence, a median of 44% had solo locoregional relapse, 37% systemic relapse, and 20% mixed

Table 14.4 Recurrence rate and median time-to-recurrence in surgery alone patients

Author [Reference]	SCC/Adenocr	Adjuvant	Lymphadenectomy	Recurrence (%)	Timing (months)
Nakagawa et al. [23]	100%/0%	66%	3-F	43%	11
Dresner et al. [46]	36%/64%	11%	2-F	48%	12
Chen et al. [21]	100%/0%	43%	2-F	49%	12
Smit et al. [52]	15%/85%	8%	2-F	59%	n.r.
Natsugoe et al. [48]	95%/5%	44%	3-F	50%	11
Kunisaki et al. [50]	n.r.	35%	2-F(75%) 3-F(25%)	43%	12
Tachibana et al. [53]	100%/0%	29%	3-F	25%	n.r.
Mariette et al. [51]	85%/15%	0%	2-F	52%	12
Kang et al. [49]	100%/0%	0%	2-F	54%	12

n.r., not reported

Table 14.5 Pattern of recurrence for the patients with relapse in surgery alone patients

Author [Reference]	Locoregional	Systemic	Mixed
Nakagawa et al. [23]	48%	44%	8%
Dresner et al. [46]	55%	37%	8%
Chen et al. [21]	54%	35%	11%
Smit et al. [52]	39%	61%	
Natsugoe et al. [48]	36%	30%	34%
Kunisaki et al. [50]	44%	36%	20%
Tachibana et al. [53]	40%	37%	23%
Mariette et al. [51]	62%	38%	n.r.
Kang et al. [49]	37%	43%	20%

n.r., not reported.

relapse. If mixed and systemic recurrences are considered together, the percentages of locoregional and systemic patterns was essentially the same.

A recent retrospective Korean study on upper thoracic SCC evaluated the pattern of failure after two-field and three-field lymphadenectomy [54]. The result of this study was a similar pattern for both groups, with an overlapping rate of cervical relapse and with locoregional relapses more frequent than systemic ones.

14.4.4 Recurrence after Neoadjuvant Therapy

The locoregional relapse rate is lower after neoadjuvant CRT, accounting for about one-third of the total recurrence rate [32, 41, 45]. A recent meta-analysis [32] found a lower locoregional recurrence rate than achieved with surgery alone, with not statistically different rates in terms of distant recurrence and all-cancer recurrence. In our personal experience with neoadjuvant CRT, the locoregional recurrence rate was 30%, compared with 70% for systemic or mixed relapse. However, even after CRT, we found a different pattern of recurrence in upper thoracic cancer, which consisted of locoregional failure in 47% of the cases, a value similar to that previously reported after surgery only [54]. Of note, a longer time-to-recurrence can probably be achieved with neoadjuvant CRT; indeed, in our database, patients who underwent chemoradiation followed by surgery had a median time-to-recurrence of 22 months, compared with the 11–12 months of surgery-only patients.

Two recent studies [45, 55] investigated the failure patterns after induction therapies, as noted in Western countries. The authors found, in both studies, a lower all-cancer recurrence after CRT than after surgery alone. These data were more significant in responders to treatment. Indeed, in one study [45] there was a trend to a lower incidence of metachronous metastases in pCR patients than in partial and non-responders; however, this difference was not confirmed by the other trial [55]. Both studies nonetheless showed a significant longer time to recurrence for pCR, and relapse was much more likely to be systemic rather than locoregional [45, 55]. A non-ignorable recurrence rate of 18–24% is seen in pCR patients, [45, 55, 56]. In our experience, the relapse rate for pCR was 18%. A very recent multicenter study [56] investigated the failure pattern for pCR alone. The authors found a significantly lower incidence of locoregional than systemic relapses, with a global recurrence rate of 23.4%.

14.4.5 Treatment of Recurrence

The best treatment for recurrences has not yet been defined, with recommendations varying depending on whether a surgical, chemotherapeutic, radiotherapeutic, or combined approach is appropriate for a particular patient [23, 46, 57, 58].

Systemic/Mixed Relapse

While mixed relapse or diffused systemic disease almost always requires non-surgical treatment (Chap. 17), an aggressive multimodal treatment involving surgery has been proposed for single distant metastases. It has been suggested that negative E-cadherin expression is a predictor of hematogenous recurrence, in particular in the liver and lung [59]; but the utility of detecting E-cadherin expression is currently only speculative.

Liver. A recent trial reported that liver recurrences represent 30% of all hematogenous relapses [48]. They are predictive of a much worse survival compared with all other types of hematogenous relapse.

Evidence for the best treatment of liver disease is still lacking. While in colorectal cancer surgical treatment for liver relapses is a well-known therapeutic procedure, for esophageal cancer there are only a few reports in the current literature. A recent trial investigated the role of liver surgery after relapse of SCC, but only two patients with esophageal cancer were enrolled [60], making it almost impossible to draw conclusions. A Japanese trial [61] investigated the efficacy of hepatic arterial infusion chemotherapy in eight patients with liver relapse of esophageal SCC, but surgical resection was not employed. Some Japanese case reports deal with surgical resection or CRT, but the paucity of data make them merely anecdotal. In summary, while there is still no defined therapy for liver recurrence, an aggressive attitude towards single liver relapses may ensure survival improvement.

Lung. Metachronous lung metastases from esophageal carcinoma account for nearly 40% of all hematogenous recurrences and for almost 8% of all-type recurrences. They are often detected as multiple lesions or in combination with extrapulmonary metastases. Hence, systemic chemotherapy is the usual approach for this disease whereas the utility of surgical metastasectomy of lung relapse is unclear and controversial [62, 63].

The results of three recent trials, each with a small sample size (5–49 patients) are shown in Table 14.6 [62-64]. Some of the patients in each trial were treated with chemotherapy, radiotherapy, or both before or after esophagectomy. The disease-free interval between esophagectomy and relapse was 14–21 months. All of the patients underwent pulmonary resection, with

Table 14.6 Pulmonary recurrence after radical surgery for thoracic SCC

Author [Reference]	N.	Previous CT or CRT	Type of surgery	DFI	OS	Relapse	Synchronous metastases
Chen et al. [64]	5	20%	Segmentectomy Wedge resection	21	24*	60%	n.r.
Shiono et al. [62]	49	36%	Segmentectomy Wedge resection Lobectomy Bilobectomy	14	30%	33%	n.r.
Ichikawa et al. [63]	23	56%	Bilateral wedge resection Wedge resections Segmentectomy Lobectomy	15	43%	66%	17%

DFI, disease-free interval expressed in months (median); *OS*, 5-year overall survival; *months (mean); *n.r.*, not reported.

different surgical modalities. Interestingly, in one study [63], 17% of the patients had synchronous extrapulmonary metastases. One trial [64] with only five patients reported a median survival of 24 months. In the other two trials [62, 63], 5-year overall survival was 30–43% but a re-recurrence rate of 33-66% was described. A disease-free interval < 12 months was shown to be an independent prognostic factor of worse outcome in multivariable analysis [62]. Moreover, univariate analysis showed that extrapulmonary metastases were an unfavorable prognostic factor [63]. Of note, in all the studies, the authors noted the extreme difficulty of distinguishing esophageal metastases from primary lung SCC, implying that some involuntary selection bias may have occurred [62, 63]. All surgical procedures were accompanied by a low morbidity (< 10%), with no mortality. Hence, the authors claimed that surgical resection is feasible and safe [62, 63]. In summary, for patients with disease-free intervals > 12 months, a metastasectomy is feasible for lung relapses involving a single node, or a single lobe not accompanied by the presence of extrapulmonary metastases. However, further studies with larger cohorts of patients are needed.

Brain. Brain metachronous metastases represent 7% of all hematological relapses [47] and < 2% of all-type recurrences [65, 66]. This could be an underestimation of the true incidence, because brain imaging is not routinely performed and asymptomatic cases can be missed [65, 67]. A significantly higher prevalence of brain metastases was encountered after chemoradiation, in contrast to surgery alone of the primary esophageal carcinoma [66].

Three studies on brain recurrence treatment, again, all small sample size trials (17–36 patients), are summarized in Table 14.7 [65, 67, 68]. In > 70% of the cases, brain relapse showed synchronous metastases at other anatomic sites. The disease-free interval between esophagectomy and brain relapse was 6–12 months. A single lesion was encountered in around half of the patients.

Table 14.7 Brain recurrence after radical surgery for thoracic SCC

Author [Reference]	N.	Single lesion	Multiple lesions	Type of treatment	DFI	OS	Synchronous metastases
Yoshida et al. [67]	17	65%	35%	Resection Resection and WBRT Radiosurgery	12	17 65 9	76%
Weinberg et al. [65]	27	48%	52%	Resection Radiotherapy Resection and WBRT Radiosurgery	6	4	70%
Ogawa et al. [68]	36	47%	53%	Resection and WBRT Radiotherapy	7	4	78%

DFI, disease-free interval expressed in months (median); *OS*, median overall survival (months); *WBRT*, whole brain radiotherapy.

The treatment consisted of resection with or without radiotherapy, radiotherapy alone, or radiosurgery. The survival of the whole population was extremely poor, with a median survival often under 6 months. Clearly, the small sample size prohibits adequate stratification and survival analysis. Nevertheless, single lesions in the absence of systemic disease probably deserve aggressive treatment [67].

Locoregional Relapse

Locoregional relapse can occur at the anastomotic site or at regional nodes. The latter can be divided into single resectable nodes and unresectable huge lymphatic masses. Unresectable masses necessitate non-surgical treatment and are dealt with in Chap. 17. Recent trials reported [57, 58, 69] a survival advantage for patients treated with an aggressive approach to resectable local recurrence, hence a strict follow-up with early detection of relapse could be reasonable.

Anastomotic relapse. This type of relapse shows up less frequently than relapse involving the nodal site and accounts for about 3% of all recurrences [70]. An American study [57] investigated recurrence at the anastomosis in an experimental study without a control group. After complete re-resection, even with a considerable morbidity-mortality, long-term survival seemed possible, with a 35% 5-year survival after re-resection for R0 patients. Noteworthy, most of the patients had adenocarcinoma of the distal esophagus and the main reconstruction type consisted of resection and re-anastomosis with the gastric conduit. An alternative was resection and anastomosis at the neck, via a coloplasty.

Resectable nodal recurrence. Two Japanese trials investigated lymph node recurrence after R0 esophageal resection for SCC only [58, 69]. Nakamura and colleagues [58] compared three types of treatment for nodal recurrence, considering retrospectively three groups of about 20 patients each: surgical resection of the recurrence, "curative" CRT, and palliation. With the limit of not being a randomized study, hence having evident selection bias, there was a statistically significant difference in survival in favor of patients treated with either surgery or CRT with respect to the palliated group. The comparison between CRT and surgery showed a trend in favor of surgery, without reaching statistical significance. Moreover, in the surgical group, lymphadenectomy proved to be useful in terms of radicality of resection, necessity of re-resection, further systemic relapses, and the survival of patients with disease involving only the nodes of the neck and thorax but not the abdominal para-aortic nodes, which should be considered systemic recurrences. The second Japanese study [69] investigated the role of "intensive" treatment for locoregional node recurrence, defined by the authors as chemoradiation or surgery, with respect to chemotherapy or best supportive care. A significant survival advantage was found for intensive care compared with palliation (41% vs. 0% 2-year overall survival). Surgery was employed in only two patients, so its exact role was not clarified in this trial. Another Japanese trial [71] reported similar results. Furthermore, in a case report study [72], two patients with lone nodal recurrence in the dorsal area of the thoracic aorta were successfully operated on via a left thoracotomy, again supporting an aggressive approach to recurrence.

A particular case is the lone cervical relapse, which is found in 5–17% of patients with recurrence [73, 74]. One study [74] reported the results of 10 patients treated with surgery followed by RT. The overall 5-year survival after resection of the recurrence was 25%. Another recent report on a small sample size [73] instead reported 2-year and 5-year survival rates after therapy of recurrence of 26 and 9%, but surgery was the treatment of choice in only one-third of the patients and no comparisons were made among the treatment possibilities. Of note, in this trial, the only prognostic factor in multivariable analysis was the presence of a single node recurrence. A third study [75] reported the results of five patients treated with resection of a cervical SCC relapse. The results for each patient were provided, without a survival analysis for the small sample size. The authors concluded that resection of a lone cervical relapse is a valuable therapeutic option.

The results of these trials, even with non-homogeneous types of treatment and with small sample size, suggest that treatment of regional nodal recurrence is feasible and confers a survival benefit over palliation. Surgery with or without CRT could be the mainstay of treatment, while surgery alone is indicated in patients previously treated with neoadjuvant CRT who have reached the maximum radiation dose.

14.5 Second Tumor and Tumor in the Gastric Tube

Relapse is a common cause of death after esophagectomy for cancer; nevertheless it has been reported [76] that long-term survivors with an initial N0 state not previously treated with neoadjuvant therapies have a higher risk of death due to second cancer than from recurrence. In the reported trial, after 3 years postoperatively, the major cause (> 50% of the patients) of death was a second malignancy.

A particular case of metachronous malignancies is a second primary tumor in the gastric tube, which is the most common conduit utilized to reconstruct the continuity of the gastrointestinal tract. The occurrence of gastric tube cancer is increasing because of improvements in patient survival. The reported incidence is about 2% [77, 78], with a mean time to recurrence of 60–100 months. A recent trial [78] reports a higher 10-year cumulative incidence (8.1%). Where attempted, surgical resection achieved poor results, with a median survival of 5 months [77], while endoscopic resection for early cancers seems promising, with an 81% 3-year survival after endoscopic resection in one study [78]. Long-term follow-up with gastroscopy can then lead to the early detection of asymptomatic patients, with increased survival.

References

1. Pedrazzani C, de Manzoni G, Marrelli D et al (2007) Lymph node involvement in advanced gastroesophageal junction adenocarcinoma. J Thorac Cardiovasc Surg 134:378-385
2. Pennathur A, Zhang J, Chen H, Luketich JD (2010) The "best operation" for esophageal cancer? Ann Thorac Surg 89:S2163-2167
3. Momma K (2010) Endoscopic diagnosis of superficial esophageal cancer. In: Society JE (ed) Endoscopic diagnosis and treatment of superficial esophageal cancer, pp 8-20
4. Stein HJ, Feith M, Bruecher BL et al (2005) Early esophageal cancer: pattern of lymphatic spread and prognostic factors for long-term survival after surgical resection. Ann Surg 242:566-573
5. Japanese Esophageal Society (2008) Japanese Classification of Esophageal Cancer, 10th edn. Kaneara & Co, Tokyo
6. Tachibana M, Hirahara N, Kinugasa S, Yoshimura H (2008) Clinicopathologic features of superficial esophageal cancer: results of consecutive 100 patients. Ann Surg Oncol 15:104-116
7. Tachibana M, Kinugasa S, Shibakita M et al (2006) Surgical treatment of superficial esophageal cancer. Langenbecks Arch Surg 391:304-321
8. Ancona E, Rampado S, Cassaro M et al (2008) Prediction of lymph node status in superficial esophageal carcinoma. Ann Surg Oncol 15:3278-3288
9. Bollschweiler E, Baldus SE, Schroder et al (2006) High rate of lymph-node metastasis in submucosal esophageal squamous-cell carcinomas and adenocarcinomas. Endoscopy 38:149-156
10. Mariette C, Piessen G, Triboulet JP (2007) Therapeutic strategies in oesophageal carcinoma: role of surgery and other modalities. Lancet Oncol 8:545-553
11. Pasini F, de Manzoni G, Pedrazzani C et al (2005) High pathological response rate in locally advanced esophageal cancer after neoadjuvant combined modality therapy: dose finding of a weekly chemotherapy schedule with protracted venous infusion of 5-fluorouracil and dose escalation of cisplatin, docetaxel and concurrent radiotherapy. Ann Oncol 16:1133-1139
12. de Manzoni G, Pedrazzani C, Pasini F et al (2007) Chemoradiotherapy followed by surgery for squamous cell carcinoma of the thoracic esophagus with clinical evidence of adjacent organ invasion. J Surg Oncol 95:261-266
13. Bedenne L, Michel P, Bouche O et al (2007) Chemoradiation followed by surgery compared with chemoradiation alone in squamous cancer of the esophagus: FFCD 9102. J Clin Oncol 25:1160-1168
14. Stahl M, Stuschke M, Lehmann N et al (2005) Chemoradiation with and without surgery in patients with locally advanced squamous cell carcinoma of the esophagus. J Clin Oncol 23:2310-2317
15. Gardner-Thorpe J, Hardwick RH, Dwerryhouse SJ (2007) Salvage oesophagectomy after local failure of definitive chemoradiotherapy. Br J Surg 94:1059-1066
16. Tachimori Y (2009) Role of salvage esophagectomy after definitive chemoradiotherapy. Gen Thorac Cardiovasc Surg 57:71-78
17. Borghesi S, Hawkins MA, Tait D (2008) Oesophagectomy after definitive chemoradiation in patients with locally advanced oesophageal cancer. Clin Oncol (R Coll Radiol) 20:221-226
18. D'Journo XB, Michelet P, Dahan L et al (2008) Indications and outcome of salvage surgery for oesophageal cancer. Eur J Cardiothorac Surg 33:1117-1123
19. Pinto CE, Fernandes Dde S, Sa EA, Mello EL (2009) Salvage esophagectomy after exclusive chemoradiotherapy: results at the Brazilian National Cancer Institute (INCA). Dis Esophagus 22:682-686
20. Tachimori Y, Kanamori N, Uemura N et al (2009) Salvage esophagectomy after high-dose chemoradiotherapy for esophageal squamous cell carcinoma. J Thorac Cardiovasc Surg 137:49-54
21. Chen G, Wang Z, Liu XY, Liu FY (2007) Recurrence pattern of squamous cell carcinoma in the middle thoracic esophagus after modified Ivor-Lewis esophagectomy. World J Surg 31:1107-1114

22. Lee SJ, Lee KS, Yim YJ et al (2005) Recurrence of squamous cell carcinoma of the oesophagus after curative surgery: rates and patterns on imaging studies correlated with tumour location and pathological stage. Clin Radiol 60:547-554
23. Nakagawa S, Kanda T, Kosugi S et al (2004) Recurrence pattern of squamous cell carcinoma of the thoracic esophagus after extended radical esophagectomy with three-field lymphadenectomy. J Am Coll Surg 198:205-211
24. Mariette C, Piessen G, Balon JM et al (2004) Surgery alone in the curative treatment of localised oesophageal carcinoma. Eur J Surg Oncol 30:869-876
25. Hsu PK, Wu YC, Chou TY et al (2010) Comparison of the 6th and 7th editions of the American Joint Committee on Cancer tumor-node-metastasis staging system in patients with resected esophageal carcinoma. Ann Thorac Surg 89:1024-1031
26. Lerut T, Nafteux P, Moons J et al (2004) Three-field lymphadenectomy for carcinoma of the esophagus and gastroesophageal junction in 174 R0 resections: impact on staging, disease-free survival, and outcome: a plea for adaptation of TNM classification in upper-half esophageal carcinoma. Ann Surg 240:962-972
27. Mariette C, Taillier G, Van Seuningen I, Triboulet JP (2004) Factors affecting postoperative course and survival after en bloc resection for esophageal carcinoma. Ann Thorac Surg 78:1177-1183
28. Law S, Kwong DL, Kwok KF et al (2003) Improvement in treatment results and long-term survival of patients with esophageal cancer: impact of chemoradiation and change in treatment strategy. Ann Surg 238:339-347
29. Thompson SK, Ruszkiewicz AR, Jamieson GG et al (2008) Improving the accuracy of TNM staging in esophageal cancer: a pathological review of resected specimens. Ann Surg Oncol 15:3447-3458
30. Altorki N, Kent M, Ferrara C, Port J (2002) Three-field lymph node dissection for squamous cell and adenocarcinoma of the esophagus. Ann Surg 236:177-183
31. Hyngstrom JR, Posner MC (2010) Neoadjuvant strategies for the treatment of locally advanced esophageal cancer. J Surg Oncol 101:299-304
32. Lv J, Cao XF, Zhu B et al (2009) Effect of neoadjuvant chemoradiotherapy on prognosis and surgery for esophageal carcinoma. World J Gastroenterol 15:4962-4968
33. Gebski V, Burmeister B, Smithers BM et al (2007) Survival benefits from neoadjuvant chemoradiotherapy or chemotherapy in oesophageal carcinoma: a meta-analysis. Lancet Oncol 8:226-234
34. Urschel JD, Vasan H (2003) A meta-analysis of randomized controlled trials that compared neoadjuvant chemoradiation and surgery to surgery alone for resectable esophageal cancer. Am J Surg 185:538-543
35. Greil R, Stein HJ (2007) Is it time to consider neoadjuvant treatment as the standard of care in oesophageal cancer? Lancet Oncol 8:189-190
36. Schneider BJ, Urba SG (2007) Preoperative chemoradiation for the treatment of locoregional esophageal cancer: the standard of care? Semin Radiat Oncol 17:45-52
37. Leers JM, Ayazi S, Hagen JA et al (2009) Survival in lymph node negative adenocarcinoma of the esophagus after R0 resection with and without neoadjuvant therapy: evidence for downstaging of N status. J Am Coll Surg 208:553-556
38. Rice TW, Blackstone EH, Adelstein DJ et al (2001) N1 esophageal carcinoma: the importance of staging and downstaging. J Thorac Cardiovasc Surg 121:454-464
39. Boffa D, Detterbeck F (2009) Neoadjuvant therapy. In: Blair A. Jobe CRT, Jr, John G. Hunter (ed) Esophageal Cancer Principles and Practice. Demos Medical, New York, pp 407-422
40. Ku GY, Illson D (2009) Preoperative therapy for esophageal cancer. In: Gastroenterology Clinics of North America, vol 38. Elsevier, pp 135-152
41. Courrech Staal EF, Aleman BM, Boot H et al (2010) Systematic review of the benefits and risks of neoadjuvant chemoradiation for oesophageal cancer. Br J Surg 97:1482-1496
42. de Manzoni G, Pedrazzani C, Laterza E et al (2005) Induction chemoradiotherapy for squamous cell carcinoma of the thoracic esophagus: impact of increased dosage on long-term results. Ann Thorac Surg 80:1176-1183

43. Verlato G, Zanoni A, Tomezzoli A et al (2010) Response to induction therapy in oesophageal and cardia carcinoma using Mandard tumour regression grade or size of residual foci. Br J Surg 97:719-725
44. Meredith KL, Weber JM, Turaga KK et al (2010) Pathologic response after neoadjuvant therapy is the major determinant of survival in patients with esophageal cancer. Ann Surg Oncol 17:1159-1167
45. Meguid RA, Hooker CM, Taylor JT et al (2009) Recurrence after neoadjuvant chemoradiation and surgery for esophageal cancer: does the pattern of recurrence differ for patients with complete response and those with partial or no response? J Thorac Cardiovasc Surg 138:1309-1317
46. Dresner SM, Griffin SM (2000) Pattern of recurrence following radical oesophagectomy with two-field lymphadenectomy. Br J Surg 87:1426-1433
47. Hsu PK, Wang BY, Huang CS et al (2011) Prognostic factors for post-recurrence survival in esophageal squamous cell carcinoma patients with recurrence after resection. J Gastrointest Surg 15:558-565
48. Natsugoe S, Matsumoto M, Okumura H et al (2010) Clinical course and outcome after esophagectomy with three-field lymphadenectomy in esophageal cancer. Langenbecks Arch Surg 395:341-346
49. Kang CH, Kim YT, Jeon SH et al (2007) Lymphadenectomy extent is closely related to long-term survival in esophageal cancer. Eur J Cardiothorac Surg 31:154-160
50. Kunisaki C, Makino H, Takagawa R et al (2008) Surgical outcomes in esophageal cancer patients with tumor recurrence after curative esophagectomy. J Gastrointest Surg 12:802-810
51. Mariette C, Balon JM, Piessen G et al (2003) Pattern of recurrence following complete resection of esophageal carcinoma and factors predictive of recurrent disease. Cancer 97:1616-1623
52. Smit JK, Pultrum BB, van Dullemen HM et al (2010) Prognostic factors and patterns of recurrence in esophageal cancer assert arguments for extended two-field transthoracic esophagectomy. Am J Surg 200:446-453
53. Tachibana M, Kinugasa S, Yoshimura H et al (2005) Clinical outcomes of extended esophagectomy with three-field lymph node dissection for esophageal squamous cell carcinoma. Am J Surg 189:98-109
54. Shim YM, Kim HK, Kim K (2010) Comparison of survival and recurrence pattern between two-field and three-field lymph node dissections for upper thoracic esophageal squamous cell carcinoma. J Thorac Oncol 5:707-712
55. Rohatgi PR, Swisher SG, Correa AM et al (2005) Failure patterns correlate with the proportion of residual carcinoma after preoperative chemoradiotherapy for carcinoma of the esophagus. Cancer 104:1349-1355
56. Vallbohmer D, Holscher AH, DeMeester S et al (2010) A multicenter study of survival after neoadjuvant radiotherapy/chemotherapy and esophagectomy for ypT0N0M0R0 esophageal cancer. Ann Surg 252:744-749
57. Schipper PH, Cassivi SD, Deschamps C et al (2005) Locally recurrent esophageal carcinoma: when is re-resection indicated? Ann Thorac Surg 80:1001-1005
58. Nakamura T, Ota M, Narumiya K et al (2008) Multimodal treatment for lymph node recurrence of esophageal carcinoma after curative resection. Ann Surg Oncol 15:2451-2457
59. Kato H, Miyazaki T, Nakajima M et al (2003) Prediction of hematogenous recurrence in patients with esophageal carcinoma. Jpn J Thorac Cardiovasc Surg 51:599-608
60. Pawlik TM, Gleisner AL, Bauer TW et al (2007) Liver-directed surgery for metastatic squamous cell carcinoma to the liver: results of a multi-center analysis. Ann Surg Oncol 14 :2807-2816
61. Nakajima Y, Nagai K, Kawano T et al (2001) Therapeutic strategy for postoperative liver metastasis from esophageal squamous cell carcinoma; clinical efficacy of and problem with hepatic arterial infusion chemotherapy. Hepatogastroenterology 48:1652-1655
62. Shiono S, Kawamura M, Sato T (2008) Disease-free interval length correlates to prognosis of patients who underwent metastasectomy for esophageal lung metastases. J Thorac Oncol 3:1046-1049

63. Ichikawa H, Kosugi S, Nakagawa S et al (2011) Operative treatment for metachronous pulmonary metastasis from esophageal carcinoma. Surgery 149:164-170
64. Chen F, Sato K, Sakai H (2008) Pulmonary resection for metastasis from esophageal carcinoma. Interact Cardiovasc Thorac Surg 7:809-812
65. Weinberg JS, Suki D, Hanbali F et al (2003) Metastasis of esophageal carcinoma to the brain. Cancer 98:1925-1933
66. Rice TW, Khuntia D, Rybicki LA et al (2006) Brain metastases from esophageal cancer: a phenomenon of adjuvant therapy? Ann Thorac Surg 6:2042-2049
67. Yoshida S (2007) Brain metastasis in patients with esophageal carcinoma. Surg Neurol 67:288-290
68. Ogawa K, Toita T, Sueyama H et al (2002) Brain metastases from esophageal carcinoma: natural history, prognostic factors, and outcome. Cancer 94:759-764
69. Kosuga T, Shiozaki A, Fujiwara H et al (2011) Treatment outcome and prognosis of patients with lymph node recurrence of thoracic esophageal squamous cell carcinoma after curative resection. World J Surg 35:798-804
70. Kato H, Tachimori Y, Watanabe H et al (1998) Anastomotic recurrence of oesophageal squamous cell carcinoma after transthoracic oesophagectomy. Eur J Surg 164:759-764
71. Shimada H, Kitabayashi H, Nabeya Y et al (2003) Treatment response and prognosis of patients after recurrence of esophageal cancer. Surgery 133:24-31
72. Kaisaki S, Kitayama J, Ishigami H, Nagawa H (2007) Solitary nodal recurrence in the dorsal area of the thoracic aorta after a curative resection of esophageal cancer: report of two cases. Surg Today 37:243-247
73. Yano M, Takachi K, Doki Y et al (2006) Prognosis of patients who develop cervical lymph node recurrence following curative resection for thoracic esophageal cancer. Dis Esophagus 19:73-77
74. Motoyama S, Kitamura M, Saito R et al (2006) Outcome and treatment strategy for mid- and lower-thoracic esophageal cancer recurring locally in the lymph nodes of the neck. World J Surg 30:191-198
75. Komatsu S, Shioaki Y, Ichikawa D et al (2005) Survival and clinical evaluation of salvage operation for cervical lymph node recurrence in esophageal cancer. Hepatogastroenterology 52:796-799
76. Sato Y, Motoyama S, Maruyama K et al (2005) A second malignancy is the major cause of death among thoracic squamous cell esophageal cancer patients negative for lymph node involvement. J Am Coll Surg 201:188-193
77. Sugiura T, Kato H, Tachimori Y et al (2002) Second primary carcinoma in the gastric tube constructed as an esophageal substitute after esophagectomy. J Am Coll Surg 194:578-583
78. Bamba T, Kosugi S, Takeuchi M et al (2010) Surveillance and treatment for second primary cancer in the gastric tube after radical esophagectomy. Surg Endosc 24:1310-1317

Treatment of Unresectable Esophageal Cancer: Indications and Long-term Results

15

Michele Pavarana and Teodoro Sava

15.1 Introduction

There is considerable debate in the literature on the appropriate preoperative treatment of esophageal squamous cell carcinoma (ESCC), with valid options being chemotherapy (CT), chemoradiotherapy (CRT), followed or not by surgery. Some authors are of the opinion that in patients with good clinical response, surgery can improve local control and minimize, in case of relapse, the need for palliative stenting; however, surgery does not seem to improve overall survival. Late surgical morbidity and mortality, even in high-volume centers, is still considerable. For this reason, definitive CRT has been proposed for patients with advanced ESCC (cT3-cT4), restricting surgery to non-responding patients (salvage surgery) [1-5].

The treatment of patients with ESCC invading resectable (cT4a) or unresectable adjacent organs (cT4b) or with bulky N+ tumors is less often discussed and the first approach is often definitive CRT. Since major responses are rare, patients with these very advanced tumors are only rarely candidates for surgery after treatment. Moreover, considering the high morbidity and mortality associated with these extended procedures, only R0 surgery should be performed. Non-radical surgery (R1-R2) does not improve local control or overall survival. [6]. The problem is how to define and then measure the response after CRT. Some authors use basal comparisons of PET-SUV, but the sensitivity and specificity are still controversial. Others have proposed endoscopic biopsy at the end of chemoradiation (suitable for T stage but not N stage), since thereafter conventional imaging (CT, MRI, echo-endoscopy) is often unable to discriminate therapy-induced fibrosis from viable residual

M. Pavarana (✉)
Oncology Unit, Borgo Trento Hospital,
Verona, Italy

G. de Manzoni (Ed.), *Treatment of Esophageal and Hypopharyngeal Squamous Cell Carcinoma*,

tumor. Regardless, it should be determined whether in patients with locally very advanced disease, salvage R0 surgery is feasible, as some studies report a 25% 5-year survival rate [6-8].

Nevertheless, the current literature does not provide any clear indications for this group of patients. Some studies include those with resectable disease (T1-T3 with N0-1), and others only patients with locally advanced unresectable cancers, but the sample size in either case is often small. In some but not all studies, patients with N1 bulky tumors are excluded. Other studies include patients with AJCC-1983 T3 tumors, corresponding to those classified as UICC-1997 T4. Cervical tumors are sometimes included; treatment doses and schedules are not homogeneous across trials (i.e., dose of radiotherapy); non-responding patients rarely are independently considered; no definitive information is available regarding prognosis; and some trials include both ESCC and adenocarcinoma.

Definitive CRT is a potential alternative to surgery and it is indicated in patients with unresectable primary tumors or inoperable disease due to medical comorbidities [6, 9-11]. Only a few studies have reported the results of definitive CRT in patients with T4b tumors invading unresectable adjacent organs: the 2-year survival was ~15%, complete response < 30%, and median survival < 12 months [12-16].

When palliation is the goal, because of the severity of symptoms, poor performance status, and survival expectations of a few months, radiotherapy with or without chemotherapy (associated with photodynamic therapy and/or endoscopic palliation) safely provides durable symptomatic relief (see Chap. 11).

15.2 Definitive Chemoradiotherapy

The curative potential of this approach has been demonstrated in trials in which unresectability was not among the eligibility criteria. The results showed that long-term survival is possible even for patients with extensive T4 primary disease [17].

In the RTOG 8501 study [18, 19], 123 patients were randomized to either 64 Gy radiotherapy alone or 50 Gy radiotherapy with 5-FU 1000 mg/m^2 on days 1–4 and cisplatin 75 mg/m^2 on day 1 every 4 weeks during radiotherapy and for two cycles every 3 weeks after radiotherapy. Eligibility criteria included localized M0 esophageal cancer. Chemotherapy improved median survival from 9.3 to 14.1 months and the 2-year survival rate from 10 to 36%. There were no 3-year survivors with radiotherapy alone whereas in the CRT arm the 5- and 10-year survival rates were 27% and 20%, respectively. The rate of isolated locoregional or persistent disease as the site of first failure was reduced from 53 to 38% and the rate of systemic failure was 30 vs. 16% when chemotherapy was added.

The ECOG study [20] compared radiotherapy (60 Gy) with or without concurrent mitomycin C 10 mg/m^2 on day 2 and 5-FU 1000 mg/m^2 day for 4 days in patients with squamous cell carcinomas: 135 patients were enrolled; resection was possible after 40 Gy of radiotherapy, and 38% of patients were selected for surgery. With the addition of chemotherapy, median survival was improved from 9.2 to 14.8 months; 2-year survival rates were 27% vs. 12% without chemotherapy.

In the phase II trial of the National Cancer Institute of Milan [21], 106 patients with ESCC were treated with cisplatin 100 mg/m^2 on day 1 and 5-FU 1000 mg/m^2 on days 1–4 for two cycles with concurrent radiotherapy (30 Gy/15 fractions); 24% of these patients also had surgery with R0 resection. The overall survival rate was 22% at 5 years and 12% at 10 years, with no differences between the two groups (surgery and no surgery).

The RTOG 94-05 (Intergroup 0123) study was a phase III randomized controlled trial [2] in which patients were randomized to high- vs. low-dose radiotherapy (64.8 vs. 50.4 Gy); infused chemotherapy was identical and consisted of two cycles of cisplatin 75 mg/m^2 on day 1 and 5-FU 1000 mg/m^2/day for 4 days concurrent with radiotherapy and two more cycles at the end of radiotherapy. A dose intensification of radiotherapy was not associated with an increase in median survival (13 vs. 18.1 months: p = n.s.), nor in 2-year survival (31% vs. 40%), nor surprisingly in locoregional control (44% vs. 48%). Thus, the standard of care for definitive chemoradiation remains 50–50.4 Gy radiotherapy by once-daily fractionation (1.8–2 Gy) with four courses of cisplatin/5-FU chemotherapy.

Two important randomized trials assessed the potential benefit of adding surgery to definitive cisplatin/5-FU based chemoradiation. To date, a survival benefit has not been demonstrated; nevertheless, the addition of surgical resection was shown to improve local control and to decrease the need for stent placement [22, 23]. The first trial, reported by Bedenne et al. [22], enrolled 444 patients to receive 5-FU and cisplatin with a concurrent continuous course of 45-Gy radiotherapy in 4.5 weeks or split-course 15-Gy radiotherapy on days 1–5 and days 22–26. Only the 230 responding patients were randomized to surgery or three additional cycles of chemotherapy with additional radiotherapy, either 20 Gy with conventional fractionation or 15 Gy over 5 days. Each chemotherapy cycle was 5-FU 800 mg/m^2/day continuous infusion and cisplatin 15 mg/m^2 1-hour infusion on days 1–5. Results for chemoradiation and trimodality therapy were a median survival of 17.7 vs. 19.3 months, a 2-year survival rate of 34% vs. 40%, and 2-year local control of 66% vs. 57% respectively. Stents were required in 5% and 32% of surgery and chemoradiation patients, respectively. The 3-month mortality rate was 9.3% with surgery and 0.8% with definitive combined modality treatment. Thus, chemoradiation alone and chemoradiation followed by surgery were equivalent in terms of survival in responding patients. Unfortunately, since non-responding patients were excluded from randomization it is unclear whether resistant tumors may benefit from surgery.

In the trial of Stahl et al. [23], 172 patients were randomized to either three cycles of induction chemotherapy with bolus 5-FU, leucovorin, and etoposide followed by one additional cycle of chemotherapy with 40 Gy radiotherapy followed by surgery or to the same induction chemotherapy followed by chemoradiation with at least 65 Gy of radiotherapy. Overall survival was equivalent in resected and non-resected patients, and the 2-year local progression-free survival rate was significantly improved with surgery (64% vs. 41%). In responding patients, the probability of 3-year survival was 50%; in non-responding patients, median survival was 9.1 months, and the 3-year survival rate was 17.9% if salvage surgery was performed (and 32% if R0 surgery could be performed) instead of 9.4% if surgery was impossible. A survival benefit with the addition of surgery might be shown from a larger study with longer follow-up.

Studies with cisplatin/5-FU-based chemotherapy supplemented with taxanes, cetuximab, and irinotecan concurrent with radiation therapy are ongoing, but no conclusive data are yet available.

From recent phase II trials, it seems that definitive chemoradiation is feasible also in elderly patients [24], with careful reductions in chemotherapy doses or radiotherapy fields. High doses of chemotherapy or radiotherapy do not seem to improve survival rates according to the data from recent small phase II trials [25].

References

1. Ishihara R, Yamamoto S, Iishi H et al (2010) Factors predictive of tumor recurrence and survival after initial complete response of esophageal squamous cell carcinoma to definitive chemoradiotherapy. Int J Radiat Oncol Biol Phys 76:123-129
2. Minsky BD, Pajak TF, Ginsberg RJ et al (2002) INT0123 phase III trial of combined-modality therapy for esophageal cancer: high-dose versus standard-dose radiation therapy. J Clin Oncol 20:1167-174
3. Cooper JS, Guo MD, Herskovic A et al (1999) Chemoradiotherapy of locally advanced esophageal cancer: long term follow-up of a prospective randomized trial. JAMA 281:1623-1627
4. Ishikura S, Nihei K, Ohtsu A et al (2003) Long-term toxicity after definitive chemoradiotherapy for squamous cell carcinoma of the thoracic esophagus. J Clin Oncol 21:2697-2702
5. Tahara M, Ohtsu A, Hironaka S et al (2005) Clinical impact of criteria for complete response of primary site to treatment of esophageal cancer. Jpn J Clin Oncol 35:316-323
6. Ariga H, Nemoto K, Miyazaki S et al (2009) Prospective comparison of surgery alone and chemoradiotherapy with selective surgery in resectable squamous cell carcinoma of the esophagus. Int J Radiat Oncol Biol Phys 75:348-356
7. Swisher SG, Wynn P, Putnam JB et al (2002) Salvage esophagectomy for recurrent tumours after definitive chemotherapy and radiotherapy. J Thorac Cardiovasc Surg 123:175-183
8. Gardner-Thorpe J, Hardwick RH, Dwerryhouse SJ (2007) Salvage oesophagectomy after local failure of definitive chemoradiotherapy. Br J Surg 94:1059-1066
9. Stahl M, Walz MK, Stuschke M et al (2007) Preoperative chemotherapy versus preoperative chemoradiotherapy in locally advanced esophagogastric adenocarcinomas: first results of a randomized phase III trial. Proc Am Soc Clin Oncol 25:4511
10. Urba SG, Orringer MB, Turrisi A et al (2007) Randomized trial of preoperative chemoradiation versus surgery alone in patients with locoregional esophageal carcinoma. J Clin Oncol 19:305-313

11. Bosset JF, Gignoux M, Tribouled JP et al (1997) Chemoradiotherapy followed by surgery compared with surgery alone in squamous-cell cancer of the esophagus. N Engl J Med 337:161-167
12. Ohtsu A, Boku N, Muro K et al (1999) Definitive chemoradiotherapy for T4 and/or M1 lymph node squamous cell carcinoma of the esophagus. J Clin Oncol 17:2915- 2921
13. Ishida K, Iizuka T, Ando N et al (1996) Phase II study of chemoradiotherapy for advanced squamous cell carcinoma of the thoracic esophagus. Jpn J Clin Oncol 26:310-315
14. Burmeister BH, Denham JW, O'Brien M et al (1995) Combined modality therapy for esophageal carcinoma: preliminary results from a large Austrialasian multicenter study. Int J Radiat Oncol Biol Phys 32:997-1006
15. Blanke CD, Choy H, Leach SD (997) Combined modality therapy for esophageal cancer. Semin Radiat Oncol 7:15-23
16. Rizk NP, Venkatraman E, Bains MS et al (2007) American Joint Committee on Cancer staging system does not accurately predict survival in patients receiving multimodality therapy for esophageal adenocarcinoma. J Clin Oncol 25:507-512
17. Nishimura Y, Suzuki M, Nakamatsu K et al (2002) Prospective trial of concurrent chemoradiotherapy with protracted infusion of 5-fluorouracil and cisplatin for T4 esophageal cancer with or without fistula. Int J Radiat Oncol Biol Phys 53:134-139
18. Herskovic A, Martz K, al-Sarraf M et al (1992) Combined chemotherapy and radiotherapy compared with radiotherapy alone in patients with cancer of the eophagus. N Engl J Med 326:1593-1598
19. al-Sarraf M, Martz K, Herskovic A et al (1997) Progress report of combined chemoradiotherapy versus radiotherapy alone in patients with esophageal cancer: an intergroup study. J Clin Oncol 15:277-284
20. Smith TJ, Ryan LM, Douglass HO Jr et al (1998) Combined chemoradiotherapy vs. radiotherapy alone for early stage squamous cell carcinoma of the esophagus: a study of the Eastern Cooperative Oncology Group. Int J Radiat Oncol Biol Phys 42:269-276
21. Bidoli P, Bajetta E, Stani SC et al (2002) Ten-year survival with chemotherapy and radiotherapy in patients with suamous cell carcinoma of the esophagus. Cancer 94:352-361
22. Bedenne L, Michel P, Bouche O et al (2007) Chemoradiation followed by surgery compared with chemoradiation alone in squamous cancer of the esophagus: FFCD 9102. J Clin Oncol 25:1160-1168
23. Stahl M, Stuschke M, Lehmann N et al (2005) Chemoradiation with or without surgery in patients with locally advanced squamous cell carcinoma of the esophagus. J Clin Oncol 23:2310-2317
24. Wakui R, Yamashita H, Okuma K et al (2010) Esophageal cancer: definitive chemioradiotherapy for elderly patients. Dis Esophagus 23:572-579
25. Hurmuzlu M, Monge OR, Smaaland R et al (2010) High-dose definitive concomitant chemioradiotherapy in non-metastatic locallyadvanced esophageal cancer: toxicity and outcome. Dis Esophagus 23:244-252

Early Results: Morbidity, Mortality, and the Treatment of Complications

16

Giovanni de Manzoni, Andrea Zanoni, and Jacopo Weindelmayer

16.1 Introduction

Despite the significant technical improvements and advances in both surgical technique and peri-operative management, esophagectomy is still associated with high morbidity and mortality [1-4]. The complication rate seems to be related to a number of factors; indeed, the characteristics and behavior of the patients as well as technical problems are often associated with an increased risk of postoperative complications following esophagectomy. Furthermore, multivariate analysis has pointed to a significantly higher risk of recurrence for patients with complications after esophagectomy than in those in whom the procedure was uneventful [5]. An accurate definition of a complication and a method to assess its severity are still lacking. Recently, a more accurate classification of surgical complications was proposed based on a cohort of 6336 patients (Table 16.1) [6].

Recent trials retrospectively evaluated the morbidity and mortality of wide cohorts of patients, from data collected in databases. The results of these studies are reported in Table 16.2 [1-4, 7, 8]. Most of the operations were carried out for malignancies (85–100%) but the surgical techniques varied greatly. Japanese authors [7] investigated the complication rate of patients with squamous cell carcinoma who were treated in a single institution, where the preferred surgical approach (three-incisional procedure) was completely different from that used in the American studies. In the multicenter Australian trial [8], open and minimally invasive esophagectomies were typically performed.

G. de Manzoni (✉)
Dept. of Surgery, Upper G.I. Surgery Division, University of Verona,
Verona, Italy

G. de Manzoni (Ed.), *Treatment of Esophageal and Hypopharyngeal Squamous Cell Carcinoma*,

Table 16.1 The Clavien-Dindo classification of surgical complications. (Modified from [6], with permission)

Grade 0	No complication
Grade 1	Deviation from normal hospital course, but no need for medication or intervention
Grade 2	Complication requiring pharmacological treatment (i.e., pneumonia, atrial fibrillation, blood transfusion, etc.)
Grade 3a	Complication requiring interventional treatment without general anesthesia (i.e., drain for empyema or abscess, drainage of pleural effusion, operative endoscopy, etc.)
Grade 3b	Any surgical re-intervention under general anesthesia
Grade 4a	Life-threatening requiring ICU admission – single organ failure
Grade 4b	Life-threatening requiring ICU admission – multi-organ failure
Grade 5	Post-operative death

Table 16.2 Morbidity and mortality in large cohorts of patients treated with different surgical approaches

Author [Reference]	N.	Operations for cancer (%)	Type of surgery (%)		Mortality (%)	Morbidity (%)
Dhungel et al. [1]	1032	96	THE Ivor-Lewis Mc Keown Other	41 20 17 22	3	50
Bailey et al. [2]	1777	85	Not reported		9.8	49
Wright et al. [3]	2315	100	THE Ivor-Lewis Mc Keown Other	18 9 2 71	2.7	57
Atkins et al. [4]	379	90	THE Ivor Lewis Mc Keown Other	36 47 4 13	5.8	64
Morita et al. [7]	1106	100	THE Ivor-Lewis Mc Keown Other	5 24 67 4	5.6	40
Zingg et al. [8]	858	100	Ivor-Lewis MIE	46 54	3.5	49

THE, Trans-hiatal esophagectomy; *MIE*, minimally invasive esophagectomy.

Overall, the reported mortality rate in these studies was between 2.7 and 9.8%, while complications occurred in 40–64% of the patients. Respiratory complications were the most important cause of morbidity (18–28%), while anastomotic leakage was reported in 11–25% of the patients, with the higher rate in the Japanese study, in which three-field dissection was performed.

Table 16.3 Factors associated and not associated with morbidity and mortality at multivariate analysis

Author [Reference]	Associated with mortality	Associated with morbidity	Not associated with mortality	Not associated with morbidity
Dhungel et al. [1]	Wound infection DM Dyspnea	DM Alcohol Smoking Transfusions	CRT	CRT Thoracotomy
Bailey et al. [2]	Age Transfusions DM Alcohol Dyspnea Smoking CRT	Age Dyspnea DM Smoking CRT	n.r.	n.r.
Wright et al. [3]	Age Cardiopathy DM Smoking	Age Cardiopathy DM Smoking	CRT	CRT
Atkins et al. [4]	Age Pneumonia	Age Pneumonia	CRT Leak	CRT
Morita et al. [7]	Age R+	n.r.	n.r.	n.r.
Zingg et al. [8]	Smoking Comorbidities	n.r.	n.r.	n.r.

DM, diabetes mellitus; *CRT*, induction chemoradiotherapy; *n.r.*, not reported; *R+*, non radical surgery.

The reported studies also investigated the role of pre- and peri-operative factors in predicting morbidity and mortality. The multivariate factors associated and not associated with morbidity and mortality are displayed in Table 16.3 [1-4, 7, 8]. Age, diabetes mellitus, dyspnea, smoking, and alcohol consumption are the most important patient characteristics related to morbidity and mortality, while intraoperative blood transfusions and post-operative pneumonia are associated with worse post-operative outcome. The use of neoadjuvant chemoradiation was not associated with increased morbidity and mortality in all but one study. One study did not find an increased risk of complications following thoracotomy [1], while in another there was no higher mortality risk in case of leak [4]. In the Japanese trial [7], incomplete resection was associated with an increased risk of in-hospital death.

In summary, these recent trials report a significant morbidity and mortality risk for patients undergoing esophagectomy, with an important impact on long-term outcome. However, some patient characteristics and behaviors should be considered and possibly corrected before or during surgery, as they significantly increase this risk.

16.2 Types of Complications

The main types of complications reported after esophageal surgery are pulmonary complications and anastomotic leaks. Atrial arrhythmias, wound infections, and sepsis are also frequent, but their incidence and therapy are similar to what occurs following all other major surgical procedures. Respiratory complications are responsible for almost one third of the total morbidity rate and for a very large part of the mortality related to esophagectomy. Anastomotic leak is an important cause of morbidity and mortality, with both acute and chronic implications.

16.2.1 Respiratory Complications

The risk of respiratory complications after esophageal surgery is higher than after other major surgical operations, including, paradoxically, lung resections. The reasons for this risk are thought to include entry into body cavities subjected to different pressures, lung edema, disruption of bronchial innervation with attenuation of sputum expectoration, postoperative pain, postoperative dysfunction of the respiratory muscles, possible recurrent laryngeal nerve injury, and discoordinated deglutition, all in the context of the patients' preoperative characteristics, i.e., advanced age, poor performance status, impaired pulmonary function before surgery, and tobacco and alcohol abuse [8-11]. Also, the duration of surgery was reported to be associated with an increased risk [9]. Despite intraoperative and postoperative techniques to reduce the frequency of pulmonary complication, they are still a major factor after esophagectomy. Indeed, pulmonary complications are in the range of 18–28% in the reported studies and are responsible for 45–88% of the deaths connected to this major surgical procedure [9, 12, 13].

Respiratory complications comprise a wide set of pathologies, ranging from pleural effusion with atelectasis to pneumonia to acute respiratory distress syndrome (ARDS) and respiratory failure requiring mechanical ventilation. The types of complications observed in the different studies are usually not well defined, making it difficult to compare results. An American trial [14] precisely defined the pattern of respiratory complications: most of the patients in the study population developed pleural effusion and atelectasis, but significant pulmonary complications occurred in one-third of the patients. Pneumonia was the most common, clinically relevant pulmonary complication, while the most severe complications, such as ARDS, developed in almost 10% of the patients. In all, 20% of the study population required prolonged mechanical ventilation.

A Japanese trial [13] investigated the risk of respiratory complications after three-field esophagectomy. Pulmonary morbidity was 50%, with 17% of the patients requiring re-intubation and tracheostomy. Some 88% of the postoperative deaths were pneumonia-related. Recurrent-nerve paralysis was seen in 28% of the patients; 18% of those suffered from aspiration pneumonia compared with a 9% rate of aspiration pneumonia in patients without recurrent-nerve injury. Furthermore, a worse 5-year overall survival was reported for patients who suffered respiratory complications in the postoperative period.

The treatment of pulmonary morbidity begins with prevention. Indeed, intense respiratory physiotherapy before surgery [15, 16], interruption of smoking and alcohol assumption, and correction of possible factors interfering with performance status, such as cachexia caused by dysphagia, might have a role in reducing the complication risk. Ongoing studies on the use of steroids and neutrophil elastase inhibitors to reduce the inflammatory response to surgical trauma and pleural effusion are promising therapeutic tools, but their efficacy is still under investigation.

Alongside preoperative prevention, intraoperative and postoperative correct care has a crucial role. Esophagectomy is burdened by an important inflammatory response, the extent of which is related to respiratory morbidity. Cytokines, particularly IL-6 and IL-8, mediate the increased extravascular lung water, which is in turn related to pneumonia and ARDS risk [17, 18]. Moreover, peri-operative instability, with the need for fluid resuscitation, contribute to the increased risk of ARDS [19].

Protective ventilation, with reduced tidal volume and introduction of positive end-expiratory pressure (PEEP) during one-lung ventilation [17], immediate extubation, early mobilization, intense respiratory physiotherapy and toilet bronchoscopies, negative fluid balance, and adequate pain control (epidural and/or patient controlled analgesia) [20] may all substantially contribute to reducing the complication rate, together with careful attention to preserving the recurrent laryngeal nerves.

16.2.2 Fluid Balance

After esophagectomy, respiratory distress due to interstitial lung edema could be related to the increased risk of pulmonary and cardiac complications, hence being life-threatening. The trauma resulting from the surgical procedure causes a severe inflammatory response syndrome [21, 22]. The related release of cytokines causes capillary leakage, loss of proteins, and a fluid shift from the intravascular space to the interstitium. Altogether, these lead to the accumulation of fluid in the body. The more intense the inflammation, the more fluid accumulates, resulting in a positive postoperative fluid balance. Accordingly, peri-operative fluid balance could be used as a marker of postoperative inflammation.

Fluid balance is calculated by subtracting the eliminated fluid from the administered fluid. The cumulative fluid balance from intraoperative to postoperative days 2–5 has been reported to be much higher in patients presenting pulmonary and cardiac complications and in those who died postoperatively [21, 22]. An anesthesiological study of the risk factors in the development of ARDS in patients admitted to the intensive care unit after major surgical procedures [23] found that in patients who received more than 20 ml/kg/h of intraoperative fluids the risk was almost fourfold higher than in patients receiving < 10 ml/kg/h. These data were confirmed by a trial specifically considering trans-thoracic esophagectomy for carcinoma [11], in which reducing intraoperative fluid administration to an infusion rate of 4-5 ml/kg/h decreased the need for bronchoscopies, while contributing to expectoration and thus reduced respiratory disturbance. A postoperative fluid administration of 1 ml/kg/h has been proposed as a safe amount for adequate hydration [24].

As mentioned above regarding respiratory complications, fluid restriction alone is not enough to improve short and long-term outcomes. Nevertheless, it plays a significant role in reducing the inflammatory response and thus improving outcome.

16.2.3 Anastomotic Leak

Anastomotic leak is defined as the leakage of luminal content from a surgical joint of two hollow viscera, through the wound and/or the drain site or creating an abscess [25]. It is the main surgical complication of esophagectomy. The reported incidence of anastomotic leaks after esophagectomy varies widely in the current literature, ranging from 5 to 25% [26-34]. Most leaks usually occur within 10 days of surgery. Mortality related to anastomotic dehiscence is still very high, in some cases reaching 40% of the deaths related to complications of esophagectomy [31, 32].

The occurrence of anastomotic leak is multifactorial, influenced by systemic and local factors [35]. Systemic factors include advanced cancer stage and poor performance status, with malnutrition as well as impaired cardiovascular and respiratory function. These act in concert to compromise blood supply, tissue oxygenation, and therefore the healing process at the anastomotic site [35]. Local factors include impaired vascularization of the esophageal stump or of the graft end, compromising either arterial supply or venous drainage, excessive mechanical tension on the anastomosis (too stretched or compressed at the thoracic inlet), and local infection, which can be both the cause and the consequence of anastomotic dehiscence. Moreover, the infiltrated margins and the intrinsic technical difficulties of performing the anastomosis can influence the occurrence of leak.

After esophagectomy, the anastomosis can be located at the neck or at the thorax in the mediastinum. Historically, it was believed that, compared with intrathoracic anastomoses, cervical anastomoses had a higher leak rate but lower complications due to dehiscence [35]. Despite the leak rate looked higher after cervical anastomosis, this was not confirmed in some studies [26, 29], which instead reported an equal or even a lower risk of leak. Furthermore, some surgeons are of the opinion that cervical anastomosis is safer because the dehiscence is confined to the neck, without involvement of the thorax. However, this was not consistent with the findings of two trials [27, 28] showing that, after trans-thoracic esophagectomy, nearly 50% of the patients with cervical dehiscence developed intrathoracic manifestations. After trans-hiatal esophagectomy, the risk was statistically significantly lower [28], probably because in the trans-thoracic approach the thoracic inlet tends to be much more widely dissected [27, 28].

Diagnosis and Clinical Presentation

A widely accepted classification of leakage is still lacking in the current literature. Some authors define a leak on the basis of radiographic findings whereas others consider the clinical impact (minor or major). The classification proposed by Schuchert et al. [33] weighs both the objective endoscopic (degree of anastomotic dehiscence) and the clinical (degree of intervention required) parameters. Urschel and co-workers [35] instead proposed a classification based on clinical presentation.

The clinical presentation of anastomotic leak ranges from an asymptomatic radiological finding to severe sepsis and shock due to necrotizing infection [34]. It depends on the ability of the surrounding tissues to contain the leak. Small contained leaks are normally asymptomatic or paucisymptomatic, whilst gastric-tube necrosis rapidly leads to the development of septic shock. Usually, anastomotic leak is associated with fever, tachycardia, high leukocyte count, outflow of gastrointestinal content from the drains, detectable presence of cervical or mediastinal abscesses, and, in the most severe cases, signs of systemic infection. Early adequate diagnosis and severity assessment are crucial, since the aggressiveness and invasiveness of the treatment should be proportional to the risk of death and to the chance to obtain healing using the least disturbing efforts for an already prostrate patient.

Considering the site of the anastomosis, a small, contained cervical leak can become clinically evident due to wound infection and/or saliva outflow from the wound or a fistula. The manifestations in this case are only local. When intrathoracic manifestations appear, either from a cervical or a thoracic leak, signs of mediastinitis might become evident, with a significant risk of both sepsis and septic shock. Limited contained mediastinal fistula may present as faded symptoms.

Routine contrast radiology is still performed by most centers before the patient is allowed oral intake, which is normally on postoperative day (POD) 7. However, there is no consensus on the timing of the examination, which can vary from POD 3 to 14. Routine screening with contrast swallow has a low sensitivity (40–87%) and good specificity (~100%) [25, 36, 37]. Thus, a normal contrast study cannot absolutely exclude a leak, whilst a positive study is fairly definitive in identifying the leak. The high number of false-negative studies is the reason why routine postoperative contrast studies are no longer warranted to identify leaks. However, patients with clinical suspicion or subtle clinical signs of sepsis must be immediately investigated: contrast swallow in these cases should be the first-line exam, as it is cheap, safe, and specific.

Recently, endoscopy with minimal air insufflation has been proposed in the diagnosis of a suspected leak [25, 34]. This test has high sensitivity and specificity (around 95–100% for both) [25, 34]; moreover, it allows direct quantification of the disrupted circumference of the anastomosis, thereby evidencing a potential conduit necrosis, and positioning of a drain or a transanastomotic nasojejunal tube.

If a leak is suspected, a computed tomography (CT) scan can be considered. CT has a sensitivity and specificity similar to that of contrast swallow, making it a second-line test in leak assessment; nevertheless, it allows the detection of signs of mediastinitis and the localization of a not drained abscess.

Treatment and Prognosis

There is no standard management for anastomotic leaks, even though some flow-charts have been proposed [34, 38]. With punctual and aggressive interventions, the vast majority of patients can be saved. Many patients with contained leaks and early diagnosis can be managed with conservative treatments: the cessation of oral intake, nasogastric tube decompression, broad-spectrum antibiotics and antifungal therapy, and parenteral or, better, enteral nutrition via an endoscopically placed fine-bore nasojejunal tube. Adequate drainage of infected peri-anastomotic fluid collections is mandatory: percutaneous drainage under CT or ultrasonographic guidance is effective for most patients.

Surgical intervention is indicated in case of extensive sepsis due to mediastinitis or peritonitis, not contained leaks with broad disruption of the anastomosis, or failure of conservative treatments. Surgery can allow better drainage of abscesses or reconstruction of the anastomosis. In case of severe cases of conduit necrosis, immediate débridement and conduit take-down with end cervical esophagostomy and placement of enteral feeding tubes is required.

In recent years, endoscopic minimally invasive treatment has gained importance in the management of anastomotic leaks. The possibilities include fibrin glue, metallic clip application, and self-expanding covered stents. However, also in such treatments, adequate drainage of external peri-anastomotic collections is absolutely necessary.

In case of smaller leaks (< 30% of the anastomotic circumference and/or a hole < 1.5 cm diameter), endoscopic clipping is indicated even if multiple endoscopic sessions are usually needed. In case of larger dehiscences, the temporary placement of a silicon-covered self-expanding stent is an effective option. Stent placement has the advantage of immediate leak occlusion in a single endoscopic session, but the stent has to be removed within 3 months to avoid long-term complications such as fistulization or upper-GI hemorrhage.

In summary, a flow-chart of the treatment of anastomotic leak can be proposed (Figs. 16.1, 16.2). Aggressive conservative treatment along with endo-

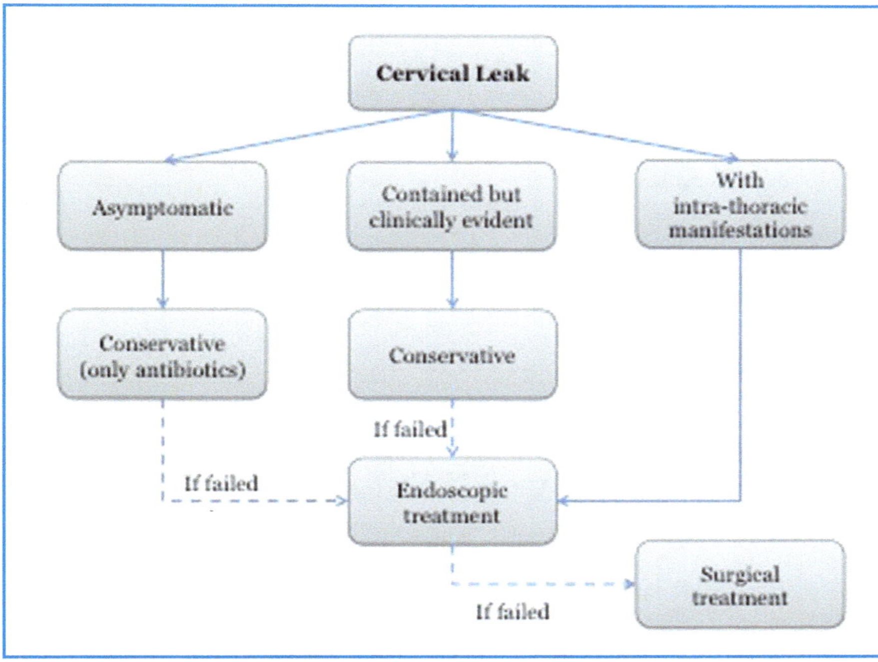

Fig. 16.1 Proposed flow-chart for the treatment of cervical leak according to the severity of the clinical manifestations

scopic treatment should be used as the first-line therapeutic option for all patients without vast disruption of the anastomosis or conduit necrosis. Surgery should be performed as the second-line option following the failure of endoscopy and conservative treatment, or as the first-line option in patients with necrosis of the conduit or disruption of the anastomosis with divergence > 70%. In this situation, stent placing is a difficult approach, yielding mixed results. Alternatively, surgical fixation of the endoscopically inserted stent along with debridement of collections might be "easier" and safer than conduit substitution.

16.3 Surgical Approaches

16.3.1 Trans-thoracic vs. Trans-hiatal Esophagectomy

Table 16.4 compares the results, in terms of morbidity and mortality, of trans-thoracic esophagectomy (TTE), with extensive mediastinal lymphadenectomy, and trans-hiatal esophagectomy (THE), with theoretically lower morbidity

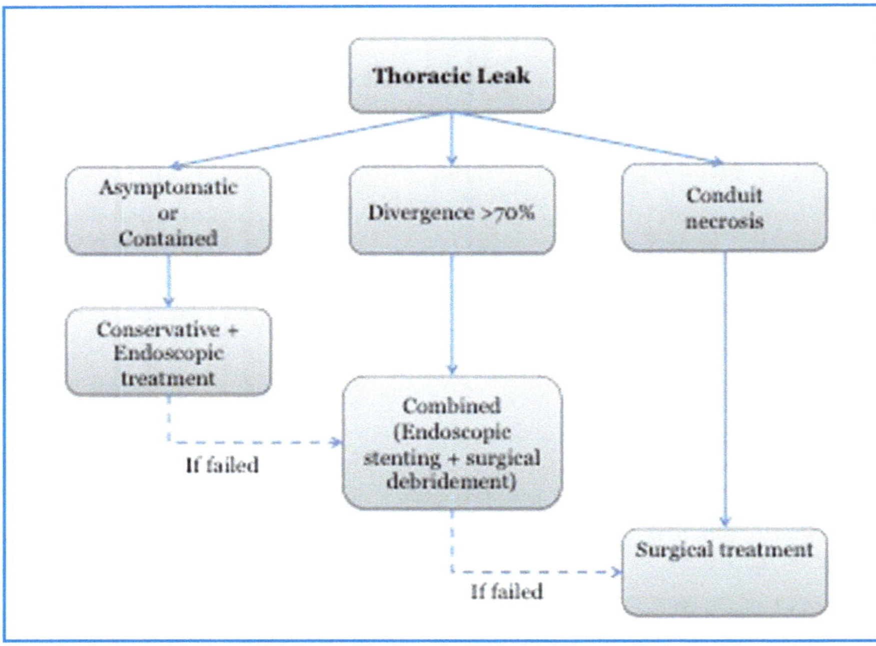

Fig. 16.2 Proposed flow-chart of the treatment of thoracic leak according to the severity of the clinical manifestations

Table 16.4 Comparison of morbidity and mortality in patients treated with trans-hiatal esophagectomy (THE) or trans-thoracic esophagectomy (TTE) for esophageal carcinoma

Author [Reference]	N.	THE	TTE	Morbidity (%)	*p*	Mortality (%)	*p*
Connors et al. [40]	17395 (not randomized)	11914	5481	THE 49 TTE 53	n.s.	8.9 8.4	n.s.
Chang et al. [39]	868 (not randomized)	225	643	THE n.r. TTE n.r.	n.s.	6.7 13.1	s
Morgan et al. [42]	151 (not randomized)	32	119	THE 59 TTE 54	n.s.	6 4	n.s.
Junginger et al. [41]	229 (not randomized)	70	159	THE 40 TTE 36	n.s.	4 8	n.s.
Renz et al. [43]	945 (not randomized)	383	562	THE 49 TTE 47	n.s.	9.9 10	n.s.

n.r., not reported; *n.s.*, not significant; *s*, significant.

[39-43]. It should be noted that all the reported studies were non-randomized, implying a selection bias for the compared arms. Chang et al., however, recorded a higher mortality for TTE, but their rate of 13.1% is the worst reported among these trials, while the 6.7% reported for THE is absolutely in line with the current literature. All the other studies failed to find any significant difference between the two approaches for either morbidity or mortality.

To date, the only randomized trial in the literature refers to adenocarcinoma alone [44]. Pulmonary complications were more pronounced in the transthoracic arm, but mortality was similar and the long-term results tended to be better in TTE.

In summary, thorax opening might be related to an increased risk of pulmonary complications, but the risks are worth considering because of the therapeutic options to control the complications and the better oncological results.

16.3.2 Ivor-Lewis Procedure

This is a frequently performed operation, especially in Western countries, where the use of three-field dissection is more highly debated. Many centers perform extended lymphadenectomy and/or an en-bloc resection, both of which are fully dealt with in Chap. 13. Studies in which an en-bloc esophagectomy with extended or complete lymphadenectomy was carried out are summarized in Table 16.5 [45-48]. In the study of Mariette and colleagues [47], SCC was the predominant histotype, which was not consistent with the other studies, in which adenocarcinoma was more frequent. The mortality rate was 2-4% in these dedicated institutions, with a morbidity rate of 18–45%. Respiratory complications were the most frequent cause of morbidity and mortality, with a median value of 15.5%. The main surgical complication was anastomotic leak, which was evident in a median 4% of the patients. Cardiac complications and bleeding were reported as other important causes of morbidity and mortality in these cohorts of patients.

Interestingly, a number of the patients in the studies of Ott et al. [45], Mariette et al. [47], and Karl et al. [48] were treated with induction chemotherapy or chemoradiotherapy. None of the three trials found any increased risk of complications between the neoadjuvant group compared with the surgery-only group. Of note, neoadjuvant-treated patients had the most advanced disease among all the included study populations. Ott and coworkers [45] investigated the complications leading to death and found that, even if very low in number in their study population, all patients with severe pulmonary complications died compared to "only" 15% of the patients who suffered from anastomotic leak. Moreover, patients whose postoperative period was uneventful had a median survival of 63 months, compared with 20 months for patients who suffered from complications ($p < 0.001$). Patients suffering from more than one complication had a higher risk of death than patients with only one complication.

Table 16.5 Morbidity, mortality and pattern of complications of patients treated with en-bloc Ivor-Lewis procedure for esophageal carcinoma

Author [Reference]	N.	Type of surgery	Mortality (%)	Morbidity (%)	Type of Complication
Ott et al. [45]	240	Ivor-Lewis en bloc (D2 + extended)	3.8	18	Respiratory 2% Leak 8%
Mariette et al. [47]	386	Ivor-Lewis en bloc (D2 + complete)	3.6	36	Respiratory 21% Leak 4%
Griffin et al. [46]	228	Ivor-Lewis en bloc (D2 + extended)	4	45	Respiratory 17% Leak 4%
Karl et al. [48]	143	Ivor-Lewis	2	29	Respiratory 14% Leak 3%

16.3.3 Two-Field vs. Three-Field Nodal Dissection

Only one randomized trial, published in 1998, compared two-field (2-F) and three-field (3-F) nodal dissection [49]. This small sample size study of Nishihira and colleagues consisted of 30 and 32 patients in the two arms. Those undergoing 2-F dissection underwent "extended" mediastinal dissection, according to the ISDE definition (Chap. 13).

Considering short-term outcome, a higher recurrent-nerve paralysis, with a significantly more frequent need of tracheostomy, was seen in the 3-F group, with an equal rate of pulmonary complications in both groups. Leakage was more frequent in the 2-F group. A retrospective Japanese trial [50] investigated the results of four types of lymphadenectomy: standard, extended, complete, and 3-F (Chap. 13). There were no differences in terms of mortality and overall morbidity, but recurrent-nerve palsy, tracheal ischemic lesions, and leakage were more frequently reported after complete and 3-F dissection.

Other non-randomized trials are reported in Table 16.6 [7, 51, 52]. Morita and co-workers [7] did not find differences in terms of mortality, while the 2-F approach was associated with much lower morbidity. No significant differences in mortality were determined by the other studies [51, 52].

In summary, 3-F dissection probably has an increased risk of pulmonary complications due to longer operating times and the higher risk of recurrent-nerve injury, but in dedicated centers these complications can be successfully managed.

16.3.4 Site of Anastomosis

Both thoracic and cervical anastomoses are widely used for gastric-tube reconstruction after esophagectomy. Cervical anastomosis should have a theoretically lower risk of fatal consequences due to anastomotic leakage, since a cervical fistula is considered to be a manageable complication [53]. A recent meta-analysis of the few randomized trials comparing cervical and thoracic anasto-

Table 16.6 Comparison of morbidity and mortality in patients treated with two-field (2-F) or three-field (3-F) lymphadenectomy for esophageal carcinoma

Authory [Reference]	N.	Two-field	Three-field	Morbidity	*p*	Mortality	*p*
Shim et al. (not randomized) [51]	91	34	57	2-F 44% 3-F 56%	n.s.	2F 0% 3F 0%	n.s.
Igaki et al. (not randomized) [52]	156	55	101	2F 71% 3F 65%	n.s.	n.r.	n.r.
Morita et al. (not randomized) [7]	1003	266	737	2F 19% 3F 47%	s	2F 3% 3F 6%	n.s.

n.r., not reported; *n.s.*, not significant; *s*, significant.

moses [53] did not find any differences between the two types with respect to mortality and respiratory complications, while cervical anastomosis was associated with a significantly higher incidence of anastomotic leakage and recurrent-nerve trauma. Nevertheless, this meta-analysis did not investigate the relationship between anastomotic leak and mortality in the two different approaches. Interestingly, it has been shown that almost half of the patients with cervical anastomotic leak have thoracic manifestations, which are more frequent after TTE than after THE [28]. It is clear that cervical anastomosis is not a risk-free procedure, and the preferred approach is still a matter of debate.

16.4 Fast-track Surgery

Fast-track surgery was first used in colon cancer patients to accelerate their recovery from surgery. The aim of this enhanced recovery program is to reduce the "stress response" caused by a surgical procedure, thus reducing morbidity, allowing a quicker return to a stable state, and reducing hospitalization. The latter two goals should, in turn, increase patient satisfaction and reduce the costs for the healthcare system. Furthermore, the charted pathways used in fast-track surgery can significantly reduce the mistakes that may occur due to staff turnover and inexperience.

Fast-track programs have been studied for a number of surgical procedures, especially colorectal operations, but only a few have focused on esophageal surgery. Traditionally, after esophagectomy, a 2-week stay is the rule, and very few centers use a charted pathway for peri-operative management. In high-volume centers, trained staff can reduce the risk of errors and enhance recovery, but the strategies are not uniform among centers.

So far, only four trials [54-57] have reported the results of fast-track programs after esophagectomy. Their aims were a quicker discharge, approximately at POD 7, oral diet, restored gastrointestinal function and ambulation, full pain relief, and high patient satisfaction. The target of the enhanced recovery program associated with fast-track surgery is the reduction of complications. Reasons for the failure of fast-track or enhanced-recovery programs are the inability of patients to follow the pathway, prolonged hospital stay, and hospital re-admission. The high peri-operative risk of esophagectomy is due to the combination of multiple-site incisions with pain and reduced thoracic motility, extended operative time with extracellular fluid shift, prolonged mechanical ventilation, and patient comorbidities.

All four studies [54-57] adopted similar pathways, which consisted of preoperative health education for the patients, with complete information and motivation programs; respiratory function exercises to augment pulmonary reserve; and a detailed daily schedule for the first 7 postoperative days. The protocol of all trials planned an immediate extubation, early mobilization (POD 1), intense respiratory physiotherapy, negative fluid balance, and adequate pain control (epidural and/or patient-controlled analgesia). In all studies, patients received jejunal tube feeding, with oral feeding introduced after the performance of a negative Gastrografin swallow on POD 4-5. Discharge was programmed in all studies between PODs 7 and 9. The surgical approach was an open Ivor-Lewis esophagectomy in two trials [54, 55] and a left abdominal approach in one [57]. One trial did not specify the type of esophagectomy [56]. An example of a fast-track protocol is provided in Table 16.7.

The protocol could be completed in 69–77% of the patients participating in the trials (Table 16.8) [54-57]. Of note, Cerfolio and colleagues [55] claimed that 75% of the patients ≥ 70 years of age failed the fast-track program due to complications, important comorbidity, or reluctance to leave the hospital. The median length of hospital stay was 7–11 days, but considering only the three studies [54-56] that more strictly adhered to the protocol, discharge was possible between POD 7 and 9. Furthermore, mortality was low, 0.3–4.4%, and morbidity was 27–45%, which was consistent with the best results obtained in high-volume dedicated hospitals. Pulmonary complications were still the main cause of morbidity, but the reported rate of 11–17% was comparable with the best results reported in the literature, as was the leak rate.

In summary, enhanced recovery programs can achieve the same or better results as obtained with traditional care. They are less operator-dependent and reduce hospitalization, with both greater patient satisfaction and reduced healthcare costs. Hence, fast-track surgery protocols should be considered as safe and feasible. They deserve further study and application.

16.5 Early Extubation

Traditionally, prophylactic overnight mechanical ventilation with extubation the morning following the surgical procedure was instituted to protect the airway from aspiration and to allow for adequate pain control. Mechanical ventilation, especially after one-lung ventilation, is associated with barotrauma,

Table 16.7 Proposed fast-track protocol after esophagectomy

	Day of surgery	POD 1	POD 2	POD 3	POD 4	POD 5	POD 6	POD 7
Treatment area	SICU	SICU	SICU	Ward	Ward	Ward	Ward	Discharge
Respiratory support	Immediate extubation	No	No	No	No	No	No	No
Physiotherapy	No	Yes	Yes	Yes	Yes	Yes	Yes	Yes
Physical activity	No	Chair	Chair	Walk	Walk	Walk	Walk	Walk
Liquids (balance)	Negative	Negative	Negative	Negative	Negative	Equal	Equal	Equal
Nutrition	No	TPN	TPN	TPN	Liquids	Semisolids	Solids	Solids
Thoracic drains	Yes	Yes	Yes	Yes	Remove	No	No	No
Urinary tube	Yes	Yes	Yes	Remove	No	No	No	No
Nasogastric tube	Yes	Yes	Yes	Remove	No	No	No	No
Central line	Yes	Yes	Yes	Yes	Yes	Remove	No	No
Blood test and ABG	Yes	Yes	Yes	Yes	Yes	Yes	Yes	Yes
Radiology	Chest	Chest	No	No	Contrast swallow and chest	No	No	No
Analgesia	Paracetamol 3 times a day + morphine on request	Paracetamol 3 times a day + morphine on request	Paracetamol 3 times a day + morphine on request	Paracetamol on request	Paracetamol on request	Paracetamol on request	Paracetamol on request	Paracetamol on request
Antibiotic	Yes	Yes	Yes	Yes	No	No	No	No
VTE prophylaxis	Yes	Yes	Yes	Yes	Yes	Yes	Yes	Yes
PPI	Yes	Yes	Yes	Yes	Yes	Yes	Yes	Yes

POD, postoperative day; *SICU*, surgical intensive care unit; *TPN*, total parenteral nutrition; *ABG*, arterial blood gas; *VTE*, venous thromboembolism; *PPI*, proton pump inhibitors.

Table 16.8 Morbidity, mortality, and length of hospital stay (LOS) of patients treated within fast-track protocols for esophageal carcinoma

Author [Reference]	N.	Type of surgery	Completion of protocol (%)	LOS (median in days)	Morbidity (%)	Pulmonary (%)	Leak (%)	Mortality (%)
Munitiz et al. [54]	74	Ivor-Lewis	69	9	31	14	7	1
Cerfolio et al. [55]	90	Ivor-Lewis	77	7	27	13	0	4.4
Low et al. [57]	340	Left-thoraco-abdominal	n.r.	11	45	17	4	0.3
Jiang et al. [56]	114	n.r.	77	7	30	11	4	2.6

n.r., not reported.

therefore continued mechanical support after surgery can be deleterious, increasing pulmonary complications and thus mortality [58-61]. If early extubation in the operating theatre were to result in equal or even lower morbidity and mortality, without any increase in failed extubation and re-intubation, it could be reasonably applied after surgery. Indeed, immediate extubation has been proposed in fast-track programs as a key step in the pathway protocol. Pain control, especially with epidural analgesia, is deemed essential in early extubation protocols. In a Chinese trial, multivariate analysis showed that the only independent factor predicting early extubation was epidural analgesia [61]. Four recent trials investigated the results of early extubation after esophagectomy, preferentially after an Ivor-Lewis procedure [58-61].

The rates of failed early extubation and re-intubation were 9–10% and 5–16%, respectively, where reported, with a pulmonary complication rate of 14–26%, consistent with the current literature on patients who underwent esophagectomy without early extubation protocols.

The theoretical advantages of reduced respiratory morbidity and mortality were not elucidated by these studies. Nevertheless, equivalent complication rates were achieved with early extubation, with tolerable rates of failed extubation and re-intubation. Thus, in summary, early extubation is feasible and safe and may offer a therapeutic choice in all medically fit patients, especially within a fast-track program.

References

1. Dhungel B, Diggs BS, Hunter JG et al (2010) Patient and peri-operative predictors of morbidity and mortality after esophagectomy: American College of Surgeons National Surgical Quality Improvement Program (ACS-NSQIP), 2005-2008. J Gastrointest Surg 14:1492-1501

2. Bailey SH, Bull DA, Harpole DH et al (2003) Outcomes after esophagectomy: a ten-year prospective cohort. Ann Thorac Surg 75:217-222
3. Wright CD, Kucharczuk JC, O'Brien SM et al (2009) Predictors of major morbidity and mortality after esophagectomy for esophageal cancer: a Society of Thoracic Surgeons General Thoracic Surgery Database risk adjustment model. J Thorac Cardiovasc Surg 137:587-595
4. Atkins BZ, Shah AS, Hutcheson KA et al (2004) Reducing hospital morbidity and mortality following esophagectomy. Ann Thorac Surg 78:1170-1176
5. Lerut T, Moons J, Coosemans W et al (2009) Postoperative complications after transthoracic esophagectomy for cancer of the esophagus and gastroesophageal junction are correlated with early cancer recurrence: role of systematic grading of complications using the modified Clavien classification. Ann Surg 250:798-807
6. Clavien PA, Barkun J, de Oliveira ML et al (2009) The Clavien-Dindo classification of surgical complications: five-year experience. Ann Surg 250:187-196
7. Morita M, Nakanoko T, Fujinaka Y et al (2011) In-hospital mortality after a surgical resection for esophageal cancer: analyses of the associated factors and historical changes. Ann Surg Oncol 18:1757-1765
8. Zingg U, Smithers BM, Gotley DC et al (2011) Factors associated with postoperative pulmonary morbidity after esophagectomy for cancer. Ann Surg Oncol 18:1460-1468
9. Law S, Wong KH, Kwok KF et al (2004) Predictive factors for postoperative pulmonary complications and mortality after esophagectomy for cancer. Ann Surg 240:791-800
10. Ferguson MK, Durkin AE (2002) Preoperative prediction of the risk of pulmonary complications after esophagectomy for cancer. J Thorac Cardiovasc Surg 123:661-669
11. Kita T, Mammoto T, Kishi Y (2002) Fluid management and postoperative respiratory disturbances in patients with transthoracic esophagectomy for carcinoma. J Clin Anesth 14:252-256
12. Whooley BP, Law S, Murthy SC et al (2001) Analysis of reduced death and complication rates after esophageal resection. Ann Surg 233:338-344
13. Kinugasa S, Tachibana M, Yoshimura et al (2004) Postoperative pulmonary complications are associated with worse short- and long-term outcomes after extended esophagectomy. J Surg Oncol 88:71-77
14. Avendano CE, Flume PA, Silvestri GA, King LB, Reed CE (2002) Pulmonary complications after esophagectomy. Ann Thorac Surg 73:922-926
15. Akutsu Y, Matsubara H (2009) Perioperative management for the prevention of postoperative pneumonia with esophageal surgery. Ann Thorac Cardiovasc Surg 15:280-285
16. Nakamura M, Iwahashi M, Nakamori M et al (2008) An analysis of the factors contributing to a reduction in the incidence of pulmonary complications following an esophagectomy for esophageal cancer. Langenbecks Arch Surg 393:127-133
17. Michelet P, D'Journo XB, Roch A et al (2006) Protective ventilation influences systemic inflammation after esophagectomy: a randomized controlled study. Anesthesiology 105:911-919
18. Morita M, Yoshida R, Ikeda K et al (2008) Acute lung injury following an esophagectomy for esophageal cancer, with special reference to the clinical factors and cytokine levels of peripheral blood and pleural drainage fluid. Dis Esophagus 21:30-36
19. Tandon S, Batchelor A, Bullock R (2001) Peri-operative risk factors for acute lung injury after elective oesophagectomy. Br J Anaesth 86:633-638
20. Saeki H, Ishimura H, Higashi H et al (2009) Postoperative management using intensive patient-controlled epidural analgesia and early rehabilitation after an esophagectomy. Surg Today 39:476-480
21. Casado D, Lopez F, Marti R (2010) Perioperative fluid management and major respiratory complications in patients undergoing esophagectomy. Dis Esophagus 23:523-528
22. Wei S, Tian J, Song X, Chen Y (2008) Association of perioperative fluid balance and adverse surgical outcomes in esophageal cancer and esophagogastric junction cancer. Ann Thorac Surg 86:266-272
23. Hughes CG, Weavind L, Banerjee A et al (2010) Intraoperative risk factors for acute respiratory distress syndrome in critically ill patients Anesth Analg 111:464-467

24. Neal JM, Wilcox RT, Allen HW, Low DE (2003) Near-total esophagectomy: the influence of standardized multimodal management and intraoperative fluid restriction. Reg Anesth Pain Med 28:328-334
25. Hogan BA, Winter DC, Broe D et al (2008) Prospective trial comparing contrast swallow, computed tomography and endoscopy to identify anastomotic leak following oesophagogastric surgery. Surg Endosc 22:767-771
26. Blewett CJ, Miller JD, Young JE et al (2001) Anastomotic leaks after esophagectomy for esophageal cancer: a comparison of thoracic and cervical anastomoses. Ann Thorac Cardiovasc Surg 7:75-78
27. Korst RJ, Port JL, Lee PC, Altorki NK (2005) Intrathoracic manifestations of cervical anastomotic leaks after transthoracic esophagectomy for carcinoma. Ann Thorac Surg 80:1185-1190
28. van Heijl M, van Wijngaarden AK, Lagarde SM et al (2010) Intrathoracic manifestations of cervical anastomotic leaks after transhiatal and transthoracic oesophagectomy. Br J Surg 97:726-731
29. Escofet X, Manjunath A, Twine C et al (2010) Prevalence and outcome of esophagogastric anastomotic leak after esophagectomy in a UK regional cancer network. Dis Esophagus 23:112-116
30. Tabatabai A, Hashemi M, Mohajeri G et al (2009) Incidence and risk factors predisposing anastomotic leak after transhiatal esophagectomy. Ann Thorac Med 4:197-200
31. Martin LW, Swisher SG, Hofstetter W et al (2005) Intrathoracic leaks following esophagectomy are no longer associated with increased mortality. Ann Surg 242:392-399
32. Alanezi K, Urschel JD (2004) Mortality secondary to esophageal anastomotic leak. Ann Thorac Cardiovasc Surg 10:71-75
33. Schuchert MJ, Abbas G, Nason KS et al (2010) Impact of anastomotic leak on outcomes after transhiatal esophagectomy. Surgery 148:831-838
34. Griffin SM, Lamb PJ, Dresner SM et al (2001) Diagnosis and management of a mediastinal leak following radical oesophagectomy. Br J Surg 88:1346-1351
35. Urschel JD (1995) Esophagogastrostomy anastomotic leaks complicating esophagectomy: a review. Am J Surg 169:634-640
36. Tirnaksiz MB, Deschamps C, Allen MS, Johnson DC, Pairolero PC (2005) Effectiveness of screening aqueous contrast swallow in detecting clinically significant anastomotic leaks after esophagectomy. Eur Surg Res 37:123-128
37. Strauss C, Mal F, Perniceni T et al (2010) Computed tomography versus water-soluble contrast swallow in the detection of intrathoracic anastomotic leak complicating esophagogastrectomy (Ivor Lewis): a prospective study in 97 patients. Ann Surg 251:647-651
38. Turkyilmaz A, Eroglu A, Aydin Y et al (2009) The management of esophagogastric anastomotic leak after esophagectomy for esophageal carcinoma. Dis Esophagus 22:119-126
39. Chang AC, Ji H, Birkmeyer NJ et al (2008) Outcomes after transhiatal and transthoracic esophagectomy for cancer. Ann Thorac Surg 85:424-429
40. Connors RC, Reuben BC, Neumayer LA, Bull DA (2007) Comparing outcomes after transthoracic and transhiatal esophagectomy: a 5-year prospective cohort of 17,395 patients. J Am Coll Surg 205:735-740
41. Junginger T, Gockel I, Heckhoff S (2006) A comparison of transhiatal and transthoracic resections on the prognosis in patients with squamous cell carcinoma of the esophagus. Eur J Surg Oncol 32:749-755
42. Morgan MA, Lewis WG, Hopper AN et al (2007) Prospective comparison of transthoracic versus transhiatal esophagectomy following neoadjuvant therapy for esophageal cancer. Dis Esophagus 20:225-231
43. Rentz J, Bull D, Harpole D et al (2003) Transthoracic versus transhiatal esophagectomy: a prospective study of 945 patients. J Thorac Cardiovasc Surg 125:1114-1120
44. Hulscher JB, van Sandick JW, de Boer AG et al (2002) Extended transthoracic resection compared with limited transhiatal resection for adenocarcinoma of the esophagus. N Engl J Med 347:1662-1669

45. Ott K, Bader FG, Lordick F et al (2009) Surgical factors influence the outcome after Ivor-Lewis esophagectomy with intrathoracic anastomosis for adenocarcinoma of the esophagogastric junction: a consecutive series of 240 patients at an experienced center. Ann Surg Oncol 16:1017-1025
46. Griffin SM, Shaw IH, Dresner SM (2002) Early complications after Ivor Lewis subtotal esophagectomy with two-field lymphadenectomy: risk factors and management. J Am Coll Surg 194:285-297
47. Mariette C, Taillier G, Van Seuningen I, Triboulet JP (2004) Factors affecting postoperative course and survival after en bloc resection for esophageal carcinoma. Ann Thorac Surg 78:1177-1183
48. Karl RC, Schreiber R, Boulware D et al (2000) Factors affecting morbidity, mortality, and survival in patients undergoing Ivor Lewis esophagogastrectomy. Ann Surg 231:635-643
49. Nishihira T, Hirayama K, Mori S (1998) A prospective randomized trial of extended cervical and superior mediastinal lymphadenectomy for carcinoma of the thoracic esophagus. Am J Surg 175:47-51
50. Fujita H, Sueyoshi S, Tanaka T et al (2003) Optimal lymphadenectomy for squamous cell carcinoma in the thoracic esophagus: comparing the short- and long-term outcome among the four types of lymphadenectomy. World J Surg 27:571-579
51. Shim YM, Kim HK, Kim K (2010) Comparison of survival and recurrence pattern between two-field and three-field lymph node dissections for upper thoracic esophageal squamous cell carcinoma. J Thorac Oncol 5:707-712
52. Igaki H, Tachimori Y, Kato H (2004) Improved survival for patients with upper and/or middle mediastinal lymph node metastasis of squamous cell carcinoma of the lower thoracic esophagus treated with 3-field dissection. Ann Surg 239:483-490
53. Biere SS, Maas KW, Cuesta MA et al DL (2011) Cervical or thoracic anastomosis after esophagectomy for cancer: a systematic review and meta-analysis. Dig Surg 28:29-35
54. Munitiz V, Martinez-de-Haro LF, Ortiz A et al (2010) Effectiveness of a written clinical pathway for enhanced recovery after transthoracic (Ivor Lewis) oesophagectomy. Br J Surg 97:714-718
55. Cerfolio RJ, Bryant AS, Bass CS et al (2004) Fast tracking after Ivor Lewis esophagogastrectomy. Chest 126:1187-1194
56. Jiang K, Cheng L, Wang JJ et al (2009) Fast track clinical pathway implications in esophagogastrectomy. World J Gastroenterol 15 :496-501
57. Low DE, Kunz S, Schembre D et al (2007) Esophagectomy—it's not just about mortality anymore: standardized perioperative clinical pathways improve outcomes in patients with esophageal cancer. J Gastrointest Surg 11:1395-1402
58. Robertson SA, Skipworth RJ, Clarke DL et al (2006) Ventilatory and intensive care requirements following oesophageal resection. Ann R Coll Surg Engl 88:354-357
59. Chandrashekar MV, Irving M, Wayman J et al (2003) Immediate extubation and epidural analgesia allow safe management in a high-dependency unit after two-stage oesophagectomy. Results of eight years of experience in a specialized upper gastrointestinal unit in a district general hospital. Br J Anaesth 90:474-479
60. Lanuti M, de Delva PE, Maher A et al (2006) Feasibility and outcomes of an early extubation policy after esophagectomy. Ann Thorac Surg 82:2037-2041
61. Yap FH, Lau JY, Joynt GM et al (2003) Early extubation after transthoracic oesophagectomy. Hong Kong Med J 9:98-102

Treatment of Recurrent and Metastatic Esophageal Cancer

17

Michele Pavarana and Teodoro Sava

17.1 Recurrence

17.1.1 Introduction

There are few studies of the treatment of relapse in patients with esophageal squamous cell cancer (ESCC). Moreover, those trials were not randomized and without convincing data. Cumulative overall 1-year and 2-year survival rates after recurrence were around 30% and 12%, respectively, with a median survival of 6 months [1]. For this reason, the goal of the treatment is usually adequate palliation instead of cure, taking into account many factors: patient characteristics (performance status, age, co-morbidity), mode of relapse (local vs. locoregional vs. systemic), site of the primary cancer (non-local recurrences are more frequent in cervical or upper thoracic cancers) [2]; site of relapse (liver recurrence is the worst prognostic site, with a median overall survival < 6 months) [3]; kinetics of relapse (indolent or aggressive, symptomatic or asymptomatic disease); and previous treatments and their toxicities.

Additionally, disease-free interval and progression-free interval are to be considered if the first-line therapy has already been administered. Disease-free interval is probably the most important factor in the choice of the proper treatment. If the relapse occurs before or after 6 months from primary treatment, the probability of response to the new treatment and survival are significantly different in terms of response rate (0 vs. 37%, respectively), median progression-free survival (2.8 vs. 4.8 months, respectively), and median overall survival (6.1 vs. 10.2 months, respectively) [4, 5].

M. Pavarana (✉)
Oncology Unit, Borgo Trento Hospital,
Verona, Italy

G. de Manzoni (Ed.), *Treatment of Esophageal and Hypopharyngeal Squamous Cell Carcinoma*,

17.1.2 Recurrence after Surgery Alone

In case of relapse in patients treated previously with surgery alone, definitive chemotherapy, radiotherapy, or both (concomitant or sequential treatment) could be considered. With this combined approach, it is sometime possible to achieve the same good results obtained in neoadjuvant setting. .

Chemoradiotherapy allows control of the disease (i.e., complete response, partial response, or stable disease) in about 20–40% of patients, but the length of the response is mostly less than 6–8 months with 1-, 2- and 3-year survival rates of 33, 15, and 12%, respectively. Clinical complete response is uncommon (< 10% of patients) [6-8]. Frequently, in case of treatment of relapse after surgery, the radiotherapy dose must be limited to 45 Gy, due to the presence of a gastric pull-up or interposed bowel in the treatment field. If dysphagia is present, radiation alone improves symptoms in approximately 60–70% of patients, chemoradiotherapy in 88% of patients, and chemotherapy alone in 20–30% of patients [6, 7].

17.1.3 Recurrence after Neoadjuvant Treatment

After neoadjuvant chemoradiotherapy, about 40% of complete responding patients develop local or distant recurrence. The prognosis of patients who fail to respond to treatment is very poor in all series, with a 2-year survival of 10% [2, 7-9].

In case of locoregional recurrence in radiotherapy fields, palliative chemotherapy can be offered in the attempt to prevent systemic disease, even though it is rarely effective for relapse because of previous radiotherapy-induced fibrosis; however, randomized trials are not available. In case of dysphagia, instead of palliative chemotherapy, endoscopic laser or stenting is indicated; in patients with endoluminal tumor growth, brachytherapy might be useful.

The role of completing doses of radiotherapy is controversial because of toxicities and small effect (increased local failure). The role of radiotherapy in extra-field relapses is palliative.

In case of systemic recurrence, first-line chemotherapy is justified.

Unfortunately many of these patients are in poor condition, with important comorbidities. Thus, most qualify only for best supportive (non-oncologic-symptom palliative) care.

17.1.4 Recurrence after Definitive Chemoradiation

As described elsewhere in this volume, few patients who have undergone definitive chemoradiation are eligible for surgery for disease relapse [4, 10, 11]. However, even though these operations are associated with high morbidity and mortality, if R0 resection is feasible, it is possible to achieve acceptable results (5-year survival rate: 25%) [11-16]. In a highly selected series of 131 recurrent patients, 24 patients with good performance status underwent surgery for local or isolated distant metastases, with a 5-year survival rate from recurrence to death of 6.7% (compared with 0, 0, and 3.9% of patients who underwent no treatment, chemotherapy only, or radiochemotherapy, respectively) [13].

17.2 Metastatic Cancer

More than two-thirds of the patients with esophageal cancer have metastatic disease at the time of diagnosis. Even patients with resectable disease or those eligible for preoperative treatment have a high rate of local and distant recurrence. The expected median survival is < 24 months, with a 5-year survival rate of < 30%. Accordingly, the goal of treatment is rarely cure but rather palliation, without compromising the patient's quality of life. This can be achieved with chemotherapy, radiation therapy, surgery, or best supportive care [17, 18].

Nevertheless, there are no conclusive literature data on the role of chemotherapy. Based on computerized (MEDLINE) and manual searches, we identified less than 100 reports of palliative chemotherapy in relapsing or metastatic patients.

In 2010, a Cochrane Library review was withdrawn [19]. Only two randomized controlled trials, with a total of 42 participants, compared chemotherapy with best supportive care for metastatic esophageal cancer. No survival benefit was shown for chemotherapy in these trials. Five randomized controlled trials with a total of 1242 patients compared different chemotherapy regimens; however, due to variations in patient population and type of chemotherapy, a pooled analysis was not possible. Nonetheless, there was no consistent benefit of any specific chemotherapy regimen. The authors concluded that there is a need for well-designed, adequately powered, phase III trials comparing chemotherapy with palliative care for patients with metastatic esophageal cancer. Chemotherapeutic drugs shown to have a good response rate and manageable toxicity were cisplatin, 5-fluorouracil, paclitaxel, docetaxel, anthracyclines, and irinotecan. The main single-agent results are summarized in Table 17.1 [20-35]. Briefly: (a) sensitivity to chemotherapy is greater in newly diagnosed patients; (b) response rates are highly variable in different studies using the same drugs; and (c) the activity of carboplatin is minimal in squamous cell cancer and it should not be a substitute for cisplatin.

Table 17.2 [36-80] summarizes the main trials with combination chemotherapy: (a) only two randomized studies comparing chemotherapy with best supportive care are available and no survival advantage for treatment was demonstrated; (b) cisplatin-based chemotherapy was the best studied combination, with more favorable activity in terms of response, although the duration

Table 17.1 Monochemotherapy in patients with metastatic esophageal cancer

Agent	Histology	N.	Response rate (%)	Author (year)
BLEO	SCC	14	0	Ravry et al. (1973) [20]
BLEO	SCC + AC	15	27	Kolaric et al. (1976) [21]
MMC	SCC	24	42	Engstrom et al. (1983) [22]
MTX	SCC	26	12	Ezdinli et al. (1980) [23]
5FU	SCC	26	15	Ezdinli et al. (1980) [23]
VDS	SCC	52	27	Bezwoda et al. (1984) [24]
VDS	SCC	34	22	Kelsen et al. (1979) [25]
ADM	SCC	20	5	Ezdinli et al. (1980) [23]
VRB	SCC	152	28	Ravry et al. (1985) [26]; Panettiere et al. (1984) [27]
VRB	SCC	30	20	Conroy et al. (1996) [28]
CDDP	SCC	35	26	Panettiere et al. (1984) [27]
CBDCA	SCC + AC	30	7	Sternberg et al. (1985) [29]
CBDCA	SCC	18	0	Queisser et al. (1990) [30]
VP16	SCC	20	0	Coonley et al. (1983) [31]
TXT	SCC + AC	52	20	Muro et al. (2004) [32]
TXL	AC	30	30	Ajani et al. (1994) [33]
	SCC	12	25	
TXT	AC	8	20	Einzig et al. (1996) [34]
VRB	SCC	17	25	Bidoli et al. (2001) [35]

AC, adenocarcinoma; *ADM*, Adriamycin; *BLEO*, bleomycin; *CBDCA*, carboplatin; *CDDP*, cisplatin; *5FU*, fluorouracil; *MMC*, mitoycin-C; *MTX*, methotrexate; *TXL* taxol; *TXT*, taxotere; *VDS* vindesine; *VP16*, etoposide; *VRB*, vinorelbine; *SCC*, squamous cell carcinoma.

of response is short (3–6 months); (c) carboplatin has less activity than cisplatin in esophageal carcinoma; and (d) taxanes and irinotecan are effective and should be incorporated into combined modality treatment [81-85].

17.3 Conclusions

Many regimens or single-drug therapies achieve a moderate response rate (30–50%), with a median duration of response of 3–6 months and a median overall survival of less than 10–12 months. Even the most intensive regimens obtained a complete response in no more than 10% of the patients, with median survival not beyond 1 year. The majority of the published studies are phase II studies or underpowered phase III studies with a small number of patients. It is therefore essentially impossible to state that one regimen is superior to others because of the different drugs with which patients were treated, the different drug combinations, and the different endpoints. Moreover, most trials did not distinguish between locally advanced and metastatic esophageal cancers.

Table 17.2 Combination chemotherapy in patients with metastatic esophageal cancer

Agent	Histology	N.	Response rate (%)	Author (year)
CDDP/BLEO/MTX	SCC	9	44	Vogl et al. (1981) [36]
CDDP/FU/ADM	SCC	21	33	Gisselbrecht et al.(1983) [37]
CDDP/BLEO	SCC	18	17	Dinwoodie et al. (1986) [38]
CDDP/BLEO/MTX	SCC	31	26	DeBesi et al. (1984) [39]
CDDP/VDS/BLEO	SCC	24	33	Kelsen et al. (1983) [40] e
CDDP/VDS/BLEO	SCC	27	29	Dinwoodie et al. (1986) [38]
CDDP/5FU/ ALLOPURINOL	SCC	37	35	DeBesi et al. (1986) [41]
CBDCA/VBL	SCC	16	0	Lovett et al. (1991) [42]
CDDP/5FU	SCC	35	34	Iizuka et al. (1992) [43]
CDDP/MTX	SCC	42	76	Ad vani et al. (1985) [44]
CDDP/5FU/LV/VP16	SCC + AC	38	45	Stahl et al. (1994) [45]
5FU/IFN	SCC	31	26	Kelsen et al. (1992) [46]; Wadler et al. (1993) [47]
VP16/MMC	AC	15	13	Braybrooke et al. (1997) [48]
CDDP/TXL	SCC	10	60	Kelsen et al. (1997) [49]
	AC	27	37	
CDDP/TXL	SCC + AC	58	52	Van der Gaast et al. (1999) [50]
CDDP/TXL	SCC + AC	44-56	41-44	Cho et al. (2005) [51], Ilson et al. (2000) [52]
5FU/ADM/MTX	SCC + AC	88	21	Webb et al. (1997) [53]
CDDP/TXL	SCC	20	40	Petrasch et al. (1998) [54]
CDDP/5FU/TXL	SCC	30	50	Ilson et al. (1998) [55]
CDDP/5FU	SCC + AC	72	30	Levard et al. (1998) [56]
Control	SCC + AC	84		
CBDCA/TXL	SCC	9	44	Philip et al. (1997) [57]
CDDP/5FU	SCC	20	55	Sekiguchi et al. (1999) [58]
CDDP/CPT11	SCC	35	36-58	Ilson et al. (1999) [59], Ajani et al. (2002) [60]
CDDP/TXL	SCC	64	52	Van der Gaast et al. (1999) [50]
CDDP/TXL/VP16	SCC	22	100	Lokich et al. (1999) [61]
EPI/CDDP/RALT	SCC + AC	21	29	Mackay et al. (2001) [62]
CDDP/5FU	SCC	42	33	Hayashi et al. (2001) [63]
CDDP/5FU	SCC	59	33	Caroli-Bosc et al. (2001) [64]
CDDP/RA/IFN	SCC	38	21	Goncalves et al. (2001) [65]
CDDP/VP16/5FU/LV	SCC	69	34	Polee et al. (2001) [66]
5FU	SCC + AC	127	16	Tebbutt et al. (2002) [67]
5FU/IFN	SCC	33	61	Bazarbashi et al. (2002) [68]
CDDP/VRB	SCC	24	34	Conroy et al. (2002) [69]

(cont.→)

Table 17.2 (*continued*)

EPI/CDDP/5FU	SCC + AC	290	42	Ross et al. (2002) [70]
MMC/CDDP/5FU	SCC + AC	290	44	
TXT/CPT11	SCC + AC	10	30-33	Govindan et al. (2003) [71]
TXT/CPT11	SCC + AC	24	12.5	Lordick et al. (2003) [72]
TXT/VRB	SCC	36	60	Airoldi et al. (2003) [73]
CDDP/GEM	SCC + AC	64	40	Urba et al. (2004) [74]
TXL/CBDCA	SCC	35	43	El-Rayes et al. (2004) [75]
CDDP/GEM	SCC + AC	36	41	Kroep et al. (2004) [76]
CDDP/CPT11	SCC + AC	39	36	Ilson et al. (2004) [77]
GEM/5FU/LV	SCC + AC	35	31	Morgan-Meadows et al. (2005) [78]
TXT/CAPE	SCC + AC	24	46	Lorenzen et al. (2005) [79]
OXA/5FU/LV	SCC + AC	35	41	Maue et al.r (2005) [80]

AC, adenocarcinoma; *MTX*, Methotrexate; *OXA*, oxaliplatin; *RA*, retinoic acid; *RALT*, raltitrexed; *SCC*, squamous cell carcinoma; *TXL*, taxol; *TXT*, taxotere; *VDS*, vindesine; *VP16*, etoposide; *VRB*, vinorelbine.

Some data suggest that the disease-free interval from primary treatment is a prognostic factor for overall survival in metastatic/recurrent ESCC, although these data remain to be confirmed in series with a higher number of recruited patients [85-87].

Liver recurrence and the absence of treatment seem to be negative prognostic factors in patients with recurrent ESCC [87]. Studies are underway investigating the therapeutic effects of anti-EGFR antibodies, the anti-angiogenic pathway, proteosome inhibitors, matrix metalloproteinase inhibitors, and cell-cycle inhibitors but definitive results have yet to be achieved.

References

1. Hsu PK, Wang BY, Huang CS et al (2011) Prognostic factors for post-recurrence survival in esophageal suamous cell carcinoma patients with recurrence after resection. J Gastrointest Surg DOI 10.1007/s11605-011-1458-1
2. Ishihara R, Yamamoto S, Iishi H et al (2010) Factors predictive of tumor recurrence and survival after initial complete response of esophageal squamous cell carcinoma to definitive chemoradiotherapy. Int J Radiat Oncol Biol Phys 76:123-129
3. Takashima A, Shirao K, Hirashima Y et al (2008) Chemosensitivity of patients with recurrent esophageal cancer receiving perioperative chemotherapy. Dis Esophagus 21:607-611
4. Nemoto K, Ariga H, Kakuto Y et al (2001) Radiation therapy for loco-regionally recurrent esophageal cancer after surgery. Radiother Oncol 61:65-168
5. Yamashita H, Nakagawa K, Tago M et al (2005) Salvage radiotherapy for postoperative loco-regional recurrence of esophageal cancer. Dis Esophagus 18:215-220

6. Maruyama K, Motoyama S, Anbai A et al (2010) Therapeutic strategy for the treatment of postoperative recurrence od esophageal squamous cell carcinoma: clinical efficacy of radiotherapy. Dis Esophagus 13:1442-1450
7. Cooper JS, Guo MD, Herskovic A et al (1999) Chemoradiotherapy of locally advanced esophageal cancer: long-term follow-up of a prospective randomized trial (RTOG 85-01). JAMA 281:1623-1627
8. Ishikura S, Nihei H, Ohtsu A et al (2003) Long-term toxicity after definitive chemoradiotherapy for squamous cell carcinoma of the thoracic esophagus. J Clin Oncol 2:2697-2702
9. Tahara M, Othsu A, Hironaka S et al (2005) Clinical impact of criteria for complete response of primary site to treatment of esophageal cancer. Jpn J Clin Oncol 35:316-323
10. Meunier B, Raoul J, Le Prise E et al (1998) Salvage esophagectomy after unsuccessful curative chemoradiotherapy for squamous cell cancer of the esophagus. Dig Surg 15:224-226
11. Swisher SG, Wynn P, Putnam JB et al (2002) Salvage esophagectomy for recurrent tumours after definitive chemotherapy and radiotherapy. J Thorac Cardiovasc Surg 123:175-183
12. Tomimaru Y, Yano M, Takachi K et al (2006) Factors affecting the prognosis of patients with esophageal cancer undergoing salvage surgery after definitive chemoradiotherapy. J Surg Oncol 93:422-428
13. Natsugoe S, Okumura H, Matsumoto M et al (2006) The role of salvage surgery for recurrence of esophageal squamous cell cancer. Eur J Surg Oncol 32:544-547
14. Ariga H, Nemoto K, Miyazaki S et al (2009) Prospective comparison of surgery alone and chemoradiotherapy with selective surgery in respectable squamous cell carcinoma of the esophagus. Int J Radiat Oncol Biol Phys 75:348-356
15. Gardner-Thorpe J, Hardwick RH, Dwerryhouse SJ (2007) Salvage oesophagectomy after local failure of definitive chemoradiotherapy. Br J Surg 94:1059-1066
16. Nishimura M, Daiko H, Yoshida J et al (2007) Gen Thorac Cardiovasc Surg 55:461-464
17. Daly JM, Karnell LH and Menck HR (1996) National cancer data base report on esophageal carcinoma. Cancer 78:1820-1828
18. Parkin D, Pisani P and Ferley J (1999) Global cancer statistics. Cancer J Clin 49:33-64
19. Cochrane Database Syst Rev. 2010. May 12: 5:CD004063
20. Ravry M, Moertel CG, Schutt AJ et al (1973) Treatment of advanced squamous cell carcinoma of the gastrointestinal tract with bleomycin. Cancer Chemother Rep 57:493-495
21. Kolari K, Marici Z, Dujmovi I et al (1976) Therapy of advanced esophageal cancer with bleomycin, irradiation and combination of bleomycin with irradiation. Tumori 62:255-262
22. Engstrom PF, Lavin PT, Klaassen DJ (1983) Phase II evaluation of mitomycin and cisplatin in advanced esophageal carcinoma. Cancer Treat Rep 67:713-725
23. Ezdinli EZ, Gelber R, Desai DV et al (1980) Chemotherapy of advanced esophageal carcinoma: Eastern Cooperative Oncology Group experience. Cancer 46:2149-53
24. Bezwoda WR, Derman DP, Weaving A et al (1984) Treatment of esophageal cancer with vindesine: an open trial. Cancer Treat Rep 68:783-785
25. Kelsen DP, Bains M, Cvitkovic E et al (1979) Vindesine in the treatment of esophageal carcinoma: a phase II study. Cancer Treat Rep 63:2019-2021
26. Ravry MJ, Moore MR, Omura GA et al (1985) Phase II evaluation of cisplatin in squamous carcinoma of the esophagus: a Southeastern Cancer Study Group trial. Cancer Treat Rep 69:1457-1458
27. Panettiere FJ, Leichman LP, Tilchen EJ et al (1984) Chemotherapy for advanced epidermoid carcinoma of the esophagus with single-agent cisplatin: final report on a Southwest Oncology Group study. Cancer Treat Rep 68:1023-1024
28. Conroy T, Etienne PL, Adenis A et al (1996) Phase II trial of vinorelbine in metastatic squamous cell esophageal carcinoma. European Organization for Research and Treatment of Cancer Gastrointestinal Treat Cancer Cooperative Group. J Clin Oncol 14:164-170

29. Sternberg C, Kelsen D, Dukeman M et al (1985) Carboplatin: a new platinum analog in the treatment of epidermoid carcinoma of the esophagus. Cancer Treat Rep 69:1305-1307
30. Queisser W, Preusser P, Mross KB et al (1990) Phase II evaluation of carboplatin in advanced esophageal carcinoma. A trial of the Phase I/II Study Group of the Association for Medical Oncology of the German Cancer Society. Onkologie 13:190-193
31. Coonley CJ, Bains M, Heelan R et al (1983) Phase II study of etoposide in the treatment of esophageal carcinoma. Cancer Treat Rep 67:397-398
32. Muro K, Hamaguchi T, Ohtsu A et al (2004) A phase II study of single-agent docetaxel in patients with metastatic esophageal cancer. Ann Oncol 15:955-959
33. Kelsen D, Ajani J, Ilson D et al (1994) A phase II trial of paclitaxel (Taxol) in advanced esophageal cancer: preliminary report. Semin Oncol 21:44-48
34. Einzig AI, Neuberg D, Remick SC et al (1996) Phase II trial of docetaxel (Taxotere) in patients with adenocarcinoma of the upper gastrointestinal tract previously untreated with cytotoxic chemotherapy: the Eastern Cooperative Oncology Group (ECOG) results of protocol E1293.Med Oncol 13:87-93
35. Bidoli P, Stani SC, De Candis D et al (2001) Single-agent chemotherapy with vinorelbine for pretreated or metastatic squamous cell carcinoma of the esophagus. Tumori 87:299-302
36. Vogl SE, Greenwald E, Kaplan BH (1981) Effective chemotherapy for esophageal cancer with methotrexate, bleomycin, and cis-diamminedichloroplatinum II. Cancer 48:2555-2558
37. Gisselbrecht C, Calvo F, Mignot et al (1983) Fluorouracil (F), Adriamycin (A), and cisplatin (P) (FAP): combination chemotherapy of advanced esophageal carcinoma. Cancer 52:974-977
38. Dinwoodie WR, Bartolucci AA, Lyman GH et al (1986) Phase II evaluation of cisplatin, bleomycin, and vindesine in advanced squamous cell carcinoma of the esophagus: a Southeastern Cancer Study Group Trial. Cancer Treat Rep 70:267-270
39. De Besi P, Salvagno L, Endrizzi L et al (1984) Cisplatin, bleomycin and methotrexate in the treatment of advanced oesophageal cancer. Eur J Cancer Clin Oncol 20:743-747
40. Kelsen D, Hilaris B, Coonley C et al (1983) Cisplatin, vindesine, and bleomycin chemotherapy of local-regional and advanced esophageal carcinoma. Am J Med 75:645-652
41. De Besi P, Sileni VC, Salvagno L et al (1986) Phase II study of cisplatin, 5-FU, and allopurinol in advanced esophageal cancer. Cancer Treat Rep 70:909-910
42. Lovett D, Kelsen D, Eisenberger M et al (1991) A phase II trial of carboplatin and vinblastine in the treatment of advanced squamous cell carcinoma of the esophagus. Cancer 67:354-356
43. Iizuka T, Kakegawa T, Ide H et al (1992) Phase II evaluation of cisplatin and 5-fluorouracil in advanced squamous cell carcinoma of the esophagus: a Japanese Esophageal Oncology Group Trial. Jpn J Clin Oncol 22:172-176
44. Advani SH, Saikia TK, Swaroop S et al (1985) Anterior chemotherapy in esophageal cancer. Cancer 56:1502-1506
45. Stahl M, Wilke H, Meyer HJ et al (1994) 5-Fluorouracil, folinic acid, etoposide and cisplatin chemotherapy for locally advanced or metastatic carcinoma of the oesophagus. Eur J Cancer 30A:325-328
46. Kelsen D, Lovett D, Wong J et al (1992) Interferon alfa-2a and fluorouracil in the treatment of patients with advanced esophageal cancer. J Clin Oncol 10:269-274
47. Wadler S, Fell S, Haynes H et al (1993) Treatment of carcinoma of the esophagus with 5-fluorouracil and recombinant alfa-2a-interferon. Cancer 71:1726-1730
48. Braybrooke JP, O'Byrne KJ, Saunders MP et al (1997) A phase II study of mitomycin C and oral etoposide for advanced adenocarcinoma of the upper gastrointestinal tract. Ann Oncol 8:294-296
49. Kelsen D, Ginsberg R, Bains M et al (1997) A phase II trial of paclitaxel and cisplatin in patients with locally advanced metastatic esophageal cancer: a preliminary report. Semin Oncol 24:S19-77-S19-81

50. Van der Gaast A, Kok TC, Kerkhofs L et al (1999) Phase I study of a biweekly schedule of a fixed dose of cisplatin with increasing doses of paclitaxel in patients with advanced oesophageal cancer. Br J Cancer 80:1052-1057
51. Cho SH, Chung IJ, Song SY et al (2005) Bi-weekly chemotherapy of paclitaxel and cisplatin in patients with metastatic or recurrent esophageal cancer. J Korean Med Sci Aug;20(4):618-23
52. Ilson DH, Forastiere A, Arquette M et al (2000) A phase II trial of paclitaxel and cisplatin in patients with advanced carcinoma of the esophagus. Cancer J 6:316-623
53. Webb A, Cunningham D, Scarffe JH et al (1997) Randomized trial comparing epirubicin, cisplatin, and fluorouracil versus fluorouracil, doxorubicin, and methotrexate in advanced esophagogastric cancer. J Clin Oncol 15:261-267
54. Petrasch S, Welt A, Reinacher A et al (1998) Chemotherapy with cisplatin and paclitaxel in patients with locally advanced, recurrent or metastatic oesophageal cancer. Br J Cancer 78:511-514
55. Ilson DH, Ajani J, Bhalla K et al (1998) Phase II trial of paclitaxel, fluorouracil, and cisplatin in patients with advanced carcinoma of the esophagus. J Clin Oncol 16:1826-1834
56. Levard H, Pouliquen X, Hay JM et al (1998) 5-Fluorouracil and cisplatin as palliative treatment of advanced oesophageal squamous cell carcinoma. A multicentre randomised controlled trial. The French Associations for Surgical Research. Eur J Surg 164:849-857
57. Philip PA, Zalupski MM, Gadgeel S et al (1997) A phase II study of carboplatin and paclitaxel in the treatment of patients with advanced esophageal and gastric cancer. Semin Oncol 24:S19-86-S19-88
58. Sekiguchi H, Akiyama S, Fujiwara M et al (1999) Phase II trial of 5-fluorouracil and low-dose cisplatin in patients with squamous cell carcinoma of the esophagus. Surg Today 29:97-101
59. Ilson DH, Saltz L, Enzinger P et al (1999) Phase II trial of weekly irinotecan plus cisplatin in advanced esophageal cancer. J Clin Oncol 17:3270-3275
60. Ajani JA, Baker J, Pisters PW et al (2002) CPT-11 plus cisplatin in patients with advanced, untreated gastric or gastroesophageal junction carcinoma: results of a phase II study. Cancer 94:641-646
61. Lokich JJ, Sonneborn H, Anderson NR et al (1999) Combined paclitaxel, cisplatin, and etoposide for patients with previously untreated esophageal and gastroesophageal carcinomas. Cancer 85:2347-2351
62. Mackay HJ, McInnes A, Paul J et al (2001) A phase II study of epirubicin, cisplatin and raltitrexed combination chemotherapy (ECT) in patients with advanced oesophageal and gastric adenocarcinoma. Ann Oncol 12:1407-1410
63. Hayashi K, Ando N, Watanabe H et al (2001) Phase II evaluation of protracted infusion of cisplatin and 5-fluorouracil in advanced squamous cell carcinoma of the esophagus: a Japan Esophageal Oncology Group (JEOG) Trial (JCOG9407). Jpn J Clin Oncol 31:419-423
64. Caroli-Bosc FX, Van Laethem JL, Michel P et al (2001) A weekly 24-h infusion of high-dose 5-fluorouracil (5-FU)+leucovorin and bi-weekly cisplatin (CDDP) was active and well tolerated in patients with non-colon digestive carcinomas. Eur J Cancer 37:1828-1832
65. Goncalves A, Camerlo J, Bun H et al (2001) Phase II study of a combination of cisplatin, all-trans-retinoic acid and interferon-alpha in squamous cell carcinoma: clinical results and pharmacokinetics. Anticancer Res 21:1431-1437
66. Polee MB, Kok TC, Siersema PD et al (2001) Phase II study of the combination cisplatin, etoposide, 5-fluorouracil and folinic acid in patients with advanced squamous cell carcinoma of the esophagus. Anticancer Drugs 12:513-517
67. Tebbutt NC, Norman A, Cunningham D et al (2002) A multicentre, randomised phase III trial comparing protracted venous infusion (PVI) 5-fluorouracil (5-FU) with PVI 5-FU plus mitomycin C in patients with inoperable oesophago-gastric cancer. Ann Oncol 13:1568-1575

68. Bazarbashi S, Rahal M, Raja MA et al (2002) A pilot trial of combination cisplatin, 5-fluorouracil and interferon-alpha in the treatment of advanced esophageal carcinoma. Chemotherapy 48:211-216
69. Conroy T, Etienne PL, Adenis A et al (2002) Vinorelbine and cisplatin in metastatic squamous cell carcinoma of the oesophagus: response, toxicity, quality of life and survival.Ann Oncol 13:721-729
70. Ross P, Nicolson M, Cunningham D et al (2002) Prospective randomized trial comparing mitomycin, cisplatin, and protracted venous-infusion fluorouracil (PVI 5-FU) With epirubicin, cisplatin, and PVI 5-FU in advanced esophagogastric cancer. J Clin Oncol 20:1996-2004
71. Govindan R, Read W, Faust J et al (2003) Phase II study of docetaxel and irinotecan in metastatic or recurrent esophageal cancer: a preliminary report. Oncology (Williston Park) 17:27-31
72. Lordick F, von Schilling C, Bernhard H et al (2003) Phase II trial of irinotecan plus docetaxel in cisplatin-pretreated relapsed or refractory oesophageal cancer. Br J Cancer 18;630-633
73. Airoldi M, Cattel L, Marchionatti S et al (2003) Docetaxel and vinorelbine in recurrent head and neck cancer: pharmacokinetic and clinical results. Am J Clin Oncol 26:378-381
74. Urba SG, Chansky K, VanVeldhuizen PJ et al (2004) Gemcitabine and cisplatin for patients with metastatic or recurrent esophageal carcinoma: a Southwest Oncology Group Study. Invest New Drugs 22:91-97
75. El-Rayes BF, Shields A, Zalupski M et al (2004) A phase II study of carboplatin and paclitaxel in esophageal cancer. Ann Oncol 15:960-965
76. Kroep JR, Pinedo HM, Giaccone G et al (2004) Phase II study of cisplatin preceding gemcitabine in patients with advanced oesophageal cancer. Ann Oncol 15:230-235
77. Ilson DH (2004) Phase II trial of weekly irinotecan/cisplatin in advanced esophageal cancer. Oncology (Williston Park) 18:22-25
78. Morgan-Meadows S, Mulkerin D, Berlin JD et al (2005) A phase II trial of gemcitabine, 5-fluorouracil and leucovorin in advanced esophageal carcinoma. Oncology 69:130-134
79. Lorenzen S, Duyster J, Lersch C et al (2005) Capecitabine plus docetaxel every 3 weeks in first- and second-line metastatic oesophageal cancer: final results of a phase II trial. Br J Cancer 92:2129-2133
80. Mauer AM, Kraut EH, Krauss SA et al (2005) Phase II trial of oxaliplatin, leucovorin and fluorouracil in patients with advanced carcinoma of the esophagus. Ann Oncol 16:1320-1325
81. Meluch AA, Hainsworth JD, Gray JR et al (1999) Preoperative combined modality therapy with paclitaxel, carboplatin, prolonged infusion 5-fluorouracil, and radiation therapy in localised esophageal cancer: preliminary results of a Minnie Pearl Cancer Research Networkphase II trial. Cancer J Sci Am 5:84-91
82. Heath EI, Burtness BA, Heitmiller RF et al (2000) Phase II evaluation of preoperative chemoradiation and postoperative adjuvant chemotherapy for squamous cell and adenocarcinoma of the esophagus. J Clin Oncol 18:868-876
83. Mauer AM, Haraf DC, Ferguson MK et al (2000) Docetaxel-based combined modality Therapy for locally advanced carcinoma of the esophagus and gastric cardia. Proc Am Soc Clin Oncol 19:954a
84. Liu An, Huang J, Cai RG et al (2008) Response af advanced esophageal cancer to chemotherapy and prognostic factors: a report of 138 cases. Ai Zheng, 27:400-406
85. Grunberger B, Raderer M, Schmidinger M, Hejna M (2007) Palliative chemotherapy for recurrent and metastatic esophageal cancer. Anticancer Res 27:2705-2714
86. Takashima A, Shirao K, Hirashima Y et al (2008) Chemosensitivity of patients with recurrent esophageal cancer receiving perioperative chemotherapy. Dis Esophagus 21:607-611

87. Hsu PK, Wang BY, Huang CS (2011) Prognostic factors for post-recurrence survival in esophageal squamous cell carcinoma patients with recurrence after resection. J Gastrointest Surg, DOI 10.1007/s11605-011-1458-1

Role of Endoscopy in Palliative Treatment 18

Luca Rodella, Francesco Lombardo, Filippo Catalano, Angelo Cerofolini,
Walid El Kheir, and Giovanni de Manzoni

18.1 Introduction

Approximately 50% of patients with esophageal squamous cell carcinoma (ESCC) have metastatic disease at presentation and are candidates for palliative therapy. The median age of these patients is 65 years such that palliative surgery has a high morbidity and mortality. The main goal of endoscopic therapy in patients with advanced cancers is the palliation of dysphagia, which contributes to improved nutritional status and quality of life. Bleeding and esophago-respiratory fistulas may also be palliated. Several endoscopic palliative treatments are available for ESCC patients, as summarized in Table 18.1.

Table 18.1 Endoscopic palliation

Mechanical	Dilatation: mechanical–hydrostatic
	Stent placement: self-expandable metallic or plastic stents, biodegradable stents
	Percutaneous endoscopic gastrostomy
Thermal	Laser therapy: Nd:YAG, KTP, diode
	Argon plasma coagulation
	Cryotherapy
	Diathermy
Chemical	Injection: sclerosants, alcohol
	Photodynamic therapy

L. Rodella (✉)
Surgical Endoscopy Unit, Borgo Trento Hospital,
Verona, Italy

G. de Manzoni (Ed.), *Treatment of Esophageal and Hypopharyngeal Squamous Cell Carcinoma*,

18.2 Mechanical Endoscopic Treatment

18.2.1 Dilatation

While esophageal dilatation is effective, the benefits are of short duration (3–4 weeks). It is often used before stent placement or tumor reduction. Perforation reduces life expectancy by half [1] and the risk is relatively high (5–8%).

18.2.2 Stents

Endoluminal esophageal stents have been widely used for over a century. Nowadays, self-expandable metallic stents (SEMS) are often chosen because of their ease of insertion and the fact that they provide rapid relief of dysphagia, with a low complication rate. The main indications and contraindications for stent are listed in Table 18.2.

Several types of self-expandable metallic (SEMS) or plastic (SEPS) stents are available. Ideally, they should have a radial force to allow a normal diet, high flexibility to adapt to angled or tortuous tumors, a low rate of migration, and be easily repositionable.

Among the SEMS, the Ultraflex stent (Boston Scientific) consists of a knitted nitinol wire tube and is available in uncovered and covered versions. In the latter, the polyurethane coating prevents tumor ingrowth. The stent has an internal diameter of 18 or 22 mm. The radial force is the lowest among the currently available types of SEMS.

The Wallstent (Boston Scientific) is made of a cobalt-based alloy; it has a lower flexibility, and a higher radial force than the Ultraflex stent. The Z-stent (Cook Europe) and the Choo stent (Mi Tech, Korea) consist of a Z-mesh of stainless steel fully covered by a polyurethane layer. The characteristics of these two stents are similar to those of the Ultraflex except for a lower flexibility.

Table 18.2 Indications and contraindications for esophageal stents

Indications
Malignant obstruction
Esophago-respiratory fistula
External esophageal compression (primary or secondary tumors of the mediastinum or lung)
Esophageal perforation (iatrogenic, traumatic, following endoscopic dilation)
Contraindications
Abnormal coagulation profile (INR > 1.5 and platelets < 50,000)
Recent (3–6 weeks) chemo/radiotherapy treatment (increased risk of hemorrhage and/or perforation)
Severely ill patients with limited life expectancy
Obstructive lesion of the stomach and/or small bowel due to peritoneal seeding
Extremely high stenoses, close to the vocal cords

SEPS stents include the Polyflex stent (Rusch), which is made of plastic and silicone and is fully covered. Nowadays, its role in advanced esophageal cancer is reduced due to its high rate of migration. Recently, this stent has been proposed for the palliation of dysphagia resulting from uncovered SEMS obstruction due to tumor ingrowth ("second stent strategy") [2].

Stent Selection

Covered stents are chosen to avoid tumor ingrowth and for the treatment of esophago-respiratory fistulas. The uncovered proximal and distal flares reduce the risk of distal migration. Totally uncovered stents may be reserved for patients with external compression or a bloated esophagus, to minimize the entrapment of fluid/semi-solid food between the stent and the esophageal wall (the "funnel phenomenon").

Vakil et al. compared 32 patients with covered and 30 patients with non-covered SEMS. Relief of dysphagia and survival were similar, but stent migration was more frequent with the covered type (12% vs. 7%), while tumor ingrowth (3% vs. 30%) requiring laser treatment or a second stent favored covered stents (0 vs. 27%) [3].

The selection of large- or small-diameter stents also has a significant influence on success rates and complications. Verschuur et al. tested three type of stents (Ultraflex, Flamingo, Z-stent) with different diameters. Recurrent dysphagia due to stent migration, tumoral overgrowth, or food impaction occurred more frequently in patients with small-diameter SEMS: Ultraflex, 42% vs. 13%; Flamingo, 37% vs. 15%; Z-stent, 27 vs. 10%. By contrast, complications of bleeding, perforation, fistula, fever, and pain occurred in 40% of the patients with large-diameter stents vs. 20% of those with small-diameter stents. Likewise, gastro-esophageal reflux was more likely with the large- rather than the small-diameter stent (9% vs. 4.1%) [4].

Results following Stent Application

Technical success in stent application is close to 100%, with a clinical success (improvement of dysphagia) rate of 95%, including patients with esophago-respiratory fistulas.

SEMS was shown to have an advantage over plastic non-expandable stents, with significant reductions of acute complications (0 vs. 43%, $p < 0.01$) and hospital stay (5.4 vs. 12.5 days, $p < 0.01$) [5].

Homs et al. [6], in a study on 209 patients treated with stent or brachytherapy (BT), reported a more rapid improvement of dysphagia after stent placement, although a better long-term effect and fewer complications were achieved after BT (stent 33% vs. BT 21%; $p = 0.02$). Recurrent dysphagia and survival were similar, while quality of life scores favored BT. These results could have been influenced by the fact that 44% of the patients in the BT group needed a stent during follow-up. Hence, a prognostic score based on sex, age, tumor length, presence of systemic metastases, and WHO performance score was developed to correctly choose between the two forms of treatment: stent or BT. A stent is probably indicated under the following circumstances: (a) expected survival < 4 or 5 months, (b) esophago-respiratory fistula, (c) recurrent dysphagia after chemo- and/or radiotherapy or BT, or (d) BT not available. The use of BT is recommended in patients (a) of young age, (b) with small tumors, (c) without metastases, (d) with good WHO performance status, (e) an expected survival > 5 months [6, 7].

After stent insertion, perforation and/or fistulization are rare. Hemorrhage, usually mild and self-limiting, is observed in 3–8% of the patients. Migration after covered stent insertion has been reported in 12–36% of patients, while occlusion (tumor, granulation tissue, or food impaction) occurs more frequently with uncovered and small-diameter stents. Chest pain is quite common in the case of large stents or in the palliation of cervical tumors. The reported mortality is 0–1.4% [1, 8].

Stents for Cervical SCC

ESCC located close to the upper esophageal sphincter is more difficult to manage because of associated pain and a "foreign body" feeling. In these patients, there is also an increased risk of complications after stent implantation, such as proximal or distal migration, perforation, trachea-esophageal fistula formation, and aspiration pneumonia. Laser treatment is also problematic because the lack of space above the tumor leads to difficulties in controlling energy delivery.

Verschuur recently reported interesting results in a group of 66 patients with tumors close to the upper esophageal sphincter (mean distance to the upper tumor margin: 4.9 ≤ 2.6 cm). Technical success was obtained in 64 patients (94%). The median dysphagia score after 4 weeks improved from 3 (liquids only) to 1 (difficult ingestion of solids), with a median patient survival of 95 days. Major complications were seen in 20% of the cases [9].

Treatment of Esophago-respiratory Fistula

Esophago-respiratory fistula develops in about 5–15% of patients with esophageal cancer and reduces life expectancy mainly because of repeated episodes of inhalation pneumonia and sepsis [10]. Shin et al. [11] reported clinical success with covered SEMS (relief of dysphagia and sealing of fistula) in 49 of 61 patients (80% of cases); half of the patients with disease recurrences (35%) were treated successfully with a second stent. There was a significant difference in survival between stent success and failure (15.1 vs. 6.2 months $p < 0.05$) [11].

A single esophageal stent is sufficient in the majority of cases. Sometimes, in case of incomplete closure of the fistula by the esophageal stent or compression of the trachea, it may be necessary to insert a second stent within the trachea. In our experience during the period 2003–2009, we used double stenting in 14 patients, with ten such procedures performed during the same session. Median dysphagia score improved from 4 (inability to swallow saliva) to 1 (dysphagia for solids only), and the median dyspnea score from 2 (severe) to 1 (slight) in all cases. Median survival was 85.2 days (range: 14–128).

18.3 Thermal Endoscopic Treatment

Thermal lasers deliver energy focused in a beam of light transmitted through a flexible glass fiber that is passed through the accessory channel of the endoscope. The laser's energy causes vaporization and coagulation necrosis of large tumors.

18.3.1 Lasers

Nd:YAG lasers have been used since the early 1980s and account for the most relevant data in the literature. However, today, the diode laser is more frequently used. The high efficacy of lasers permits rapid recanalization, with technical success in more than 95% of treated patients but relief from dysphagia in only 70–85% [12]. The short-term efficacy often forces patients to be treated every 4–6 weeks. Laser is ideal for tumors located in the mid-esophageal tract and of short length (< 6 cm). It may be difficult to treat tumors longer than 6 cm, located close to the upper esophageal sphincter, or in sharply angled sites, such as the esophago-gastric junction, because of the glass fiber's stiffness. Pre-dilatation is often necessary and the duration of the procedure is longer than in stent application (118 vs. 38 min). These problems, together with the need for frequent repeat treatment, may restrict the use of lasers, especially in elderly or terminally ill patients. Overall, complications occur in less than 5% of patients and the risk of perforation is low (2%), including in patients with prior radiotherapy. There is also little risk of hemorrhage (0.5–1%). Equipment costs are relatively high for Nd-YAG lasers, but lower and acceptable for diode lasers.

18.3.2 Argon Plasma Coagulation

In this therapeutic technique, monopolar electrocoagulation is delivered using a stream of ionized argon gas ignited by a high-voltage discharge at the tip of a flexible catheter probe. APC is a suitable alternative to the laser due to the quick learning curve, the added effect of good treatment at sharply angled sites (esophago-gastric junction), the homogeneous depth of penetration (3–5 mm) and, consequently, the low risk of perforation. In addition, APC can be used for the treatment of cancer ingrowth involving the stent [13].

18.3.3 Cryotherapy

The local application of extremely cold temperatures by means of cryogens sprayed through the working channel of the endoscope enables the treatment of large surface tumors of the esophagus. The effects of cryotherapy are of two types, immediate and delayed, and include the following: failure of cellular metabolism, damage to cell membranes due to intracellular ice formation and, finally, vascular stasis with subsequent edema. The first case was reported by Cash et al. in a patient with recurrent ESCC after chemoradiotherapy: complete remission for 2 years was achieved [14]. Four other patients with T1/T2 esophageal carcinoma had a complete response after 3–11 months of cryotherapy with between three and seven treatments [15]. The widespread application of cryotherapy is still limited by factors such as patient discomfort and difficult operator control of the endoscopic settings.

18.4 Ablation Therapies vs. SEMS Procedures

The optimal palliative method does not exist and the different techniques have to be tailored according to the needs of the particular patient. Stent insertion and ablation therapies could be jointly used for better palliation. In a randomized controlled trial comparing different palliative treatments, Shenfine et al. reported similar results in dysphagia improvement at 1 month, while quality of life was worse in SEMS patients equally after 1 and 6 weeks [16], probably due to the more severe complications and higher mortality. In contrast, the higher cost of stents was balanced by the high number of hospital admissions for laser treatment [17, 18]. It has to be considered that salvage stent therapy for dysphagia relief might be necessary in about 77% of the patients previously treated with laser or BT [16].

18.5 Chemical Endoscopic Treatment: Photodynamic Therapy

A photosensitizing agent consisting of a hematoporphyrin derivate is administered intravenously and is selectively retained in tumor cells. Its activation by a wavelength-specific endoscopically delivered laser light produces necrosis through a cytotoxic effect mediated by singlet oxygen.

PDT is indicated in severely narrowed stenoses or in those located close to the upper esophageal sphincter, where laser or stent application may be difficult or impossible. Palliation is equivalent to Nd:YAG laser, with a reduced risk of perforation and a prolonged effect. However, the widespread use of PDT is limited by severe complications (sunburn, chest pain, atrial fibrillation, fever), the necessity for treated patients to stay in dark areas for long times, and the high cost [19, 20]. Recently, Yano et al. used salvage PDT in the treatment of a group of patients who relapsed after definitive chemoradiotherapy but had refused esophagectomy: 19 out of 22 patients (73%) obtained a complete response, with 1-year and 2-year survival rates of 77 and 60%, respectively [21].

18.6 Relief of Dysphagia during Neoadjuvant Treatment

Malnutrition, a known risk factor for postoperative complications and survival, is reported in 79% of patients with ESCC prior to any treatment [22]. Esophagitis and mucositis during chemo/radiotherapy may worsen dysphagia, with nutritional support necessary in half of the patients to avoid weight loss and immune system failure [23].

Laser recanalization or temporary stent placement may serve as a bridge until surgery, as long as neoadjuvant treatment is provided [6, 17].

Lecleire et al. showed improved dysphagia scores in 89% of the 120 inoperable patients treated with esophageal stents, although without improvement in nutritional parameters and WHO performance index after 1 month [24]. Bower et al. [25] compared the treatment of dysphagia in a group of patients who subsequently underwent preoperative chemo/radiotherapy: group 1 (25 patients) was treated with silicone stents, group 2 (21 patients) with feeding-tube nutrition, and group 3 (12 patients) with oral diet alone. The first group showed better tolerance of chemo/radiotherapy, decreased percentage of weight loss (1.5% vs. 5.4% vs. 5.7%), and greater improvement in albumin levels [25]. Siddiqui et al. reported similar rates of dysphagia improvement (5/5 patients, 100%) with a mean weight gain of 6 kg but with three cases of stent migration [26]. Stent migration is the most frequently observed adverse event (about 22% of the cases) as tumor shrinkage due to neoadjuvant treatment can impair stent anchorage. In most cases, migration of the stent can be solved by its endoscopic removal; however, early and late perforations necessitating acute surgery are reported (5–6%), reducing the chance of subsequent curative resection [27, 28].

An alternative role is played by laser recanalization. Between 2000 and 2008, 88 patients with esophageal cancer were treated with laser in our unit before they received neoadjuvant therapy. An improvement in the dysphagia score was obtained in 85 patients (96.6%) without severe complications (2 perforations: 2.3%). A gain of body weight (median: 5 kg) and an increase in the serum albumin level (median: 0.8 mg/dl) were also obtained.

References

1. Leiper K, Morris AL (2002) Treatment of esophago-gastric tumours. Endoscopy 34:139-145
2. Conio M, Blanchi S, Filiberti R, De Ceglie A (2010) Self-expanding plastic stent to palliate symptomatic tissue in/overgrowth after self-expanding metal stent placement for esophageal cancer. Dis Esophagus 23:590-596
3. Vakil N, Morris AI, Marcon N et al (2001) A prospective, randomized, controller trial of covered expandable metal stents in the palliation of malignant esophageal obstruction at the gastroesophageal junction. Am J Gastr 96:1791-1796
4. Verschuur EM, Steyerberg EW, Kuipers EJ et al (2007) Effect of stent size on complications and recurrent dysphagia in patients with esophageal or gastric cardia cancer. Gastrointest Endosc 65:592-601

5. Knyrim K, Wagner H, Bethge N et al (1993) A controlled trial of an expansible metal stent for palliation of esophageal obstruction due to inoperable cancer. N Engl J Med 329:1302-1307
6. Homs MYV, Steyerberg EW, Eijkenboom WMH et al (2004) Single-dose brachytherapy versus metal stent placement for the palliation of dysphagia from esophageal cancer: multicentre randomised trial. Lancet 364:1497-1504
7. Steyerberg EW, Homs MY, Stokvis A, et al (2005) Stent placement or brachytherapy for palliation of dysphagia from esophageal cancer: a prognostic model to guide treatment selection. Gastrointest Endosc 62:333-340
8. Kozarek RA, Ball TJ, Brandabur JJ et al (1996) Expandable versus conventional esophageal prostheses: easier insertion may not preclude subsequent stent-related problem. Gastrointest Endosc 43:204-208
9. Verschuur EML, Kuipers EJ, Siersema PD (2007) Esophageal stents for malignant strictures close to the upper esophageal sphincter. Gastrointest Endosc 66:1082-1090
10. Boyce HW (1984) Palliation of advanced esophageal cancer. Semin Oncol 11:186–195
11. Shin JH, Song HY, Ko GY et al (2004) Esophagorespiratory fistula: Long-term results of palliative treatment with covered expandable metallic stents in 61 Patients. Radiology 232:252
12. Brown S, Hawes R, Mattewson K et al (1987) Endoscopic laser palliation for advanced malignant dysphagia. Gut 28:799-807
13. Dumot JA, Greenwald BD (2008) Argon plasma coagulation, bipolar cautery, and cryotherapy: ABC's of ablative techniques. Endoscopy 40:1026-1032
14. Cash BD, Johnston LR, Johnston MH (2007) Cryospray ablation (CSA) in the palliative treatment of squamous cell carcinoma of the esophagus. World J Surg Oncol 5:34
15. Greenwal BD, Cash BD (2007) Cryotherapy ablation of early stage esophageal cancer. Gastrointest Endosc 65:AB276
16. Shenfine J, McNamee P, Steen N, Bond J, Griffin SM (2009) A randomized controlled clinical trial of palliative therapies for patients with inoperable esophageal cancer. Am J Gastroenterol 104:1674-1685
17. Dallal HJ, Smith GD, Grieve DC et al (2001) A randomized trial of thermal ablative therapy vs expandable metal stents in the palliative treatment of patients with esophageal carcinoma. Gastrointest Endosc 54:549-557
18. Sihvo EIT, Pentikainen T, Luostarinen ME et al (2002) Inoperable adenocarcinoma of the oesophagogastric junction: a comparative clinical study of laser coagulation versus self-expanding metallic stents with special reference to cost analysis. Eur J Surg Oncol 28:711-715
19. Heier SK, Rothman KA, Heier LM, Rosenthal WS (1995) Photodynamic therapy for obstructing esophageal cancer: light dosimetry and randomized comparison with Nd:YAG laser therapy. Gastroenterology 109:63-72
20. Saidi RF, Marcon NE (1998) Non thermal ablation of malignant esophageal strictures: Photodynamic therapy, endoscopic intratumoral injection and novel modalities. Gastrointest Endosc Clin N Am 8:465-491
21. Yano T, Muto M, Minashi K et al (2010) Phase II study of photodynamic therapy (PDT) for local failure after chemoradiotherapy (CRT) in patients with esophageal squamous cell carcinoma (ESCC). Gastroenterology 138:S758-S759
22. Riccardi D, Allen K (1999) Nutritional management of patients with esophageal and esophagogastric junction cancer. Cancer Control 6:64-72
23. Stockeld D, Fagerberg J, Granstrom L et al (2001) Percutaneous endoscopic gastrostomy for nutrition in patients with oesophageal cancer. Eur J Surg 167:839-844
24. Lecleire S, Di Fiore F, Antonietti M (2006) Undernutrition is predictive of early mortality after palliative self-expanding metal stents insertion in patients with inoperable or recurrent esophageal cancer. Gastrointest Endosc 64:479-484
25. Bower MR, Martin RCG (2009) Nutritional management during neoadjuvant therapy for esophageal cancer. J Surg Oncol 100:82-87

26. Siddiqui AA, Loren D, Dudnick R, Kowalski T (2007) Expandable polyester silicon-covered stent for malignant esophageal structures before neoadjuvant chemoradiation: a pilot study. Dig Dis Sci 52:823-829
27. Vleggar FP (2009) Stent placement in esophageal cancer as a bridge to surgery (Editorial). Gastrointest Endosc 70:620-622
28. Langer FB, Schoppmann SF, Prager G et al (2010) Temporary placement of self-Expanding oesophageal stents as bridging for neoadjuvant therapy. Ann Surg Oncol 17:470-475

Follow-up and Quality of Life after Esophagectomy

19

Giovanni de Manzoni, Francesco Casella, and Andrea Zanoni

19.1 Follow-up

While follow-up programs after curative resection for esophageal cancer are normally performed, neither guidelines nor widely accepted protocols are available in the current literature. Follow-up programs are aimed at the detection of disease recurrence or new neoplasms, the management of nutritional disorders, and the treatment of benign complications, but they are also able to offer psychological support [1]. Despite these many advantages, the cost effectiveness of follow-up programs is still debated, due at least in part to a lack of definitive studies confirming the benefits. In addition to the controversy regarding the adoption of follow-up programs, there is also the question of their timing and which tests should be included, two issues that are strongly debated.

The treatment of benign symptoms and nutritional disorders can be accomplished by the general practitioner and, if necessary, with the assistance of the endoscopist. However, the role of follow-up in detecting recurrence or a second primary tumor is still controversial. Indeed, if no treatment were possible after recurrent disease detection, the role of follow-up, and thus its costs, would be minimal. However, if early detection was confirmed to have a positive impact on survival or quality of life (QoL), then cost effectiveness discussions would favor the support of follow-up programs.

The early detection of recurrence is the focus of increasing attention, as the treatment of relapse has become possible in selected cases involving localized disease (see Chaps 14 and 15). In fact, early detection could guarantee curative treatment in single relapses, before the disease is able to spread and curative treatment is no longer possible. Moreover, studies comparing palliation with surgical resection or chemoradiation therapy (CRT) report significantly

G. de Manzoni (✉)
Dept. of Surgery, Upper G.I. Surgery Division, University of Verona,
Verona, Italy

G. de Manzoni (Ed.), *Treatment of Esophageal and Hypopharyngeal Squamous Cell Carcinoma*,

better survival when treatment is more aggressive [2]. Moreover, if started early, palliation would achieve better control of symptoms, with improved quality of residual life for the patient.

Recurrence may be suspected based on symptoms or, in clinically asymptomatic patients, on elevated disease markers or the findings on imaging and endoscopy. A recent American retrospective trial [3] reported the results of follow-up examination for adenocarcinoma of the esophagogastric junction in terms of detection of recurrence and survival. When clinical symptoms were evident, the most frequent were dysphagia, bone pain, bowel obstruction, neurological deficits, and weight loss. In such patients, the probability of detecting advanced and untreatable disease is fairly high.

Among the potential markers of disease recurrence, carcinoembryonic antigen (CEA) elevation may be a very early indicator of relapse. However CEA is only rarely elevated and is not reliable due to its low sensitivity [1].

Endoscopy (gastroscopy and bronchoscopy) is the mainstay in the detection of early relapse, but it also plays a significant role in revealing second primary tumors in the aerodigestive tract, which are the main cause of death in longtime survivors of esophageal cancer. Thus, the early detection of a new cancer is particularly important in these high-risk patients, to assure curative treatment.

CT scans and cervical region ultrasonography allow the detection of locoregional recurrence and metastatic disease at the most frequent sites of relapse: mediastinum, neck, liver, and lungs. Brain scans are not routinely performed but if brain involvement is suspected, CT is a reliable tool. PET-CT can confirm relapse and is particularly useful in the detection of bone metastases. However, the cost effectiveness of PET-CT and the potentially harmful effects of routine scans during follow-up make it a second-line option in follow-up protocols [1].

The correct timing of the follow-up examination has not been definitively established. Most recurrences appear within the first 2 years after surgery [1, 3-7]. The aforementioned American trial [3] reported a median overall time-to-recurrence of 11 months, with more than 90% of the relapses detected within 33 months. Beyond the third postoperative year and until the seventh year, the annual percentage of recurrence was 2–3%. As perhaps expected, earlier and more frequent recurrence was observed in patients with advanced disease or with scarce or a null response to neoadjuvant treatment. The authors therefore recommended a follow-up program of 7 years duration. Very frequent controls during the first few years, for instance, every 3 months for the first 2 years, have been advocated by some authors [4] whereas annual check-ups are considered sufficient by others [6, 7]. We suggest follow-up examinations every 6 months for the first 5 years, followed by annual controls for the subsequent 5 years. This schedule is aimed at the detection of early relapse and/or second primary tumors and is feasible for most healthcare systems.

In summary, although there are no definitive data supporting the benefits of early detection of recurrence and no guidelines have been created, in current

Table 19.1 Proposed follow-up protocol after esophagectomy for squamous cell carcinoma

1 month after surgery	• Hospital visit to: – Obtain pathological report – Assess nutritional status – Check surgical wounds healing
4 months after surgery	• Blood tests • Gastroscopy (no bronchoscopy) • CT of neck, thorax and abdomen • Neck US • Hospital visit
6 months after last follow-up	• Blood tests • Gastroscopy and tracheobronchoscopy • CT of neck, thorax and abdomen • Neck US • Hospital visit
6 months after last follow-up	• Blood tests • Gastroscopy • CT of neck, thorax and abdomen • Neck US • Hospital visit
Every 6 months for the first 5 years, then annual follow-up for further 5 years. tracheobronchoscopy should be performed once a year.	

practice most centers systematically adopt follow-up protocols. Table 19.1 is a suggested follow-up program for patients who have undergone esophagectomy. Four weeks after surgical resection, a hospital visit is carried out to obtain the pathological report, assess the patient's nutritional status, and check surgical wound healing. The second control visit takes place 4 months after surgery and consists of gastroscopy, CT scans of the neck, chest, and abdomen, neck ultrasound and blood tests. From then on, the same exams are performed every 6 months, adding a tracheobronchoscopy once a year. After 5 years and until the tenth year after surgical resection, annual check-ups with the same tests are performed. After 10 years, the follow-up program ends and the patient is discharged back to the general practitioner for periodic controls, aimed especially at detecting new primary tumors since recurrence is less probable after this long protocol.

19.2 Quality of Life after Esophagectomy

An esophagectomy greatly impacts the quality of residual life and thus represents a challenge for both the patient and the surgeon. QoL is a very important factor, mainly due to the dismal prognosis of the great majority of patients with esophageal squamous cell carcinoma (SCC). Indeed, QoL issues influence the patient's remaining lifetime as well as surgical decision-making.

Eating habits and physical activity change significantly after this highly tissue-destructive procedure. Eating and digestive disorders, some of which persist for only a short period of time while others are permanent, commonly occur after surgery involving the upper digestive tract. There are no restrictions on the type of food eaten, although some foods, such as milk, can cause nausea and diarrhea. Importantly, the patient should avoid carbonated drinks and the simultaneous consumption of solids and liquids for the remainder of his or her life. In addition, new eating habits must be adopted, consisting of small and frequent meals. An overly rich meal might cause food stagnation in the neo-esophagus, with subsequent nausea, bloating, and vomiting, while rapid food passage may determine a "dumping syndrome." Shortages of iron, B12, and D vitamin are common and often need pharmacological supplementation. Anastomotic stenosis can slow food transit, causing dysphagia and vomiting. Such cases normally require endoscopic dilations. In our institution, the median rate of strictures 6 months after esophagectomy is 20%, which declines to 3.5% at 1 year in patients treated with endoscopic dilatations.

A randomized clinical trial by Johansson et al. [8] investigated the use of proton pump inhibitors (PPIs) in reducing the incidence of benign anastomotic strictures after esophagectomy with gastric tube reconstruction. The results showed that the prophylactic use of PPIs for one year indeed reduced the rate of benign anastomotic strictures compared to a no-treatment group (13% vs. 45% $p = 0.002$).

Patients may also complain of biliary or acid reflux associated with a significant deterioration in the quality of life that persists during the follow-up period. Even if completely different in terms of pH, the two types of reflux show similar clinical features.

Reflux disease is considered an unavoidable consequence of esophageal resection due to the removal of all normal anti-reflux mechanisms, such as the lower esophageal sphincter, the intra-abdominal position of the stomach, the diaphragmatic hiatus, and the muscle fibers of the crus. Pyloroplasty, while on the one hand allowing better gastric emptying and reducing acid reflux, on the other hand exposes the esophagus to increased pancreato-biliary secretion reflux.

Mucosal damage from acid and bile exposure affects approximately half of the patients, but usually there is no correlation between symptoms and mucosal damage. When present, reflux esophagitis shows a progression from inflammation to erosion, with the possible development of columnar metaplasia. Prevention and treatment are still debated. No specific drugs exist for the treatment of biliary reflux, while acid reflux can be treated with PPIs and prokinetics. However, neither surgical management with anti-reflux repair nor medical therapy with PPIs and prokinetics guarantees symptom relief or mucosal defense. Proper dietary habits and elevation of the head to about 30° during sleep seem to be the best means to control symptoms.

The return to normal physical activity, with full recovery, ranges from 3 to 6 months in young and otherwise healthy patients to around 18 months in weaker and older patients. A prolonged recovery is to be expected in patients who have undergone cervical esophagectomy, especially after pharyngo-laryngo-esophagectomy (PLE). However, even in those treated with a larynx-preserving procedure a lengthy rehabilitation is required to avoid food aspiration. However, light exercise, if started early, even during the hospital stay, accelerates full recovery and allows patients to cope with the more intensive demands of daily life and to return to previous activities, including work.

Patients' QoL can be assessed at follow-up through the European Organization for Research and Treatment of Cancer (EORTC) [9] questionnaire (EORTC QLQ-C 30), which is among the most widely used means to assess QoL in oncology patients. In esophageal cancer patients, along with this core questionnaire, key functions, such as physical, emotional, and social well-being, can be evaluated using a site-specific module, the QLQ OES 18 [10].

Health-related quality of life (HRQL) has been studied extensively during the first year following esophagectomy in terms of prognostic value and short-term outcomes. In a review by Parameswaran, the retrospective evaluation of HRQL questionnaires showed their relevant role in surgical decision-making for patients newly diagnosed with esophageal SCC. However, despite well-performed studies of HRQL after esophagectomy, there are currently no methods to inform patients of the impact of surgery on HRQL [11].

Evidence suggests that pre-treatment QoL scores are independently prognostic of survival in patients with cancer, but the role of QoL data in predicting short-term outcome after surgery is uncertain. A British study [12] examined the association between QoL scores and short-term outcomes after surgery for esophageal cancer. The QoL scores supplemented standard staging procedures by providing prognostic information, but they did not contribute to peri-operative risk assessment.

In a Dutch trial, QoL data were collected before and after potentially curative surgical resection, to predict survival. Preoperative (physical symptoms) and postoperative (social functioning, pain, and activity level) subscales were shown to be independent predictors of survival in potentially curable patients with esophageal adenocarcinoma [13]. Interestingly, patients with adenocarcinoma were at lower risk for poor HRQL than their counterparts with SCC [14].

Preliminary evidence indicates that patients with worse baseline dyspnea and patients who do not have improved physical function, pain, and fatigue scores within 6 months after potentially curative treatment have a significantly increased risk of shorter survival, mainly due to early disease recurrence [15, 16].

The literature addressing QoL for long-term survivors is limited. Some cross-sectional studies, using validated instruments, indicated that patients who survive beyond 2–5 years after esophagectomy have QoL scores similar to those of the general population [17-19]. By contrast, in a population-based study by Djarv and colleagues, HRQL at 3 years was similar to that at 6 months postoperatively and worse than in the general population [20]. This reduced QoL in long-term survivors after esophagectomy was confirmed by an

Irish trial, in which swallowing dysfunction was the main factor associated with compromised QoL [21].

Studies on the type of surgery have indicated that the QoL after trans-thoracic esophagectomy is comparable to that achieved with trans-hiatal resection [22].

Neoadjuvant therapy has a significant, albeit transient effect on HRQL, with recovery to baseline within 5–7 weeks after completion of induction therapy. HRQL decreases again after surgery, returning to baseline levels within 3 months, according to Saffieddine and coworkers [23].

In a Norwegian study, two groups of patients were evaluated: those receiving neoadjuvant CRT + surgery and those treated with surgery alone. The neoadjuvant group had a worse QoL than the surgery alone group. The exceptions were laryngectomized patients, who had nearly the same QoL as the neoadjuvant group. The QoL of the surgery alone group did not differ from that of the general population [24].

In a Japanese retrospective study comparing the QoL of patients undergoing surgery vs. definitive CRT for advanced SCC, CRT was superior to surgery in terms of QoL, although the CRT group had a larger number of patients with poorer prognostic factors [25].

A retrospective Taiwanese study showed that control of dysphagia in cervical esophageal cancer was better after radical surgery, including total PLE, than after definitive CRT, whilst the global QoL scores were comparable [26].

In summary, good QoL seems to correlate with better short- and long-term outcome, even though the data are not unanimous. The impact of CRT and surgical technique on QoL has yet to be completely elucidated. Nevertheless, a return to a QoL similar to that before the disease and its treatment is of utmost importance for the patient, underlining the need for careful attention to the treatment strategy, peri-operative period, and post-operative education to correct alimentary and behavioral habits.

References

1. Moyes LH, Anderson JE, Forshaw MJ (2010) Proposed follow up programme after curative resection for lower third oesophageal cancer. World J Surg Oncol 8:75
2. Nakamura T, Ota M, Narumiya K et al (2008) Multimodal treatment for lymph node recurrence of esophageal carcinoma after curative resection. Ann Surg Oncol 15:2451-2457
3. Abate E, DeMeester SR, Zehetner J et al (2010) Recurrence after esophagectomy for adenocarcinoma: defining optimal follow-up intervals and testing. J Am Coll Surg 210:428-435
4. Chen G, Wang Z, Liu XY, Liu FY (2007) Recurrence pattern of squamous cell carcinoma in the middle thoracic esophagus after modified Ivor-Lewis esophagectomy. World J Surg 31:1107-1114
5. de Manzoni G, Pedrazzani C, Pasini F et al (2003) Pattern of recurrence after surgery in adenocarcinoma of the gastro-oesophageal junction. Eur J Surg Oncol 29:506-510
6. Dresner SM, Griffin SM (2000) Pattern of recurrence following radical oesophagectomy with two-field lymphadenectomy. Br J Surg 87:1426-1433
7. Nakagawa S, Kanda T, Kosugi S et al (2004) Recurrence pattern of squamous cell carcino-

ma of the thoracic esophagus after extended radical esophagectomy with three-field lymphadenectomy. J Am Coll Surg 198:205-211
8. Johansson J, Oberg S, Wenner J et al (2009) Impact of proton pump inhibitors on benign anastomotic stricture formations after esophagectomy and gastric tube reconstruction. Ann Surg 250:667-673
9. Aaronson NK, Ahmedzai S, Bergman B et al (1993) The European Organization for Research and Treatment of Cancer QLQ-C30: a quality-of-life instrument for use in international clinical trials in oncology. J Natl Cancer Inst 85:365-376
10. Blazeby JM, Alderson D, Winstone K et al (1996) Development of an EORTC questionnaire module to be used in quality of life assessment for patients with oesophageal cancer. The EORTC Quality of Life Study Group. Eur J Cancer 32A:1912-1917
11. Parameswaran R, McNair A, Avery KN (2008) The role of health-related quality of life outcomes in clinical decision making in surgery for esophageal cancer: a systematic review. Ann Surg Oncol 15:2372-2379
12. Blazeby JM, Metcalfe C, Nicklin J et al (2005) Association between quality of life scores and short-term outcome after surgery for cancer of the oesophagus or gastric cardia. Br J Surg 92:1502-1507
13. van Heijl M, Sprangers MA, de Boer AG et al (2010) Preoperative and early postoperative quality of life predict survival in potentially curable patients with esophageal cancer. Ann Surg Oncol 17:23-30
14. Djarv T, Blazeby JM, Lagergren P (2009) Predictors of postoperative quality of life after esophagectomy for cancer. J Clin Oncol 27:1963-1968
15. Djarv T, Metcalfe C, Avery KN et al (2010) Prognostic value of changes in health-related quality of life scores during curative treatment for esophagogastric cancer. J Clin Oncol 28:1666-1670
16. Healy LA, Ryan AM, Moore J et al (2008) Health-related quality of life assessment at presentation may predict complications and early relapse in patients with localized cancer of the esophagus. Dis Esophagus 21:522-528
17. Courrech Staal EF, van Sandick JW, van Tinteren H et al (2010) Health-related quality of life in long-term esophageal cancer survivors after potentially curative treatment. J Thorac Cardiovasc Surg 140:777-783
18. Deschamps C, Nichols FC, 3rd, Cassivi SD et al (2005) Long-term function and quality of life after esophageal resection for cancer and Barrett's. Surg Clin North Am 85:649-656
19. Moraca RJ, Low DE (2006) Outcomes and health-related quality of life after esophagectomy for high-grade dysplasia and intramucosal cancer. Arch Surg 141:545-549
20. Djarv T, Lagergren J, Blazeby JM, Lagergren P (2008) Long-term health-related quality of life following surgery for oesophageal cancer. Br J Surg 95:1121-1126
21. Donohoe CL, McGillycuddy E, Reynolds JV (2011) Long-Term Health-Related Quality of Life for Disease-Free Esophageal Cancer Patients. World J Surg. doi:10.1007/s00268-011-1123-6
22. de Boer AG, van Lanschot JJ, van Sandick JW et al (2004) Quality of life after transhiatal compared with extended transthoracic resection for adenocarcinoma of the esophagus. J Clin Oncol 22:4202-4208
23. Safieddine N, Xu W, Quadri SM et al (2009) Health-related quality of life in esophageal cancer: effect of neoadjuvant chemoradiotherapy followed by surgical intervention. J Thorac Cardiovasc Surg 137:36-42
24. Hurmuzlu M, Aarstad HJ, Aarstad AK et al (2011) Health-related quality of life in long-term survivors after high-dose chemoradiotherapy followed by surgery in esophageal cancer. Dis Esophagus 24:39-47
25. Yamashita H, Okuma K, Seto Y et al (2009) A retrospective comparison of clinical outcomes and quality of life measures between definitive chemoradiation alone and radical surgery for clinical stage II-III esophageal carcinoma. J Surg Oncol 100:435-441
26. Chou SH, Li HP, Lee JY et al (2010) Radical resection or chemoradiotherapy for cervical esophageal cancer? World J Surg 34:1832-1839

Section IV

Operative Techniques

Carcinoma of Thoracic and Cervical Esophagus: Technical Notes

20

Giovanni de Manzoni, Simone Giacopuzzi, and Gerardo Mangiante

20.1 Surgical Approach

Historically, surgeons have controversially discussed the merits of one surgical approach over another. According to Orringer, for example, every patient in need of an esophagectomy for malignant disease is a potential candidate for trans-hiatal esophagectomy (THE). Other surgeons claim the superiority of the trans-thoracic approach (TTE), performed in two or three phases depending on whether the tumor is above or below the carina. TTE has the advantage of a more radical resection and lymphadenectomy. The majority of the published trials report a higher incidence of anastomotic leakage and vocal cord paralysis after THE, while TTE more often results in pulmonary complications and greater peri-operative blood loss [1, 2]. The most recent Dutch randomized trial, dealing only with adenocarcinoma and already discussed in previous chapters, showed a higher complication rate in the TTE group while no difference was reported in mortality; additionally, a survival advantage was noted for patients with tumors located in the distal esophagus [3]. In a recent international survey, 52% of the surgeons were found to prefer TTE and 26% THE [4].

The surgical approach to cervicothoracic cancer at the thoracic inlet is completely different. Surgical decision-making in these cases can be very challenging since these tumors may involve not only the esophagus but also the high retrosternal trachea and extend longitudinally to the larynx. In these patients, a cervical exenteration was proposed by Grillo [5], with a pharyngo-laryngo-esophagectomy and removal of the medial clavicles, upper manubrium, and adjacent medial first and second ribs and the construction of an ante-

G. de Manzoni (✉)
Dept. of Surgery, Upper G.I. Surgery Division, University of Verona,
Verona, Italy

G. de Manzoni (Ed.), *Treatment of Esophageal and Hypopharyngeal Squamous Cell Carcinoma*,

rior mediastinal tracheostomy. Fortunately, the improved results obtained with combined multimodal treatments (chemoradiotherapy) have reduced the need for employing the exenterations technique; however, salvage surgery is still an indication in these patients when there is persistent or recurrent local disease [6, 7].

Based on the above, it is clear that centers specialized in esophageal surgery must offer a diversified approach, one that takes into account the physiological factors and tumor characteristic of each patient.

20.2 Location of the Anastomosis

While thoracic and cervical anastomoses are used worldwide for reconstruction after esophagectomy, they have been compared in only four randomized trials [8-11]. The meta-analysis of these trials suggested that cervical anastomoses are more frequently associated with anastomotic leaks and recurrent nerve palsy while there are no differences with respect to pulmonary complications, mortality, and benign stricture of the anastomosis. Thus, at present, no significant advantage of one type of anastomosis over the other can be claimed [12].

20.3 Type of Anastomosis

There is a high degree of personal preference and opinion regarding the most appropriate anastomotic method. Cervical anastomoses are more frequently fashioned using the hand-sewn technique while a stapled technique is generally preferred in intrathoracic anastomoses [4]. In our randomized trial comparing manual and mechanical cervical anastomoses, we did not find any difference in outcome [13]. These results were confirmed by Urschel et al. in a meta-analysis of randomized controlled trials, which showed that hand sewn and circular stapled esophagogastric anastomotic techniques yielded similar results for anastomotic outcomes, such as leaks and strictures [14].

In both cervical and intrathoracic anastomoses, the end-to-side anastomotic technique is applied more often, in 50% and 64% of the cases, respectively, according to a recent international survey involving the most important specialized centers [4].

20.4 Type of Esophageal Conduit

Ideally, the transposed organ should preserve as many as functions of the normal esophagus as possible (transport, barrier to reflux and aspiration, provision for vomiting and belching, etc.). The decision regarding conduit reconstruction is often dictated by tumor location, morbidity and mortality associated with the procedure, and previous surgical operation [6, 7].

Roux-en-Y jejunal reconstruction, for example, are reserved for patients in whom the stomach or colon is not available and are limited to lower-third lesions, even though with the technique proposed by Kasai the anastomosis can be made above the level of pulmonary vein [15]. A free jejunal graft transposed to the neck, where the artery and vein are anastomosed with microvascular techniques to suitable vessels in the cervical area, can be used for reconstruction of the pharynx and hypopharynx, especially with proximal lesions [6].

The stomach is the most commonly used post-resection conduit, routinely applied in more than 90% of the cases worldwide [4]. Although it must always be kept in mind that, after the left and short gastric vessels have been divided, vascularization of the fundus depends only on the submucosal microvascular channels, the stomach nonetheless has a reliable blood supply, is easily adaptable, and reconstruction is accomplished by a single anastomosis. Recognized drawbacks include loss of the gastric reservoir and an increased risk of acid reflux due to the valveless joining of the esophagus and stomach. A gastric tube created along the greater curvature, with excision of the upper two-thirds of the lesser curvature in continuity with the celiac nodes and esophagus, is routinely applied by 90% of the surgeons in Europe, 80% in North America, and 79% in Asia. The routine use of the whole stomach is reported more frequently in Asia and North America than in Europe (22% and 21% vs. 11%) [4-7].

Colon reconstruction has the advantage of providing an isoperistaltic substitute, thus preserving the gastric reservoir and reducing post-resection reflux symptoms. These properties are a function of the colon's mucous shield and the peristaltic rush in response to acid reflux. The disadvantages of colon reconstruction include a much longer and more complex operation involving three anastomoses, increased risk of internal hernia, and a tendency for the tube to become tortuous and dilated over time. The most popular technique uses the left and transverse colon based on the ascending branch of the left colic artery, after controlling for the adequacy of communications between the left and midcolic vessels [6, 7]. The colon is the first choice as a substitute when the stomach has been truncated by caustic burn, scar, or ulceration; its use is mandatory in case of squamous cell carcinoma in patients who have undergone prior gastrectomy for peptic ulcer disease or for gastric cancer. This is a not rare situation (3.4% in a very large Chinese series) since gastrectomy (especially the Billroth I) has been shown to precipitate subsequent chronic gastroesophageal reflux and to induce the development of squamous dysplasia and carcinoma at multiple locations in the esophagus [16].

20.5 Route of the Esophageal Conduit

Ideally, the substitute organ should lie in a straight line. The posterior mediastinal route in the bed of the resected esophagus is used in the majority of the cases. This route is short and direct, allowing both anastomoses to be positioned along the axis of the conduit. As an alternative, the retrosternal route can be used when the posterior mediastinum is frozen or when adhesions block safe crossing of the pleural space. This route is created by blunt separation of connections between the sternum in front and the pericardium, thymus gland and innominate vein behind. The disadvantage of this approach is that the swallowing route is not direct, with a possible angle at the manubrium in the neck and at the xyphoid at the lower end [6, 7].

20.6 Pyloric Drainage after Reconstruction with a Gastric Conduit

This is another area in which there is no general agreement among surgeons: a pyloroplasty is routinely performed by 40% but never done by 38% [4]. Urschel et al., in their meta-analysis published in 2002, showed a non-significant trend favoring pyloric drainage with respect to gastric emptying and nutritional status, while for the late outcome of bile reflux, there was a non-significant trend favoring the no-drainage group. Thus, the published results seem to suggest that pyloric drainage procedures reduce the occurrence of early symptoms of gastric outlet obstruction but they have little effect on other early and late patient outcomes [17].

20.7 Transthoracic Esophagectomy with Intrathoracic Esophagogastric Anastomosis

20.7.1 Indications

Most esophageal squamous cell cancers (SCCs) are located in the intrathoracic portion, with the majority of these occurring in the middle (about 60%) and lower (around 20%) thoracic segments. The most widely used approach in these cases was described by Lewis, who proposed an abdominal phase and then a right thoracotomy involving an anastomosis with the proximal esophagus at the apex of the pleural cavity.

In our institution, all patients with SCCs located in the middle and lower thoracic esophagus, below the carina, undergo Ivor-Lewis esophagectomy, regardless of preoperative chemoradiotherapy. In case of T1 cancer, a standard mediastinal dissection is performed, while for advanced cancers a two-field extended lymphadenectomy is the preferred approach.

The esophageal reconstruction is made according to the personal technique proposed by Prof. Claudio Cordiano.

20.7.2 Surgical Technique

Access to the abdominal cavity is obtained by a laparotomy, using a median approach. After separation of the greater omentum, starting from the level of the

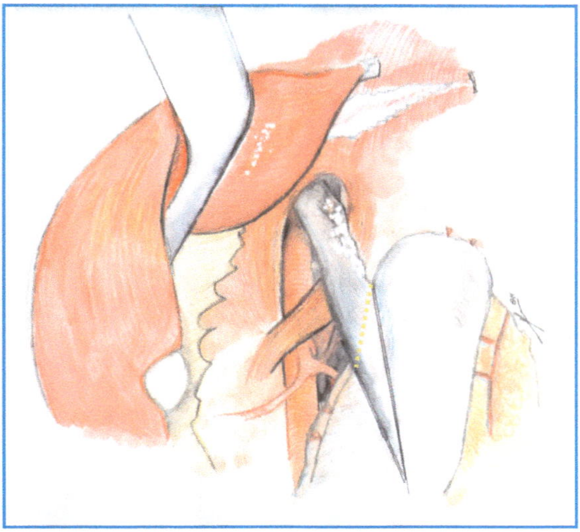

Fig. 20.1 Exposure and division of the abdominal esophagus using a linear stapler along the dotted line

pylorus and at least 1–2 cm from the right gastroepiploic arch, and completion of a Kocher maneuver, the left gastroepiploic and short gastric vessels are ligated.

Once the greater curvature of the stomach has been mobilized, the abdominal esophagus is completely exposed, with sections of the anterior and posterior trunks of the vagus nerve and the esophagus divided using a GIA 60 linear stapler at the esophago-gastric junction level (Fig. 20.1). The surgeon then constructs the gastric tube along the greater curvature, using multiple serial firings of the linear staplers (GIA 60 and 80). The procedure starts at the top, at the angle of His, with division of the stomach parallel to the greater curvature for 5–6 cm and then in the direction of the lesser curvature (Fig. 20.2). In the second step, sectioning is started at the distal part, on the lesser curvature, parallel to the greater curvature, arriving up to 5 cm from the upper section (Fig. 20.3). This results in an access pouch that will be used for entry of the circular stapler (Fig. 20.4).

The transverse diameter of the gastric conduit should not exceed 4 cm in order to reduce the space occupied in the mediastinum and to ensure a perfect vascularization of the organ. Extramucosal pyloroplasty is performed and the esophageal hiatus is opened to free the lower esophagus and to complete lower mediastinal node dissection. A D2 lymph node dissection is then carried out , after which the gastric tube is attached to the esophageal stump, the abdominal cavity is closed, and the patient repositioned in left lateral decubitus.

A right anterolateral thoracotomy allows entry into the chest at either the fourth or fifth intercostal space. The mediastinal pleura is incised, the azygos vein is isolated and divided, and the esophagus is encircled with a Penrose drain and dissected downwards to the lower esophagus and then towards the upper thoracic esophagus (Fig. 20.5). A two-field extended lymph node dissec-

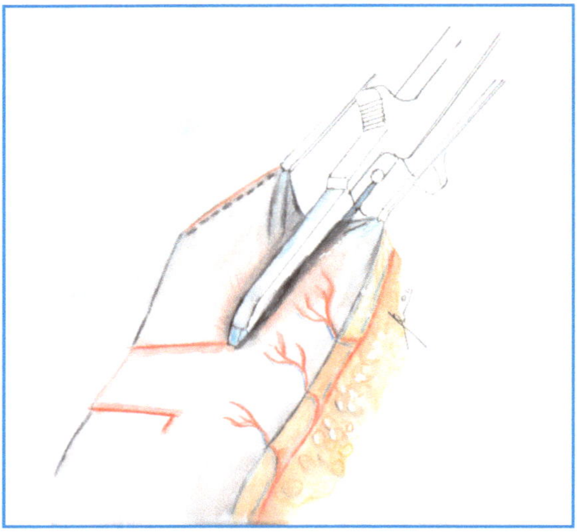

Fig. 20.2 Division of the stomach for 5-6 cm parallel to the greater curvature and then in the direction of the lesser curvature

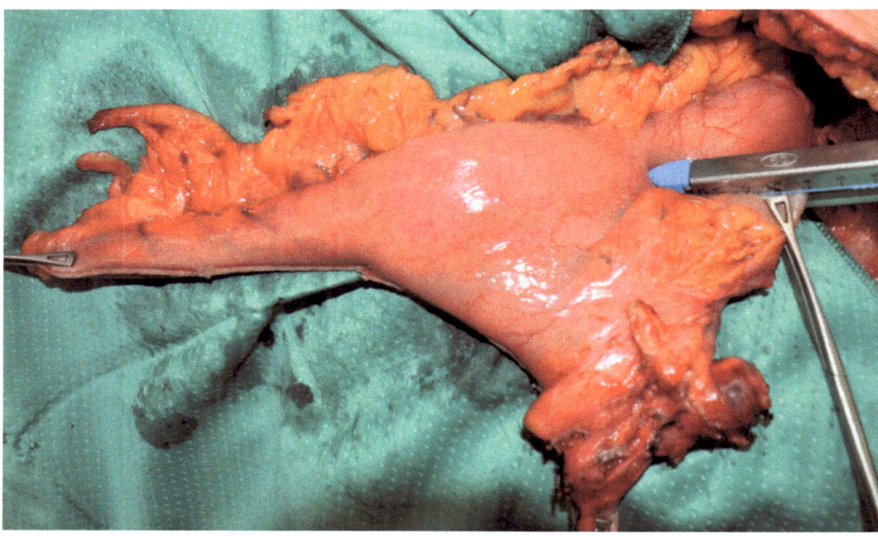

Fig. 20.3 Section starting at the distal part of the lesser curvature 2 cm from the pylorus

tion is then performed (Figs. 20.6, 20.7). The esophagus is divided 2–3 cm above the azygos vein and the gastric conduit is transposed in the chest cavity. A 25-mm anvil is placed in the esophageal stump and secured with a purse-string suture; a second purse-string is created at the top of the conduit (Fig. 20.8). The circular stapler is inserted through a gastrotomy, performed on the access

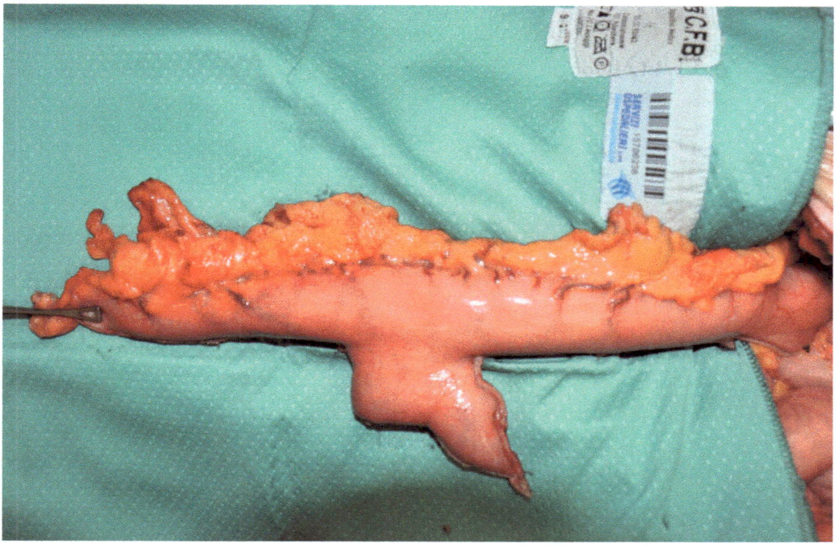

Fig. 20.4 Completion of the access pouch for the circular stapler

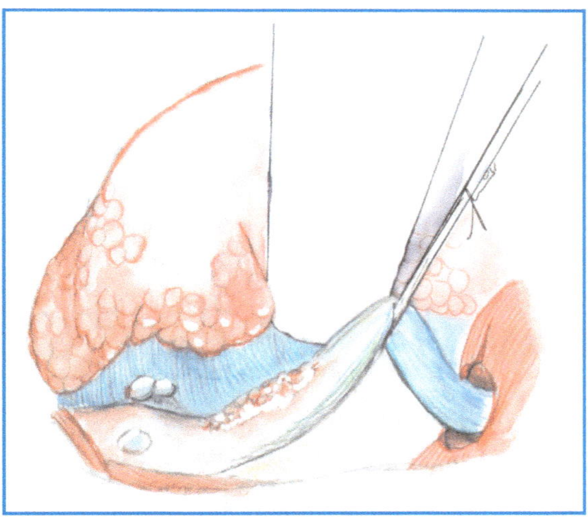

Fig. 20.5 Esophagus encircled with a Penrose drain

pouch, and advanced through the gastric conduit until the tip emerges from the purse-string, at the top of the tube. The cartridge on the circular stapler is attached to the anvil placed in the esophageal stump and a circular stapled end-to-end anastomosis is created (Fig. 20.9). The access pouch is closed with a linear TIA 45 stapler and the anastomosis is oversewn with a running suture (Fig. 20.10). A nasogastric tube is positioned through the anastomosis under direct vision, with the distal end immediately upstream of the pyloroplasty.

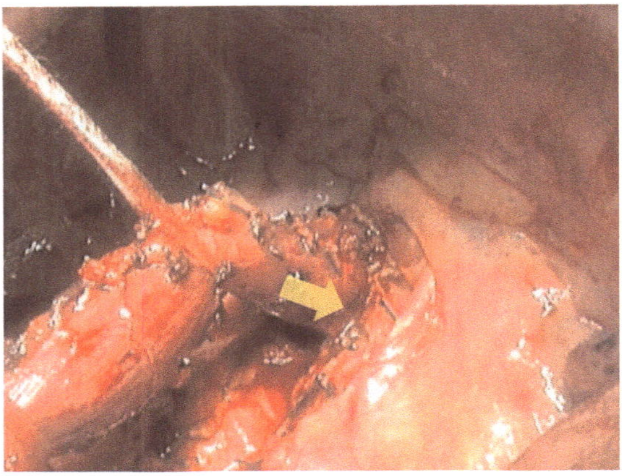

Fig. 20.6 Lymphadenectomy of the right intrathoracic recurrent nerve chain

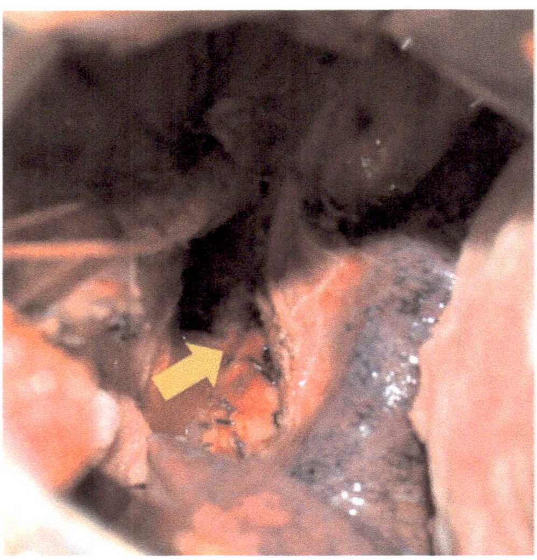

Fig. 20.7 Lymphadenectomy of the sub tracheal carina lymph-nodes

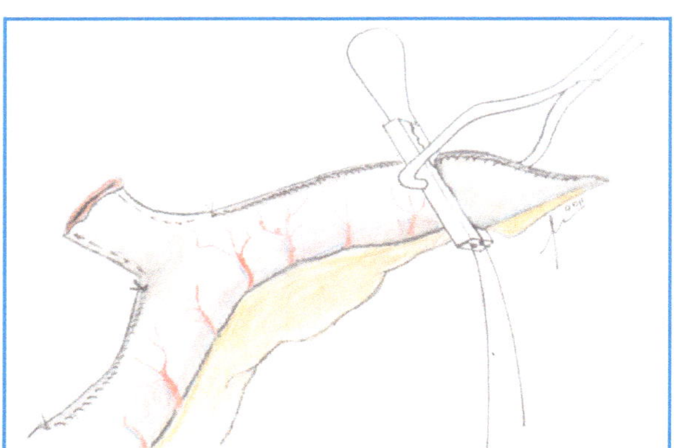

Fig. 20.8 Purse-string suture at the top of the conduit to allow passage of the circular stapler

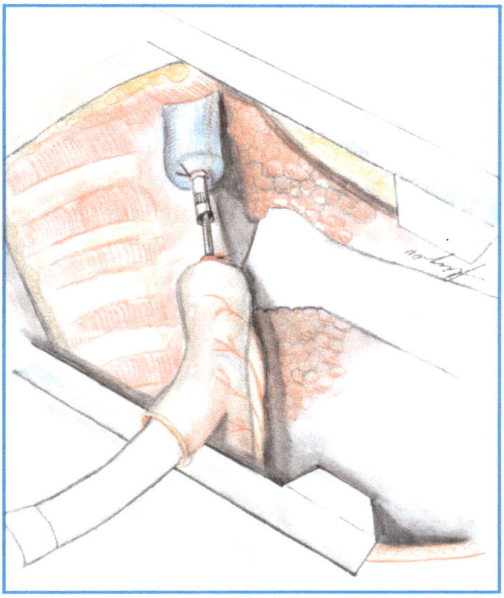

Fig. 20.9 The circular stapler is inserted through the gastrostomy on the access pouch and advanced through the upper part of the conduit to create a circular stapled end-to-end anastomosis

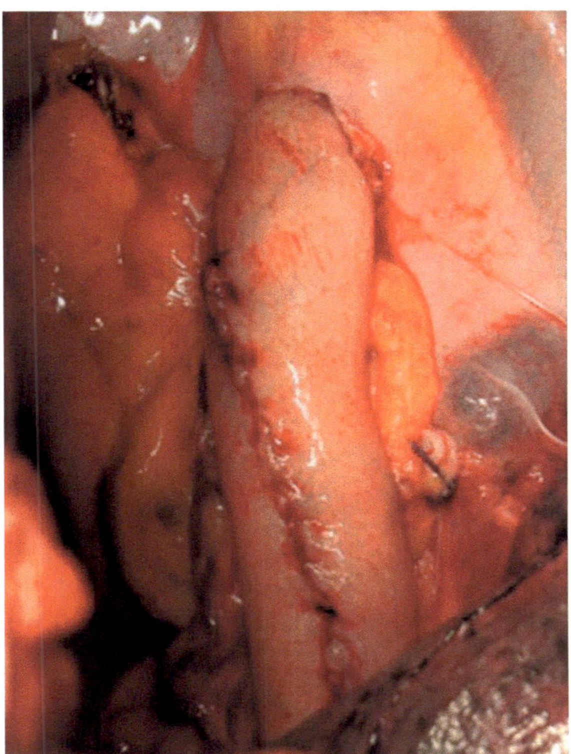

Fig. 20.10 The access pouch is closed using a TIA 45 stapler; both the resection line and the anastomosis are oversewn with a running suture

20.8 Three-phase Esophagectomy

20.8.1 Indications

For tumors located in the thoracic esophagus above the carina, an anastomosis placed in the neck is necessary to obtain sufficient proximal resection margins. In this case, resection is best carried out via a three-phase approach (right thoracotomy followed by abdominal and neck incisions). In case of cancer ≥ T1sm, a three-field lymphadenectomy is indicated.

20.8.2 Surgical Technique

The operation is carried out in three stages. In the first step, a right thoracotomy is performed to excise the esophagus and to allow a complete mediastinal lymphadenectomy. The second step consists of an abdominal stage, identical to that in the above-described two-stage procedure, with the only difference being that the gastric tube does not require an access pouch (Fig. 20.11). Finally, a collar cervical incision is made through which a bilateral neck nodal dissection (compartments II, III and IV, with the recurrent chain) and the esophago-gastric anastomosis are performed.

Depending on the diameter of the esophagus and mainly on the location of the tumor there are several different choices for the neck anastomosis. In patients with cervico-thoracic cancer, to be sure of the resection margin, a manual end-to-end esophago-gastric anastomosis is preferred. The cancer located in the upper thoracic esophagus allows a choice between two possibilities:

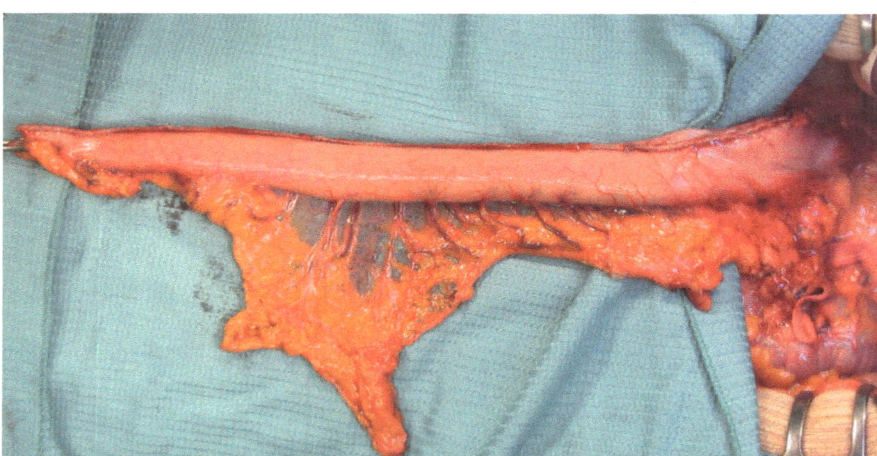

Fig. 20.11 Completion of the gastric tube

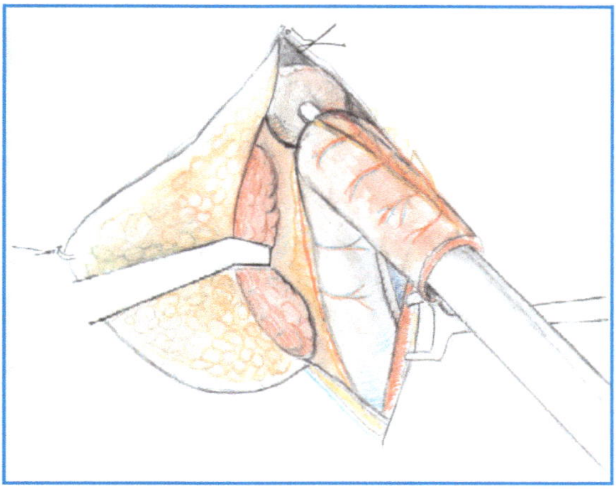

Fig. 20.12 End-to-side stapled anastomosis. The anvil is placed in the esophageal stump and the circular stapler is inserted through the gastrotomy to the top of the conduit

End-to-side stapled anastomosis. A 21-mm circular stapler anvil is placed in the esophageal stump, just below the upper esophageal sphincter. The EEA stapler is then inserted through the transected end of the gastric tube and advanced through the gastric conduit for 4–5 cm, with the tip emerging from the posterior wall of the gastric tube. The cartridge on the circular stapler is attached to the anvil placed in the esophageal stump and the anastomosis is created (Fig. 20.12); the gastrotomy is closed using a linear mechanical stapler.

Side-to-side stapled anastomosis. The posterior walls of the esophagus and the gastric tube are aligned using a seromuscular over-running suture 5 cm long on both sides. The endoGIA 3.0-3.5 staple cartridge is inserted into two small holes made on the posterior walls of the esophagus and the gastric tube (in the center between the linear stapler and the vascular line), with the thinner jaw inserted in the esophagus and the thicker jaw in the gastric tube (Fig. 20.13). With one additional firing of the 60 GIA, the esophagus and the tip of the gastric tube are sectioned and removed, mechanically closing the anterior site of the anastomosis (Fig. 20.14).

20.9 Trans-hiatal Esophagectomy

20.9.1 Indications

For patients with limited cardiopulmonary reserve who are not candidates for thoracotomy, a trans-hiatal esophagectomy (THE) may be performed. In these patients, adequate thoracic lymphadenectomy is not possible. We reserve this approach for patients with SCC of the lower esophagus, in whom the pleural cavity cannot be entered due to adhesions or if there is insufficient pulmonary reserve to tolerate a thoracotomy.

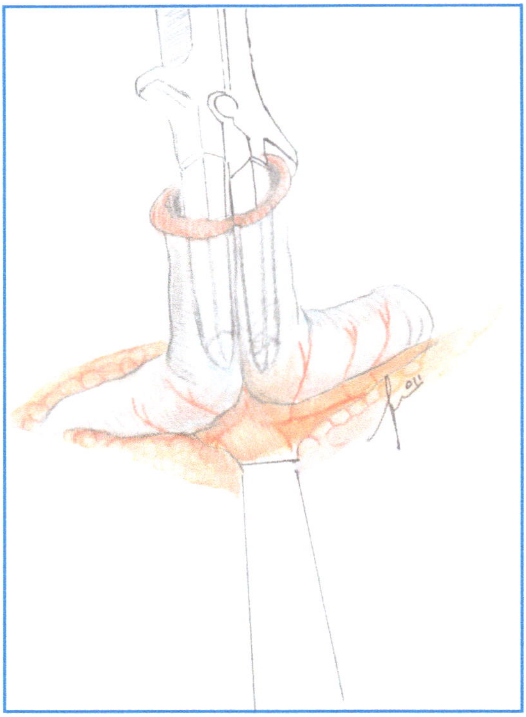

Fig. 20.13 Side-to-side stapled anastomosis. The posterior walls of the esophagus and gastric tube are aligned and the endoGIA is inserted into two small holes

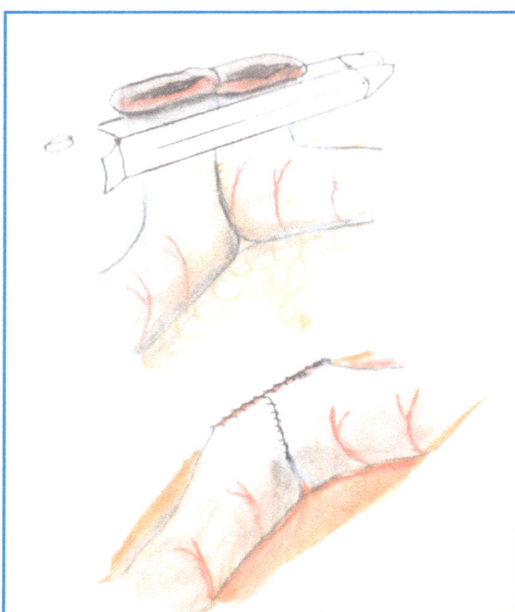

Fig. 20.14 An additional GIA firing closes the hole that has been formed previously, creating a completely mechanical anastomosis

20.9.2 Surgical Technique

The abdominal phase and cervical esophago-gastric anastomosis are the same as described above, with the difference being the blind esophagectomy. The distal 10 cm of the esophagus is mobilized from the posterior mediastinum and the esophageal dissection is done to at least the level of the carina. It is very important to confirm that the tumor of the lower esophagus is not fixed to adjacent mediastinal structures, which precludes a THE. The trans-hiatal dissection is carried out along the posterior wall of the esophagus following the prevertebral fascia, with one hand inserted through the hiatus and the other through the cervical incision. After posterior dissection, dissection along the anterior surface of the esophagus avulses the attachment to the posterior trachea; then the remaining lateral esophageal attachments are divided. When the entire thoracic esophagus has been mobilized, the gastric tube, previously ligated to the lower esophagus, is transposed to the cervical region and anastomosed to the esophagus.

20.10 Esophagectomy for Hypopharyngeal, Cervical and Cervicothoracic Esophageal Cancer

20.10.1 Cervicothoracic Cancer

The approach we use in patients with cervicothoracic cancer was first described by Cordiano in 1982 [6]: (1) thoracotomy in the 3rd intercostal space to determine resectability, dissect the thoracic esophagus, and perform a lymphadenectomy of the medium and upper mediastinum; (2) laparotomy with gastric tube preparation as described above; (3) after a bilateral long collar incision, a lateral neck dissection (levels II, III, and IV), with mobilization of the larynx, pharynx, and cervical esophagus and sectioning of the digestive tract.

Unless the tumor is intraoperatively discovered on the surgical margin or involves the trachea, laryngeal preservation is required and the pharyngeal wall must be sectioned obliquely: from the hypopharyngeal wall (posterior and left side) to the first 1–2 cm of the cervical esophagus (anterior and right side) (Fig. 20.15). The hand-sewn anastomosis is then performed with the gastric conduit (Figs. 20.16, 20.17). A temporary tracheostomy is then necessary to avoid postoperative "ab ingestis" pneumonias due to the transitory uncoordinated swallowing that affects these patients.

20.10.2 Cervical and Hypopharyngeal Cancer

In patients with advanced cancer of the hypopharynx or cervical esophagus, the first approach is through a cervical incision, in order to evaluate the

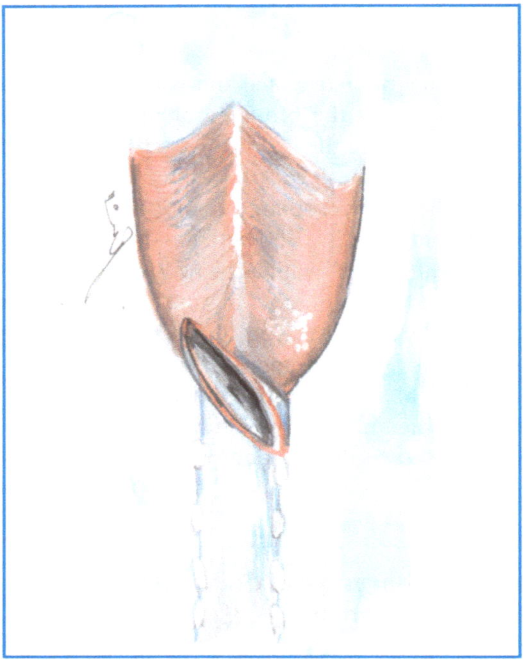

Fig. 20.15 Oblique section from the posterior and left side of the hypopharyngeal wall to the anterior and right side of the cervical esophagus

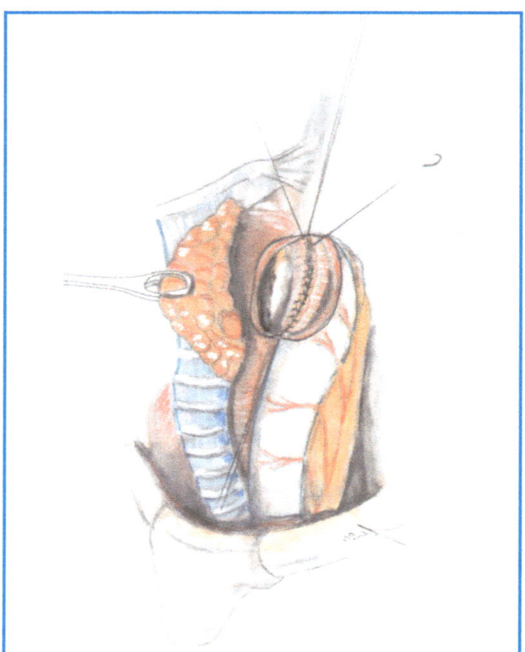

Fig. 20.16 Hand-sewn anastomosis involving the hypopharynx and esophagus

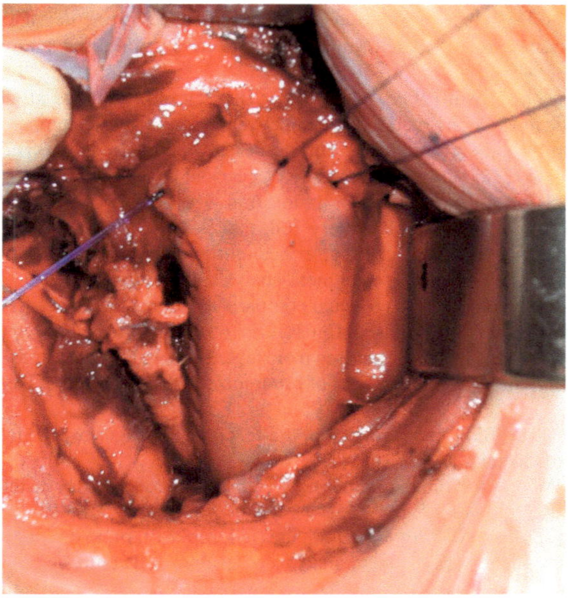

Fig. 20.17 Final view of the anastomosis

resectability of the cancer. If operable, a pharyngo-laryngo-esophagectomy is performed, accompanied by functional cervical node dissection. As described above for THE, the gastric tube previously ligated to the lower esophagus is transposed to the cervical region. In patients with multiple comorbidities and previous radiotherapy, the anastomosis can be a particular technical challenge. We perform a hand-sewn termino-terminal anastomosis at the base of the tongue with two layers of interrupted sutures along the complete circumference of the anastomosis. This is followed by a definitive tracheostomy.

References

1. Battocchia A, Laterza E (2002) Le malattie del'esofago. Diagnosi e Terapia. Piccin Editore, Padova
2. Orringer MB, Marschall B, Chang AC et al (2007) Two thousand transhiatal esophagectomies: changing trend , lessons learned. Ann Surg 246: 363-372
3. Hulscher JB, van Sandick JW, De Boer AG et al (2002). Extended transthoracic resection compared with limited transhiatal resection for adenocarcinoma of the esophagus. New Engl J Med 347:1662-1669
4. Boone J, Livestro DP, Elias SG et al (2009) International Survey on esophageal cancer: part I surgical techniques. Dis Esophagus 22:195-202
5. Grillo HC, Mathisen DJ (1990) Cervical Exenteration. Ann Thor Surg 49:401-408
6. Cordiano C, Stipa V, Tendella E (1982) Chirurgia dell'Esofago e dell'ipofaringe Trattato di tecnica chirurgica (a cura di C. Cordiano) Volume V/2. Piccin Editore, Padova
7. Cordiano C, Nardi G (1989) Color Atlas of Gastrointestinal Surgery. Piccin Editore, Padova.
8. Chasseray VM, Kiroff GK, Buard JL et al (1989) Cervical or thoracic anastomosis for esophagectomy for carcinoma. Surg Gynecol Obstet 169:55-62

9. Ribet M, Debrueres B, Lecomte HM (1992) Resection for advanced cancer of the thoracic esophagus: cervical or thoracic anastomosis ? late results of a prospective randomised study. J Thorac Cardiovasc Surg 103:784-789
10. Walther B, Johansson J, Johnson F et al (2003) Cervical or thoracic anastomosis after esophageal resection and gastric tube reconstruction: a prospective randomized trial comparing sutured neck anastomosis with stapler intrathoracic anastomosis. Ann Surg 238: 803-812
11. Okuyama M, Motoyama S, Suzuki H et al (2007) Hand-sewn cervical anastomosis versus stapled intrathoracic anastomosisfor esophagectomy for middle or lower thoracic esophageal cancer: a prospective randomized controlled trial. Surgery Today 37:947-952
12. Biere SSAY, Maas KW, Cuesta MA, van der Pet (2011) Cervical or thoracic anastomosis after esophagectomy for cancer: a systematic review and meta-analysis. Dig Surg 28: 29-35
13. Laterza E, de Manzoni G, Veraldi GF et al (1999) Manual compared with mechanical cervical oesophagogastric anastomosis: a randomised trial. Eur J Surg 165:1051-1054
14. Urschel JD, Blewett CJ, Bennett WF et al (2001) Handsewn or stapled esophagogastric anastomoses after esophagectomy for cancer: meta-analysis of randomized controlled trials. Dis Esophagus 14:212-217
15. Kasai M, Abols SI, Makino K et al (1965) Reconstruction of the cervical esophagus by a pedicled jejunal graft. Surg Gynecol Obstet 121:102-106
16. Li HH, Zhang QZ, Xu L, Hu JW (2008) Clinical outcome of esophageal cancer after distal gastrectomy: a prospective study. Int J Surg 6:129-135
17. Urschel JD, Blewett CJ, Young JE et al (2002) Pyloric drainage (pyloroplasty) or no drainage in gastric reconstruction after esophagectomy: a meta-analysis of randomized controlled trials. Dig Surg 19:160-164

Minimally Invasive Esophagectomy: General Problems and Technical Notes

21

Ichiro Uyama, Simone Giacopuzzi, Jun Isogaki, and Giovanni de Manzoni

21.1 Introduction

Despite its wide acceptance in colorectal surgery, minimally invasive esophagectomy (MIE) in esophageal cancer (EC) is still controversial. The first report of MIE dates back to 1993, when Cuschieri et al. and Collard et al, reported the feasibility of thoracoscopic mobilization of the esophagus and consensual lymphadenectomy in EC patients [1, 2]. The latter work described 12 cases (2 conversions), including seven involving en-bloc resection and the removal of up to 51 nodes [2]. De Paula et al., in 1995, reported the first series of trans-hiatal esophagectomy (THE) using a laparoscopic approach, applied almost exclusively to benign disease [3]. In a series of six patients with EC, Jagot et al., in 1996, were the first to describe a laparoscopic approach for mobilization of the stomach, which was followed by thoracotomy [4]. Since then, many techniques have been developed: hybrid MIE (thoracoscopy/laparotomy; laparoscopy/thoracotomy) or totally MIE (laparoscopy/thoracoscopy). The first case of totally MIE was reported by Luketich et al., in 1998 [5], while Watson et al., in 1999 [6], were the first to describe an Ivor-Lewis subtotal esophagectomy, entirely thoracoscopic and laparoscopic, carried out in two patients and including manual intrathoracic esophagogastric anastomosis.

21.2 Minimally Invasive Surgery vs. Open Surgery

In the UK, the use of MIE has increased from 0.6% of the cases in 1996/1997 to 16.0% of those in 2007/2008 [7]. Recently, in many high-volume centers

G. de Manzoni (✉)
Dept. of Surgery, Upper G.I. Surgery Division, University of Verona,
Verona, Italy

G. de Manzoni (Ed.), *Treatment of Esophageal and Hypopharyngeal Squamous Cell Carcinoma*,

the number of minimally invasive procedures performed has exceeded the number of open operations [8]. Unfortunately, the majority of the studies published are single-center series, with low number of cases, or they propose new techniques. Comparative studies between open esophagectomy (OE) and minimally invasive surgery based on appropriate numbers of patients are few and the majority are retrospective, with selection bias and seldom differentiating between hybrid and totally MIE [9, 10]. Moreover, despite meta-analysis that sought to clarify the more controversial issues [11-13], there is still a need for prospective randomized trials comparing the two approaches.

21.2.1 Surgical Outcomes

Initially, MIE was reserved for patients with early-stage cancer or Barrett's high-grade dysplasia but nowadays specialized centers use this approach in the treatment of advanced EC [5, 14-16].

The reported percentage of conversion differs widely in the literature and is strictly dependent on the surgeon's experience. Thus, in high-volume centers the conversion rate is 0–7.3% [5, 14, 17-19], while in low volume series the rates are in the range of 10–36% [11, 20-23].

The duration of the procedure is undeniably longer in MIE (220-470 min) [11] but there is a significant reduction in intraoperative blood loss [11, 12]. Tsujimoto et al. showed that patients undergoing laparoscopic treatment have a reduced systemic inflammatory response, based on an analysis of systemic inflammatory response syndrome (SIRS) criteria, although a clear influence on postoperative morbidity could not be established [24].

21.2.2 Short-term Results

Morbidity and Mortality

In the above cited meta-analysis, systemic complications were shown to be lower after MIE than after open surgery [11-13]. This was especially the case with respiratory complications, which seem to be more frequent due to the thoracotomy and manipulation of the lung or to the need for single-lung ventilation. During totally MIE, lung manipulation is minimal, especially when the patient is placed in the prone or hemi-prone position, which allows good view with low levels of intrathoracic insufflation. In Nagpal's meta-analysis, there were significantly fewer respiratory complications after totally MIE ($p = 0.04$) or hybrid ($p = 0.03$) than after OE; however, the author pointed out the selection bias in the examined studies due to the exclusion of patients with bulky tumors and to the inclusion of series in which THE was used, i.e., without the need to exclude or manipulate the lung [12]. Butler [11], analyzing only case series, reported a respiratory morbidity rate of 31.7%, significantly higher than in open trans-thoracic esophagectomy (TTE) [25].

Anastomotic leakage is the most serious surgical complication and the results reported in the different MIE series are highly variable, with very large differences (2.2–52.9%) [11]. This variability could be related not only to the different techniques used for the anastomosis (intrathoracic/cervical, manual/mechanical; side-to-side, end-to-end, end to side), but also to the different detection methods (clinical suspicion, routine contrast X-ray, endoscopy). In an evaluation of comparative studies, a significant difference was reported in favor of MIE ($p = 0.02$) [13], but the positive result shown for the hybrid technique was actually influenced by a single paper in which the anastomotic leak after open surgery was suspiciously high (62%) [9]. By contrast, in a recent series [8], the anastomotic leak rate was 17% and 20% for totally and hybrid MIE, respectively, compared to 11% for OE. Necrosis of the gastric tube is a catastrophic complication requiring takedown of both the anastomosis and the intrathoracic stomach, cervical esophagostomy, and the insertion of a feeding tube. The spectrum of conduit ischemia is broad and includes cases involving anastomotic leak or stricture as well as those in which there is frank graft necrosis. Wormuth [26], in a review of this topic, reported that the rate of postoperative conduit ischemia after OE is 1–3%, similar to our experience (1%). This dramatic complication seems to be higher after MIE, reaching 3–10% [5, 8, 27], which probably explains why some authors have suggested alternative techniques, such as ischemic conditioning [28] or extracorporeal preparation of the gastric conduit [14]. Among the factors identified as correlating with the risk of ischemia are: (a) length of the conduit, (b) intracorporeal gastric tubulization that, without adequate stretching of the organ during stapling, could cause a shortening of the tube, and (c) an insufficient Kocher maneuver, which could prevent its adequate elevation to the neck.

Postoperative mortality after MIE ranges from 0 to 5.9%, which is lower than the rate reported by Hulscher et al. in a historical meta-analysis of OE that was published in 2001 (9.2% TTE and 7.2% THE) [11, 25]. However, at present, the mortality reported in high-volume centers for open surgery ranges from 4% to 8% [29-31] and in our experience is even lower (1.6%).

The two meta-analyses of comparative studies did not show any difference in mortality between open and minimally invasive surgery [11, 13].

Hospital Stay and Quality of Life

Health-related quality of life (HRQL) is a key index used to evaluate outcomes in neoplastic disease. Following surgery for EC, patients require up to one year to regain their basic level of HRQL, which clearly cannot be achieved if their expected survival is less than 2 years [32]. A less invasive approach could, theoretically, improve quality of life, at least in the early postoperative period. A recent prospective study on 55 patients undergoing MIE showed a marked deterioration of HRQL 6 weeks after surgery, with progressive improvement after 3 months. The baseline condition was reached after 6 months and remained steady up to one year after surgery [33]. Nafteux et al., in a comparative study between open and minimally invasive surgery, confirmed these data, reporting a better outcome for MIE after 1–3 months ($p = 0.02$), but with an equalization after 6 months [34].

Comparative studies on the length of hospital stay determined a slight reduction in hospitalization in MIE (9–16 days) compared to OE (11–23) [10, 15, 17, 35]. In the meta-analysis of Nagpal, there was a significant advantage of MIE, in terms of both ICU and hospital stay [12].

21.2.3 Oncological Results

Resection Margins

Positive resection margins after MIE are reported in 0–14% of cases [11], with higher percentages for circumferential margins (CRM), especially in bulky tumors [36]. Smithers et al. were unable to show any significant differences in positive margins (19%, 14%, and 20% R1 in OE, hybrid, and totally MIE, respectively) even if in patients not receiving neoadjuvant therapy there was greater involvement of the CRM in open surgery than in the hybrid technique (15% vs. 8%) [10]. A recent series [8] reported a higher rate of positive CRM after open surgery (47%) and hybrid MIE (55%) than with totally MIE (39%), but bulky cancers were excluded from treatment using the minimally invasive approach.

Nodes Retrieval

As reported in Chap. 13, the number of nodes retrieved during esophagectomy correlates directly with long-term survival, with a possible cut-off of 23 nodes [37]. Butler reported a range of removed nodes between 5 and 29 [11]. According to the results of individual trials, the findings of only two were consistent with this cut-off [38, 39]. A recent study in the UK did not identify differences in methods, showing an average number of nodes between 12 and 15 depending on the technique [8]. In the meta-analyses of Sgourakis [13] and of Nagpal [12], there were no differences in the number of lymph nodes removed with respect to the different techniques, even if the number of retrieved nodes per patient in the reported series was rarely appropriate. This result was confirmed by a paper from Japan, in which a very good median number of nodes was removed [40]. The authors did not find a difference between the thoracoscopic and thoracotomic approaches (mean number 33.9 vs. 32.8) [40]. It is likely that the magnification obtained with minimally invasive procedures provides a better view, allowing clear identification of nodal stations and the preservation of delicate structures such as the recurrent nerves.

Prognosis

To analyze the impact of MIE on prognosis is extremely difficult, due to the broad heterogeneity among the various studies, which prevents a proper meta-analysis. Smithers et al. found no significant prognostic difference, after stratification for stage and response to neoadjuvant therapy, between totally MIE, hybrid MIE, and OE (5-year survival 22%, 41%, and 16%, respectively) [10]. Lee et al. reported equal median survival for open vs. minimally invasive surgery (38 months and 42 months, respectively), also distinguishing early from advanced stages [41].

In their evaluation of recurrence, Thompson et al. reported a rate of 57.6% for open transthoracic surgery (TTE) vs. 67.9% for assisted thoracoscopic surgery ($p = 0.10$). In their study, the only independent prognostic factors for local recurrence were positive margins and number of positive nodes, and for systemic recurrence T stage, length of tumor > 6 cm, tumor differentiation and number of positive nodes. In other words, surgical approach was not a prognostic factor for recurrence [42].

21.2.4 Conclusions

Many problems regarding MIE in esophageal cancer remain to be solved. There are no randomized clinical trials in the literature comparing MIE and OE, except for the TIME trial, which is a currently ongoing randomized trial with the primary objective of assessing the rate of pulmonary complications and surgery-related events [43]. Also, in the majority of the studies conducted thus far, patients who underwent MIE usually had earlier-stage disease and relatively few co-morbidities.

Another issue is whether preoperative chemoradiotherapy is a restriction for the thoracoscopic approach. A recent study [44] evaluated 41 patients treated with 5-FU, cisplatin, and 4500 rads of radiation followed by MIE: 76% subsequently underwent thoracoscopy, 17% thoracoscopy with eventual mini-thoracotomy to perform the anastomosis, and only one patient treated by thoracotomy. In almost all the cases (95%), R0 resection was possible, with a median of 15 nodes excised. The feasibility of the thoracoscopic approach in patients with locally advanced tumors (cT4) who undergo surgery after chemoradiation therapy (CRT) is debated, as the structures in the proximity of the lesion (trachea, bronchi, pericardium) are commonly involved by a thick inflammation, with the need for wide resection to ensure safe margins.

There are also problems for the surgeon with respect to the learning curve. Safranek showed a significant reduction in anastomotic stenosis in patients treated after the first 20 similar cases, with a decrease in hospitalization time and rate of anastomotic fistulas [8]. Osugi et al. observed a significant reduction in operation time and blood loss after the first 36 patients [40]. Given the technical difficulties of the surgical procedures involved, training should begin with small tumors in patients with earlier-stage disease that should not be treated with neoadjuvant CRT. Based on these rules, it will take about 2 years in a high-volume center to properly train a surgeon.

21.3 Minimally Invasive Esophagectomy: Technical Notes

21.3.1 Introduction

Thoracoscopic esophagectomy for esophageal cancer may have, as reported above, several advantages, in particular a lower morbidity rate and a shorter hospital stay than is the case with the open procedure [45-48]. However, the technical complexity of thoracoscopic surgery has limited its wider acceptance. A modification of the procedure, in which the patient is placed in the prone position, was introduced and its benefits claimed over those of the left lateral position [49, 50]. We adopted this maneuver in 2006 and in the following report we describe our experience over the last 5 years.

21.3.2 Patients and Methods

The diagnosis of esophageal cancer is confirmed by endoscopy, pathological examination of the biopsy specimen, endoscopic ultrasound, and computed tomography of the chest and abdomen. The esophageal tumor is clinically staged according to the Japanese Classification of Esophageal Carcinoma [51]. Indications for thoracoscopic esophagectomy in the treatment of esophageal cancer are: (1) clinically T1b~T3, (2) < N2, and (3) the patient's ability to tolerate one-lung ventilation.

21.3.3 Prone Position

The patient is intubated using a double-lumen endotracheal tube and managed under one-lung ventilation during the thoracoscopic part of the operation. While on the operating table, the patient is shifted to a left semi-prone position. The patient's right arm is elevated, the left arm is placed alongside the body, and the right side is elevated slightly (Fig. 21.1). Subsequently, the body position is changed to completely prone, which is accomplished by table rotation. If an emergency thoracotomy is required, the body position can be changed to left lateral only by rotation of the table.

We use the four-ports technique, with each port having a diameter of 12 mm. The first port is placed in the seventh intercostal space (ICS) on the posterior axial line. An artificial pneumothorax is established using 6 mmHg carbon dioxide gas insufflation. The right lung collapses due to the intrathoracic positive pressure and one-lung ventilation. The second port is placed in the fifth ICS on the posterior axial line, the third port at the third ICS along the middle axial line, and the fourth port in the ninth ICS slightly dorsal to the posterior axial line. The ports in the fifth and seventh ICS are for the surgeon; the port in the third ICS is for the surgical assistant, and the one in the ninth ICS is for the camera (Fig. 21.2).

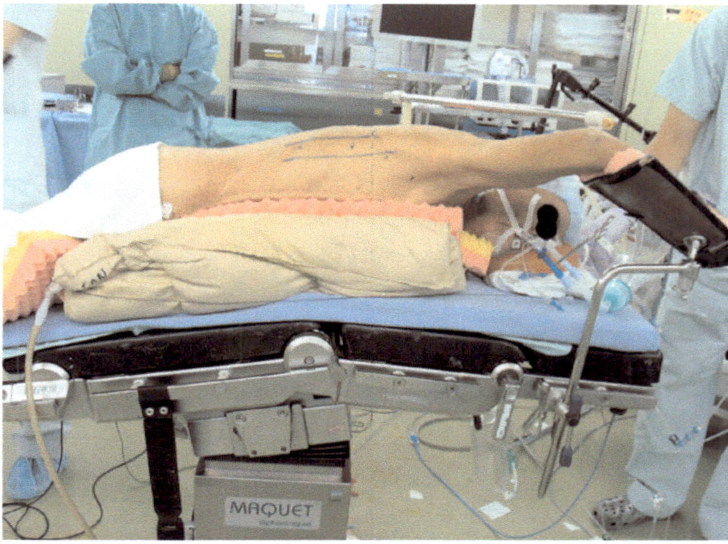

Fig. 21.1 With the patient on the operating table and intubated, the body position is changed to left semi-prone. The right arm is elevated, the left arm is placed alongside the trunk of the body, and the right side of the patient is elevated slightly. The body position is changed to complete prone by bed rotation

The surgeon, the assistant, and the camera operator stand at the patient's right side. The video monitor is at the patient's left side. The surgeon holds the dissecting forceps in the right hand and the grasping forceps in the left. The surgeon arbitrarily replaces the forceps in the right hand with the LigaSure vessel sealing system (VSS) (Valleylab, Boulder, CO, USA) and the SonoSurg laparoscopic coagulating shears (LCS) (Olympus, Tokyo, Japan). The assistant uses the grasping forceps with gauze to hold down the lung and mediastinal organs in order to maintain the surgical field.

Our procedure for esophageal cancer consists of three stages: (1) manipulation under the thoracoscope, (2) dissection of the abdominal esophagus under laparoscope and preparation of the gastric conduit, and (3) the cervical part of the procedure, in which the gastric conduit is raised up to the neck and an anastomosis between the cervical esophagus and the gastric conduit is made.

21.3.4 Thoracoscopic Manipulation of the Thoracic Esophagus

The pleura is incised along with the middle thoracic esophagus. The anterior incision line is along the dorsal pericardium and the posterior line along the anterior margin of the vertebra. Each incision line is extended caudally, with the two incisions merging near the esophageal hiatus of the diaphragm. The incision is extended cranially. The azygos vein is exposed and divided using a

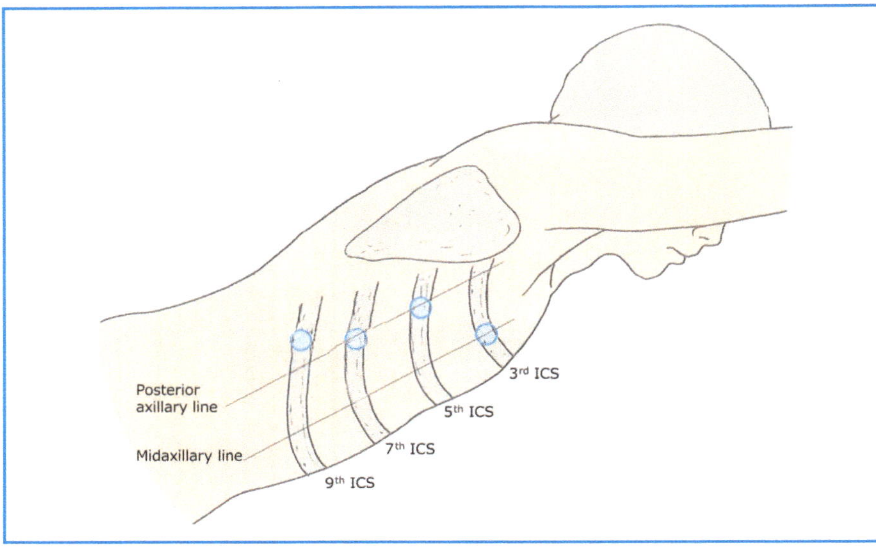

Fig. 21.2 The port position during the thoracic manipulation according to the four ports technique. The first port is placed at the seventh intercostal space (ICS) and the second at the fifth ICS, both on the posterior axial line. The third port is placed at the third ICS on the midaxial line and the forth at the ninth ICS on the slightly dorsal side of the posterior axial line

linear stapler (ETS, ENDOPATH ETS Flex, Ethicon Endo-Surgery, Cincinnati, OH, USA). The right bronchial artery is identified and preserved. The anterior incision line of the pleura is extended up to the thoracic inlet, along the right vagus nerve. The assistant uses forceps with gauze to hold down the pleura over the superior vena cava, thus maintaining the surgical field (Fig. 21.3).

Near the right subclavian artery, the right recurrent laryngeal nerve is identified and the lymph node along with this nerve (station 106recR) is dissected (Fig. 21.4). The esophagus is mobilized from the membranous trachea and the upper thoracic vertebra. The thoracic duct is identified and preserved. The esophagus is divided using the linear stapler at the proximal side of the lesion. Mobilization of the distal esophagus is extended to the carina. The assistant holds down the right bronchus, such that the membranous trachea faces the surgeon and a sufficient surgical field in the middle mediastinum is maintained. The right vagus nerve is transected just distal from the bifurcation of its pulmonary branch. The subcarinal and main bronchial lymph nodes (stations 107 and 109) are dissected, followed by mobilization of the esophagus to the caudal side up to the diaphragmatic hiatus.

The assistant depresses the trachea to maintain the surgical field in the left upper mediastinum. The connective tissue in the left side of the trachea is separated from the tracheal wall. This tissue contains the left recurrent laryngeal nerve and the left recurrent nerve lymph node (station 106recL) (Fig. 21.5). The recurrent laryngeal nerve is identified and the lymph node dissection

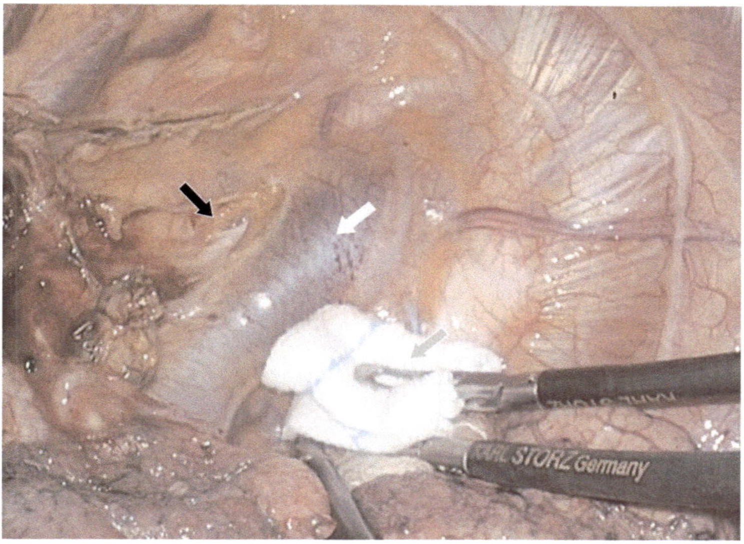

Fig. 21.3 The assistant uses forceps and gauze (*gray arrow*) to hold down the pleura over the superior vena cava (*white arrow*). This maneuver maintains the surgical field around the right vagal nerve (*black arrow*) and the right recurrent laryngeal nerve

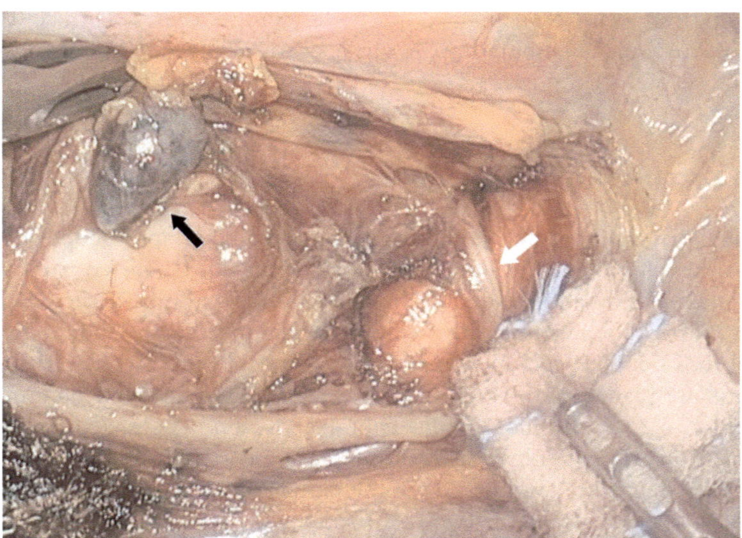

Fig. 21.4 The right recurrent laryngeal nerve (*white arrow*) is located near the right subclavian artery, and the lymph node along with this nerve (station no. 106recR) (*black arrow*) is dissected

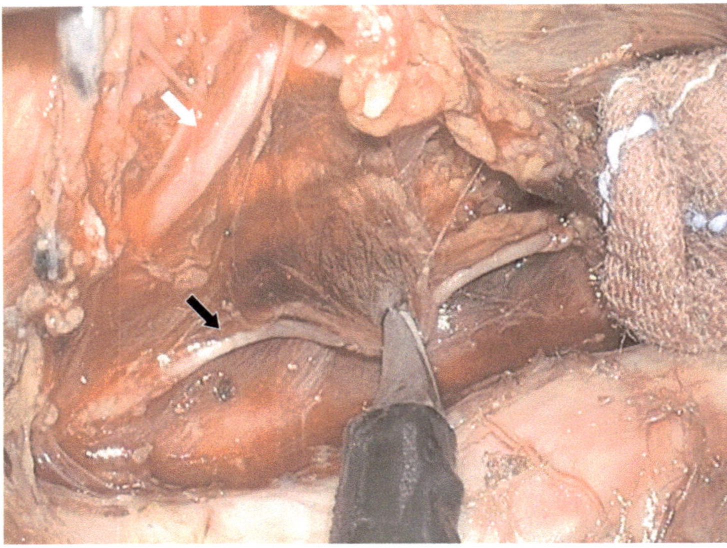

Fig. 21.5 The connective tissue on the left side of the trachea is separated from the tracheal wall. This tissue contains the left recurrent laryngeal nerve (*white arrow*) and the left recurrent nerve lymph node (station no. 106recL). The cardiac branch of the sympathetic nerve (*black arrow*) is identified and preserved

around this nerve continued to the hilum of the left lung, with simultaneous dissection of the left main bronchial lymph node (station 109L). This completes the thoracoscopic manipulation. A chest drain is placed through the puncture of the seventh ICS port.

21.3.5 Laparoscopic Manipulation

In the following, dissection of the abdominal esophagus under laparoscope and preparation of the gastric conduit are described. The patient is shifted from a prone to a supine position and the double-lumen endotracheal tube is replaced with a single-lumen tube. We use the five-port technique for the abdominal part of the procedure. The camera port is inserted at the umbilicus and the other four ports are placed as follows: two ports at the bilateral hypochondriac regions and two at both sides of the lateral abdomen. The specimen is removed and the gastric conduit formed through the enlarged umbilical incision. The surgeon stands at the right side of the patient and the assistant at the left. The camera operator stands between the patient's legs. The lateral segment of the liver is elevated using Nathanson's liver retractor (Mediflex Surgical Products, NY, USA). The 10-mmHg pneumoperitoneum is created. The dissection starts at the gastrocolic ligament, preserving the right and left gastroepiploic vessels along the greater gastric curvature. The roots of the left gastroepiploic vessels are identified and divided. The short gastric vessels and gastrophrenic ligament are divided using the VSS up to the esophageal hiatus. The lesser omentum is dissected and the assistant elevates the gastropancreatic fold. The roots of the left gastric vein and artery are divided and the lymph nodes around the left gastric artery (station 7) are dissected. If the cancer is located in the abdominal part of the esophagus, the lymph nodes along the common hepatic, celiac, and proximal splenic arteries (stations 8, 9 and 11p) are also dissected. The thoracic esophagus is extracted through the abdominal cavity, and the esophagus and stomach are removed through the enlarged umbilical incision. The small-diameter (3-cm) gastric conduit is created extracorporeally using a liner stapler. A pyloroplasty is not performed.

21.3.6 The Cervical Part of the Procedure

This is performed through a collar incision in the neck. The gastric conduit is elevated through the mediastinum up to the neck, guided by cotton tape tied to the distal stump of the esophagus. A single-layer esophagogastric end-to-end anastomosis is created using the triangular anastomosis method, which, as reported by Fukunaga et al. [52], is useful to prevent problems with the anastomosis. No drain is placed in either the neck or the abdomen.

21.3.7 Conclusions

Esophagectomy still plays a central role in surgically resectable esophageal cancer. Placing the patient in the prone position alleviates some of the technical difficulty of thoracoscopic esophagectomy [49, 50]. This procedure provides excellent exposure of the operative field and better ergonomics for the surgical team. Even in the left deep mediastinal space, the organs are displaced to the ventral side by gravity and a sufficient operative field is maintained.

References

1. Cuschieri A (1993) Endoscopic subtotal oesophagectomy for cancer using the right thoracoscopic approach. Surg Oncol 2 Suppl 1:3-11
2. Collard JM, Lengele B, Otte JB et al (1993) En bloc and standard esophagectomies by thoracoscopy. Ann Thorac Surg 56:675-679
3. DePaula AL, Hashiba K, Ferreira EA et al (1995) Laparoscopic transhiatal esophagectomy with esophagogastroplasty. Surg Laparosc Endosc 5:1-5
4. Jagot P, Sauvanet A, Berthoux L et al (1996) Laparoscopic mobilization of the stomach for oesophageal replacement. Br J Surg 83:540-542
5. Luketich JD, Nguyen NT, Weigel T et al (1998) Minimally invasive approach to esophagectomy. JSLS 2:243-247
6. Watson DI, Davies N, Jamieson GG (1999) Totally endoscopic Ivor Lewis esophagectomy. Surg Endosc 13:293-297

7. Lazzarino AI, Nagpal K, Bottle A et al 2010) Open versus minimally invasive esophagectomy: trends of utilization and associated outcomes in England. Ann Surg 252:292-298
8. Safranek PM, Cubitt J, Booth MI (2010) Review of open and minimal access approaches to oesophagectomy for cancer. Br J Surg 97:1845-1853
9. Braghetto I, Csendes A, Cardemil G et al (2006) Open transthoracic or transhiatal esophagectomy versus minimally invasive esophagectomy in terms of morbidity, mortality and survival. Surg Endosc 20:1681-1686
10. Smithers BM, Gotley DC, Martin I et al (2007) Comparison of the outcomes between open and minimally invasive esophagectomy. Ann Surg 245:232-240
11. Butler N, Collins S, Memon B et al (2011) Minimally invasive oesophagectomy: current status and future direction. Surg Endosc 25:2071-2083
12. Nagpal K, Ahmed K, Vats A et al (2010) Is minimally invasive surgery beneficial in the management of esophageal cancer? A meta-analysis. Surg Endosc 24:1621-1629
13. Sgourakis G, Gockel I, Radtke A et al (2010) Minimally invasive versus open esophagectomy: meta-analysis of outcomes. Dig Dis Sci 55:3031-3040
14. Palanivelu C, Prakash A, Senthilkumar R et al (2006) Minimally invasive esophagectomy: thoracoscopic mobilization of the esophagus and mediastinal lymphadenectomy in prone position—experience of 130 patients. J Am Coll Surg 203:7-16
15. Bresadola V, Terrosu G, Cojutti A et al (2006) Laparoscopic versus open gastroplasty in esophagectomy for esophageal cancer: a comparative study. Surg Laparosc Endosc Percutan Tech 16:63-67
16. Dapri G, Himpens J, Cadière GB (2008) Minimally invasive esophagectomy for cancer: laparoscopic transhiatal procedure or thoracoscopy in prone position followed by laparoscopy? Surg Endosc 22:1060-1069
17. Nguyen NT, Roberts P, Follette DM et al (2003) Thoracoscopic and laparoscopic esophagectomy for benign and malignant disease: lessons learned from 46 consecutive procedures. J Am Coll Surg 197:902-913
18. Berrisford RG, Wajed SA, Sanders D et al (2008) Short-term outcomes following total minimally invasive oesophagectomy. Br J Surg 95:602-610
19. Tinoco R, El-Kadre L, Tinoco A et al (2007) Laparoscopic transhiatal esophagectomy: outcomes. Surg Endosc 21:1284-1287
20. Bann S, Moorthy K, Shaul T et al (2005) Laparoscopic transhiatal surgery of the esophagus. JSLS 9:376-381
21. Sanders G, Borie F, Husson E et al (2007) Minimally invasive transhiatal esophagectomy: lessons learned. Surg Endosc 21:1190-1193
22. Robertson GS, Lloyd DM, Wicks AC et al (1996) No obvious advantages for thoracoscopic two-stage oesophagectomy. Br J Surg 83:675-678
23. Van den Broek WT, Makay O, Berends FJ et al (2004) Laparoscopically assisted transhiatal resection for malignancies of the distal esophagus. Surg Endosc 18:812-817
24. Tsujimoto H, Ono S, Sugasawa H et al (2010) Gastric tube reconstruction by laparoscopy-assisted surgery attenuates postoperative systemic inflammatory response after esophagectomy for esophageal cancer. World J Surg 34:2830-2836
25. Hulscher JB, Tijssen JG, Obertop H et al (2001) Transthoracic versus transhiatal resection for carcinoma of the esophagus: a meta-analysis. Ann Thorac Surg 72:306-313
26. Wormuth JK, Heitmiller RF (2006) Esophageal conduit necrosis. Thorac Surg Clin 16:11-22
27. Veeramootoo D, Parameswaran R, Krishnadas R et al (2009) Classification and early recognition of gastric conduit failure after minimally invasive esophagectomy. Surg Endosc 23:2110-2116
28. Berrisford RG, Veeramootoo D, Parameswaran R et al (2009) Laparoscopic ischaemic conditioning of the stomach may reduce gastric-conduit morbidity following total minimally invasive oesophagectomy. Eur J Cardiothorac Surg 36:888-893
29. Dimick JB, Wainess RM, Upchurch GR et al (2005) National trends in outcomes for esophageal resection. Ann Thorac Surg 79:212-216
30. Begg CB, Cramer LD, Hoskins WJ et al (1998) Impact of hospital volume on operative mortality for major cancer surgery. JAMA 280:1747-1751

31. Santin B, Kulwicki A, Price P (2008) Mortality rate associated with 56 consecutive esophagectomies performed at a "low-volume" hospital: is procedure volume as important as we are trying to make it? J Gastrointest Surg 12:1346-1350
32. Zieren HU, Jacobi CA, Zieren J (1996) Quality of life following resection of oesophageal carcinoma. Br J Surg 83:1772-1775
33. Parameswaran R, Blazeby JM, Hughes R et al (2010) Health-related quality of life after minimally invasive oesophagectomy. Br J Surg 97:525-531
34. Nafteux P, Moons J, Coosemans W et al (2011) Minimally invasive oesophagectomy: a valuable alternative to open oesophagectomy for the treatment of early oesophageal and gastro-oesophageal junction carcinoma. Eur J Cardiothorac Surg Apr 21. Epub ahead of publishing
35. Fabian T, Martin JT, McKelvey AA et al (2008) Minimally invasive esophagectomy: a teaching hospital's first year experience. Dis Esophagus 21:220-225
36. Martin DJ, Bessell JR, Chew A, Watson DI (2005) Thoracoscopic and laparoscopic esophagectomy: initial experience and outcomes. Surg Endosc 19:1597-1561
37. Peyre CG, Hagen JA, DeMeester SR et al (2008) The number of lymph nodes removed predicts survival in esophageal cancer : an international study on the impact of extent of surgical resection. Ann Surg 284:549-556
38. Böttger T, Terzic A, Müller M et al (2007) Minimally invasive transhiatal and transthoracic esophagectomy. Surg Endosc 21:1695-1700
39. Kawahara K, Maekawa T, Okabayashi K et al (1999) Video-assisted thoracoscopic esophagectomy for esophageal cancer. Surg Endosc 13:218-222
40. Osugi H, Takemura M, Higashino M et al (2003) A comparison of video-assisted thoracoscopic oesophagectomy and radical lymph node dissection for squamous cell cancer of the oesophagus with open operation. Br J Surg 90:108-113
41. Lee JM, Cheng JW, Lin MT et al (2011) Is there any benefit to incorporating a laparoscopic procedure into minimally invasive esophagectomy? The impact on perioperative results in patients with esophageal cancer. World J Surg 35:790-797
42. Thomson IG, Smithers BM, Gotley DC et al (2010) Thoracoscopic-assisted esophagectomy for esophageal cancer: analysis of patterns and prognostic factors for recurrence. Ann Surg 252:281-291
43. Biere SS, Maas KW, Bonavina L et al (2011) Traditional invasive vs. minimally invasive esophagectomy: a multi-center, randomized trial (TIME-trial). BMC Surg 11:2
44. Ben-David K, Rossidis G, Zlotecki RA et al (2011) Minimally invasive is safe and effective following neoadjuvant chemoradiation therapy. Ann Surg Oncol Apr 9 doi: 10.1245/s10434-011-1702-7
45. Fabian T, Martin J, Katigbak M et al (2008) Thoracoscopic esophageal mobilization during minimally invasive esophagectomy: a head-to-head comparison of prone versus decubitus positions. Surg Endosc 22:2485-2491
46. Zingg U, McQuinn A, DiValentino D et al (2009) Minimally invasive versus open esophagectomy for patients with esophageal cancer. Ann Thorac Surg 87:911-919
47. Verhage RJ, Hazebroek EJ, Boone J et al (2009) Minimally invasive surgery compared to open procedures in esophagectomy for cancer: a systematic review of the literature. Minerva Chir 64:135-146
48. Biere SS, Cuesta MA, Van Der Peet DL (2009) Minimally invasive versus open esophagectomy for cancer: a systematic review and meta-analysis. Minerva Chir 64:121-133
49. Cuschieri A (1994) Thoracoscopic subtotal oesophagectomy. Endosc Surg Allied Technol 2:21-25
50. Palanivelu C, Rangarajan M, Senthilkumar R et al (2008) Combined thoracoscopic and endoscopic management of mid-esophageal benign lesions: use of the prone patient position: thoracoscopic surgery for mid-esophageal benign tumors and diverticula. Surg Endosc 22:250-254
51. Kuwano H, Nishimura Y, Ohtsu A et al (2008) Guidelines for diagnosis and treatment of carcinoma of the esophagus April 2007 edition: part II edited by the Japan Esophageal Society. Esophagus 5:117-132

52. Furukawa Y, Hanyu N, Hirai K et al (2005) Usefulness of automatic triangular anastomosis for esophageal cancer surgery using a linear stapler (TA-30). Ann Thorac Cardiovasc Surg 11:80-86

Subject Index

MIX
Papier aus verantwortungsvollen Quellen
Paper from responsible sources
FSC® C105338

If you have any concerns about our products,
you can contact us on
ProductSafety@springernature.com

In case Publisher is established outside the EU,
the EU authorized representative is:
Springer Nature Customer Service Center GmbH
Europaplatz 3, 69115 Heidelberg, Germany

Printed by Libri Plureos GmbH
in Hamburg, Germany